101 Sports Medicine Tips/Facts: Vol.1—Understanding the Basics

Barry Boden, MD
Francis O'Connor, MD, MPH
Robert Wilder, MD

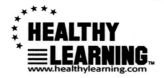

HEALTHY LEARNING
www.healthylearning.com

ISBN: 978-1-58518-055-4
Library of Congress Control Number: 2007931405
Cover design & book layout: Roger W. Rybkowski
Front cover photo: Andy Mead/Icon SMI/ZUMA Press
Back cover photos: ©2007 Jupiterimages Corporation

Healthy Learning
P.O. Box 1828
Monterey, CA 93942
www.healthylearning.com

Dedication

This book is dedicated to those coaches who help promote physical fitness, team play, and integrity in their efforts to make participating in sports a positive experience for everyone involved. We also want to express our gratitude to our wives and children—whose love and support helped make this book a reality.

Acknowledgments

We would like to thank the medical and health/fitness professionals with whom we have had the opportunity to interact over the years. Their feedback, advice, guidance, and suggestions have had a profound impact not only on our interest in developing the "101 Sports Medicine" book series, but also our ability to do so in a thoughtful manner.

Table of Contents

Introduction

101 Sports Medicine Tips and Facts: Vol. 1—Understanding the Basics is designed to be an informative resource that can help both new and experienced coaches be better prepared to understand and deal with the various sports medicine-related problems that can affect their athletes. The book features targeted, up-to-date information written by some of the top medical professionals in their particular field of interest.

As physicians, parents, and volunteer coaches, we firmly believe in the value of sports participation. Athletics have real merit and real consequences. To the extent that the easy-to-understand and easy-to-apply advice and guidelines presented in this book can serve as a roadmap to help coaches make sports a more injury-free experience for everyone involved, then the collective efforts to develop this book (and the series) will have been worthwhile.

1

The Preparticipation Examination

Francis G. O'Connor, MD, FACSM

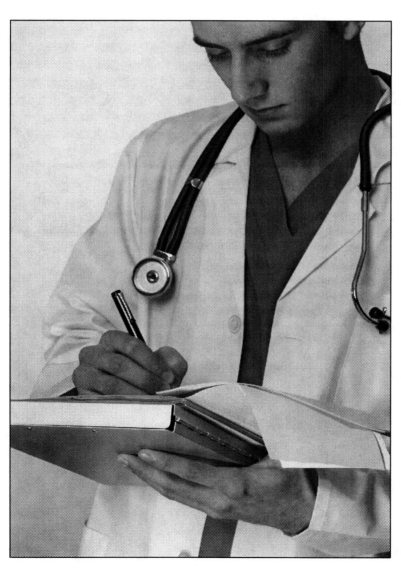

TIP/FACT #1
Any meaningful commitment to prevent sports injuries will involve a preparticipation examination.

The preparticipation examination (PPE) should be the cornerstone of the relationship between the medical personnel who work with a particular sports team and that team's coaching staff. Although traditionally thought of as a yearly height, blood-pressure check, and quick physical examination, a properly performed PPE is the fundamental sports-medicine endeavor to prevent injuries. While this annual process can serve many functions, first and foremost, it is designed to ensure safe participation for those athletes who will be taking part in sports. In other words, its principal purpose is to help maintain the health and safety of the athlete in both training and competition. A list of additional primary and secondary objectives for the PPE is provided in Table 1-1. Although some people may question the value of the PPE (in particular, the cost and man-hours necessary to complete these examinations), the numerous benefits of this annual preseason procedure far outweigh any perceived or actual limitations.

Objectives of the Preparticipation Examination
Primary Objectives
Detect conditions that may predispose to injury
Detect conditions that may be life-threatening or disabling
Meet legal and insurance requirements
Secondary Objectives
Determine general health
Counsel on health-related issues
Assess fitness level for specific sports

Table 1-1. Objectives of the preparticipation examination

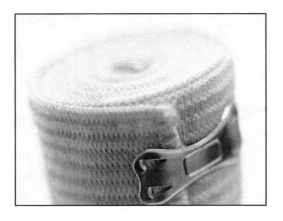

TIP/FACT #2
The preparticipation examination (PPE) should be comprehensive, performed by trained personnel, and concentrate on areas that are of relatively high risk to competitive athletes.

The foremost concern of the PPE process should be the qualifications of the healthcare professional who performs the examination. A very strong argument can be advanced that this responsibility should be with a physician. On the other hand, it is a fact that each individual state determines who has the authority to perform a PPE within that state. In many states, non-physician providers are allowed to perform PPEs. As such, it is the responsibility of the particular school or institution to be totally familiar with relevant state laws governing who may perform athletic PPEs. In that regard, coaches and the athletic training staff (if the institution has one) should share in the responsibility of ensuring that only qualified personnel perform PPEs.

The exact components of the PPE vary greatly across the United States, which is one of the principal reasons that many authorities are calling for a uniform examination process. Strong support exists among leading sports-medicine organizations in the United States that the PPE should include both a written questionnaire and an actual physical examination prior to permitting an individual to participate in an athletic endeavor. The written phase of the PPE should include a personal medical history, a family history, and a detailed list of questions concerning present day health that might prompt the provider to ask more questions (e.g., have you ever passed out while exercising?). In that regard, the American Heart Association has developed guidelines that specifically address questions and examination techniques that attempt to identify a young athlete possibly at risk for sudden death.

An individual's family history should include a specific inquiry for a family history of premature coronary-artery disease, diabetes mellitus, hypertension, sudden death, syncope, significant disability from cardiovascular disease in relatives younger than age 50, hypertrophic cardiomyopathy (HCM), arhythmogenic right ventricular dysplasia (ARVC), Marfan's syndrome, prolonged QT syndrome, or significant arrhythmias.

The athlete's personal past history should include specific inquiries that would otherwise help a provider detect a heart murmur, diabetes mellitus, hypertension, hyperlipidemia, smoking, or on the presence of HCM, ARVC, Marfan's syndrome, prolonged QT syndrome, or significant arrhythmias. Recent history inquiries should include a history of syncope, near syncope, profound exercise intolerance, exertional chest discomfort, dyspnea, or excessive fatigue.

The physical exam should specifically address those relatively identifiable factors that might place the athlete at individual risk, such as hypertension, heart rhythm, cardiac murmur, and the findings of unusual facies or body habitus associated with a congenital cardiovascular defect, especially Marfan's syndrome. The cardiac (heart) examination should be performed in a quiet, well-lighted environment. Cardiac auscultation (using a stethoscope) should be performed in the supine and standing positions, while murmurs should be assessed with Valsalva (i.e., forcefully bearing down by holding one's breath) and position maneuvers when indicated. Femoral pulses should be assessed and blood pressure measured with an appropriately sized cuff in a sitting position.

Blood pressure measurements can frequently be obtained by an allied health professional prior to the provider's examination. This assessment can be done with either a conventional blood pressure cuff or an automated machine. A key point is that the athlete needs to be seated for five minutes prior to the blood pressure assessment being performed, and that within the hour before the examination, the athlete must neither ingest caffeine nor smoke, as both of which may falsely elevate the individual's blood pressure. Coaches should remind their athletes of this fact to avoid them being falsely labeled as having high blood pressure, thereby requiring multiple follow-up visits.

As anyone can quickly see, these examinations, if done properly, cannot be conducted effectively in a crowded, poorly lit locker room at a rate of one athlete per minute, if they are to be performed in a safe, effective manner. The staff should ensure an adequate environment for the provider, and expect that a proper examination be performed. While the PPE can be completed quite effectively in a matter of minutes, providers who "crank-out" 100 examinations in an hour should raise suspicion, rather than praise.

TIP/FACT #3
The preparticipation examination should be performed six weeks prior to the onset of an athlete's season.

The consensus recommendation of every reputable medical organization in the United States that is concerned with an athlete's health and safety (e.g., the American Academy of Family Physicians, American Academy of Pediatrics, American Medical Society of Sports Medicine, American Medical Society of Sports Medicine, American Orthopedic Society of Sports Medicine, and the American Osteopathic Academy of Sports Medicine) is that the PPE be performed ideally six weeks prior to the start of the preseason practices. This scheduling allows adequate time to facilitate the medical evaluation process that may be required (e.g., an echocardiogram for a suspicious heart murmur, rehabilitation of an injured body part, etc.). If the process is completed well before the six-week mark, coaches should remind their athletes of each player's responsibility to subsequently report any injuries or illnesses that might have occurred to the medical team.

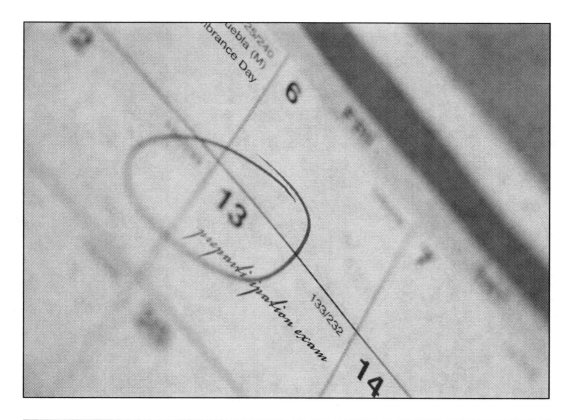

TIP/FACT #4
The frequency of sports preparticipation examinations is subject to regional rules.

How often an athlete should undergo a PPE has been a topic of considerable controversy within both the medical and athletic communities, with recommendations ranging from requiring a single PPE prior to the start of each competitive season to conducting no PPEs at all. Recently, however, the American Heart Association (AHA) has endorsed two position statements/guidelines on the frequency of the PPE. The AHA recommends that a complete personal and family history and a physical examination be done for all athletes. The physical examination should focus on identifying those cardiovascular conditions known to cause sudden death. Furthermore, a complete preparticipation examination should be performed for all high school athletes every two years, and for all collegiate athletes upon entering the institution. A history and blood-pressure measurement should be obtained in the interim years, and any abnormalities identified by these requirements should be further investigated. The key point, however, is that the final determination for the frequency of examinations is dependent upon the rules and regulations that govern a particular team/league.

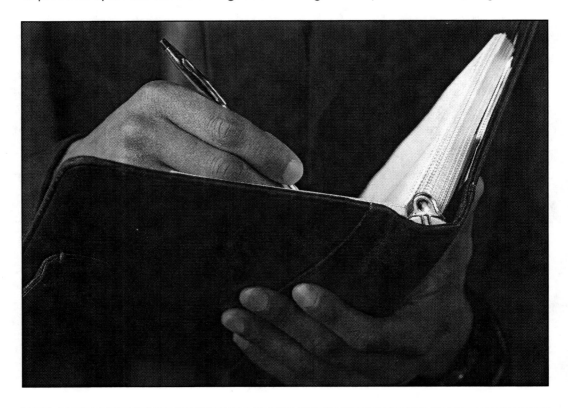

TIP/FACT #5
The preparticipation examination can be done in a physician's office or in a station-based setting.

Two principal means exist by which preparticipation examinations are completed—the office setting or station-based. In the office-based PPE, the ideal procedure would be to have the athlete's personal primary-care physician perform the PPE. This approach tends to facilitate continuity of care for the athlete, since that physician frequently has been the individual's long-term healthcare provider. Given the likelihood that athletes would be more likely to trust an individual who has provided them with ongoing care, an opportunity for the player to ask questions and receive counsel on health-related issues that may otherwise not be discussed would be created. Among the factors may otherwise make this particular method inadequate or undesirable are the expense involved, the possibility that the athlete's personal primary-care provider might have limited sports medicine knowledge, and the fact that not all athletes have an established relationship with a primary-care provider.

Because station-based PPEs, on the other hand, do not have the basic disadvantages of PPEs conducted in an office setting, they are commonly employed in the United States. For example, station-based PPEs are often more cost-efficient. They frequently incorporate the skills of a number of providers, who more often than not will volunteer their time. This type of examination also has the advantage in that athletes, trainers, coaches, and medical providers can communicate "on the spot." Another advantage of station-based PPEs is that they provide the opportunity for multiple stations, including fitness assessments that can be administered by the coaching staff (refer to Table 1-2).

One of the disadvantages of station-based PPEs is that a substantial diminishment of continuity of care may occur, since the examining provider may lose touch with any follow-up that might be necessary for a particular athlete. These examinations also require excellent coordination among everyone involved in the PPE process, since running several hundred athletes through an evening (or morning) of examinations is no small task (at best). As a rule, a team's coaches are key to the process of conducting station-based PPEs, because they will be responsible for coordinating the timing of the PPEs (with any and all medical personnel involved), communicating with their athletes, and (not infrequently) assisting in administering the actual PPEs.

Required and Optional Stations and Personnel for Station-Based Preparticipation Physical Evaluations	
Required Stations	**Personnel**
Sign-in	Ancillary staff
Height,weight	Ancillary staff
Vital signs	Ancillary staff
Vision	Ancillary staff
Physical examination	Physician
History review and clearance	Physician
Optional Stations	**Personnel**
Nutrition	Dietician
Dental	Dentist
Injury evaluation	Physician
Flexibility	Trainer, therapist
Body Composition	Trainer, physiologist, therapist
Strength	Trainer, physiologist, therapist, coach
Speed, agility, power, endurance, balance	Trainer, physiologist, coach

Table 1-2. Required and optional stations and personnel for station-based preparticipation physical evaluations

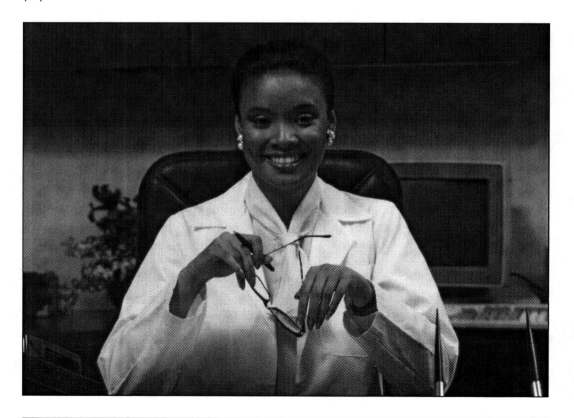

TIP/FACT #6
No requirement exists that a preparticipation examination must include a laboratory analysis or special tests.

Over the years, medical providers have grown accustomed to utilizing various laboratories tests when they conduct the annual physical examination of their patients (adults and children alike). In the process, the practice of utilizing these tests (in situations where their use may or may not be warranted) has been widespread. In fact, the preparticipation examination often includes several routine laboratory tests, depending on the circumstances attendant to the test, such as the location of the test (office or field), the philosophy of those involved with the process (primary care providers, athletic staff, parents, etc), and regional considerations. Among the tests that have commonly been incorporated into the PPE are CBC (complete blood count), UA (urinalysis), echocardiogram, and EKG (electrocardiogram). The use of laboratory tests, however, can be a double-edged sword. In addition to being expensive, they may provide a false-positive result. In other words, while a particular test may show an abnormality, the athlete who has been tested may be fine and may suffer only from a test result that is misleading. Accordingly, because all tests have limitations, the use of routine screening tests is not recommended.

On the other hand, while routine screening tests are not recommended, medical providers may incorporate diagnostic tests to help clarify a symptom or make a diagnosis. For example, it would be highly appropriate to obtain a complete blood count (CBC) in a female athlete, who may be complaining of fatigue, in order to diagnose whether she has anemia, or have an athlete who has a recent history of mononucleosis undergo an abdominal ultrasound to evaluate for an enlarged spleen. Table 1-2 (refer to Tip/Fact #5) provides a list of several of the numerous fitness tests and/or skill stations that could be added to the PPE if circumstances warranted it.

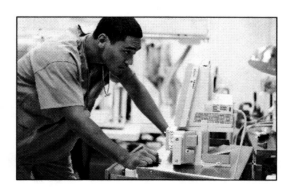

TIP/FACT #7
No "easy" answer exists regarding how to screen for athletes who may be at risk for sudden death on an athletic field.

One particularly sensitive area of controversy attendant to the PPE involves whether to screen young athletes to determine whether they are risk for sudden cardiac death by the routine incorporation of electrocardiography and echocardiography. An electrocardiogram is obtained by applying leads to the chest wall to obtain an electrical tracing of the heart's rhythm. An echocardiogram involves having a camera-like transducer run over a patient's chest to reproduce an image of the individual athlete's heart on a video screen. Both tests are considered to be noninvasive to the athlete (in other words, they don't cause any pain, and they don't involve needles or catheters).

While these tests may sound useful, they have the same problem that plagues all screening tests…a low probability of finding disease. While sudden death in an athlete is catastrophic, it's exceedingly rare, estimated at 1:200,000 athletes each year. In fact, a much greater opportunity exists to mislabel an athlete who is normal as abnormal, than there is to literally identify the proverbial "needle in the haystack." As a result, leading cardiologists recommend against the routine use of these tests. On the other hand, for any athlete with a suspicion or question of cardiac-related disease, their use as a diagnostic tool is strongly endorsed.

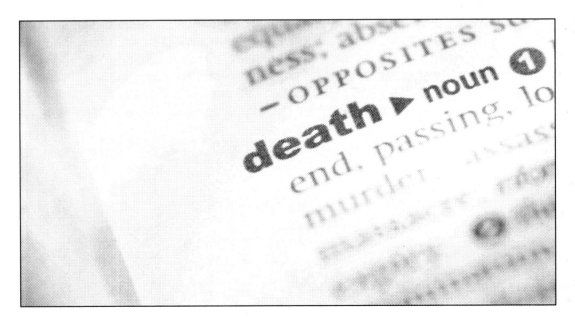

TIP/FACT #8
Neurpsychometric testing may have a role for athletes who may be at risk for concussion.

Neuropsychometric testing is relatively new on the horizon. This form of testing is especially useful in athletes who may be at risk for head injury. These tests are principally computer-based and are used to establish a baseline for brain function. When an athlete has a head injury, these tests are then utilized to ensure that an athlete has returned to normal, prior to returning to play. While these tests may sound great, they can be both time-consuming to perform and expensive. Because their routine use remains under study, their utility and appropriateness are still in question.

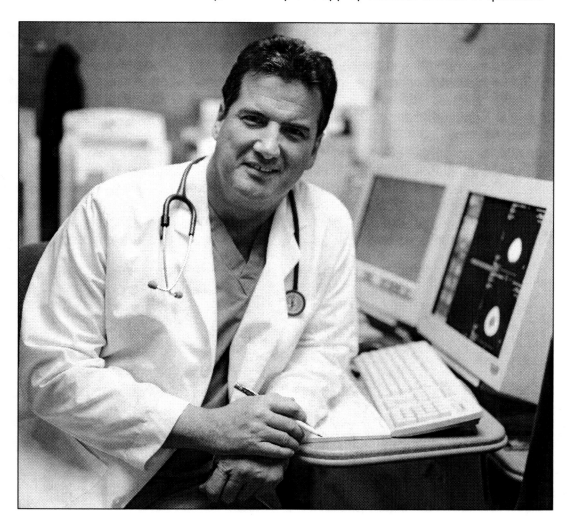

TIP/FACT #9
Medical clearance is ultimately the responsibility of the team physician.

The most important decision involving the PPE process is that of clearance. Providers are often led to believe that, with regard to the PPE and whether individuals are approved to participate, athletes are either "cleared" or "not cleared." However, this perception is not the case. Providers should keep in mind that they have essentially three options with regard to participation clearance for a particular athlete: (1) cleared for all sports; (2) cleared for only certain sports, but restricted from others; or (3) cleared for participation, but only after satisfying specified requirements.

In the latter instance, the provider must specifically state what needs to be done to satisfy clearance requirements, as well as identify what the athlete can do in the interim. An example would be an athlete who wants to play basketball who has just had a severe ankle sprain. This athlete can be cleared only after demonstrating normal strength, range of motion, and sports-specific function in the affected ankle. However, he may be allowed to participate in certain rehabilitation activities, ride a stationary cycle, and engage in basketball-related activities that do not place undue stresses on the ankle, e.g. practice free throws. A track athlete, on the other hand, who has been passing out during his quarter-mile repeats, should be cleared only after seeing a cardiologist. He should be prohibited from all physical activity, pending this evaluation. Coaches, trainers, and providers all have an inherent and absolute obligation to respect the importance of the final clearance recommendation, and must always remember to focus on treating the injured individual as a patient first and as an athlete second.

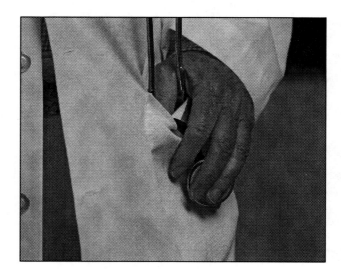

TIP/FACT #10
Everyone will not always agree on the findings of the preparticipation process.

Instances will occur when an athlete (or a coach for that matter) does not concur with the provider's determination (e.g., a heart condition leading to a lack of clearance to participate). The legal system in the United States has supported the concept that every athlete has the right to participate against medical advice. On the other hand, the courts have also determined that schools and institutions have a right to decide who may play, based upon sound medical opinions that are derived from established guidelines. In all cases where there is a disagreement, legal counsel is recommended before allowing an athlete to participate, with or without a waiver from the individual. Once again, the paramount factor should be to treat the individual as a patient first and as an athlete second.

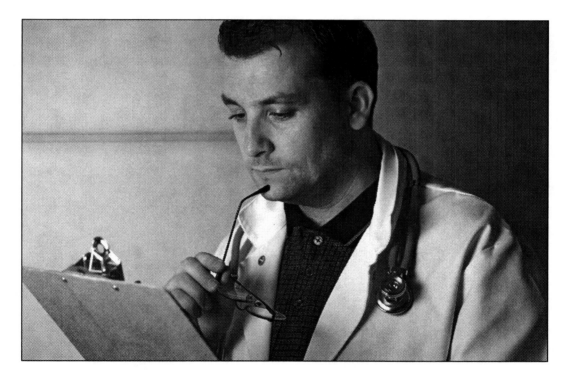

References:

American Academy of Family Physicians, American Medical Society for Sports Medicine, American Orthopedic Society for Sports Medicine, American Osteopathic Academy of Sports Medicine (1996) *Preparticipation Physical Evaluation,* 2nd ed. McGraw-Hill, New York, NY.

American Heart Association (1998) Cardiovascular preparticipation screening of competitive athletes: An Addendum. *Circulation* **97**: 2294.

Maron, BJ, Thompson, PD, Puffer, JC, McGrew, CA, Strong, WB, Douglas, PS, Clark, LT, Mitten, MJ, Crawford, MH, Atkins, DL, Driscoll, DJ, Epstein, AE (1996) Cardiovascular preparticipation screening of competitive athletes: a statement for health professionals from the sudden death committee (clinical cardiology) and congenital cardiac defects committee (cardiovascular disease in the young), American Heart Association. *Circulation* **94**: 850-856.

O'Connor FG, Kugler, JP, Oriscello, RG (1998) Sudden Death in Young Athletes: Screening for the Needle in the Haystack. *American Family Physician* **57**: 2763.

——(1994) 26th Bethesda Conference. Recommendations for determining eligibility for competition in athletes with cardiovascular abnormalities. *American Journal of Cardiology* **24**: 845-899.

2

Common Sports-Related Problems
Thomas M. Howard, MD

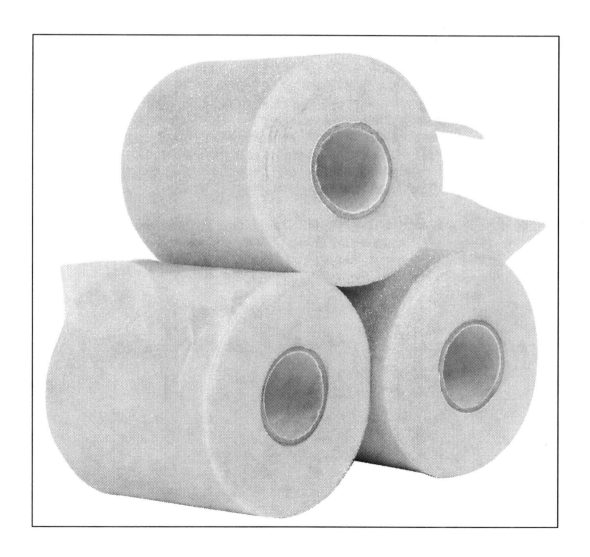

TIP/FACT #11
Proper foot care can help prevent blisters.

Blisters are a result of friction from ill-fitting equipment and moisture that make the skin more susceptible to friction. The most common locations for blisters are the feet for most athletes, followed by the hands. Blisters often occur over bony prominences or under existing calluses. Excessive moisture, repetitive motions, and ill-fitting equipment (e.g., shoes) contribute to the development of these nagging and sometimes serious injuries if they become infected.

Strategic measures to prevent blisters often begin with the proper fit of athletic shoes and break-in periods for new shoes prior to their extensive use in practice or games. Another strategy includes managing calluses and controlling moisture. Calluses should be pared down with an emery board, pumice stone, or paring blade. Using antiperspirant spray, polypropylene socks, or a polypropylene sock liner under a game sock to control moisture can also be an effective measure to help prevent blisters. Athletes with a tendency toward friction blisters over a particular bony prominence can pre-treat the area with a lubricant, like petroleum jelly or a moisturizer like Aquaphor. Some athletes (e.g., ultramarathoners) have been known to treat "hotspots" with tincture of benzoine and duct tape while competing.

Athletes should monitor themselves for the early development of "hot spots," which involve an early inflammation of the skin prior to blister formation. Addressing these hotspots with padding, a moleskin doughnut, or an adjustment of equipment may also alleviate the development of painful blisters.

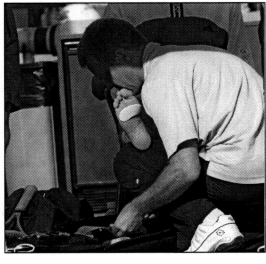

Art Seitz / ZumaPress

TIP/FACT #12
Proper nail trimming can prevent ingrown toenails.

Ingrown nails often occur on the great toenail. They occur from pressure along the nail bed on the inside and outside part of the nail that forces the nail into the surrounding tissue. This pressure causes irritation and may lead to infection and pain.

Among the most effective strategies for preventing an ingrown toenail are proper trimming of the nail, avoiding tight fitting shoes, and the early treatment of symptoms. The nail should be trimmed straight across from one side to the other.

The athlete should avoid trimming back the nail folds along the side of the nail, because doing so will encourage growth into the surrounding soft tissue. In addition, athletes should ensure that their shoes have adequate room in the toe box. Their shoes should be snug, but should enable the athlete to be able to easily wiggle their toes. When symptoms of an ingrown toenail develop, the athlete should first initiate warm soaks in water or Epsom salts to reduce irritation. Attempts to free up the in-growing portion of the nail may also alleviate symptoms. If the condition exhibits any signs of infection, medical attention should be sought.

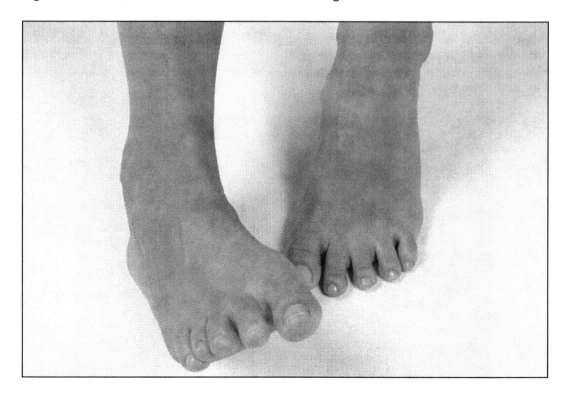

TIP/FACT #13
Athletes should wear shower shoes in public showers to prevent athlete's foot.

Athlete's foot is caused by a superficial fungal infection of the feet. A warm, moist environment favors the growth of these fungi. Prevention strategies should address controlling the environment of the feet, avoiding exposure, and prompt management of early symptoms.

Athletes should avoid walking barefoot in public places and wear shower shoes in public showers. In addition, athletes should not share shoes. After bathing or swimming, feet should be dried thoroughly, especially between the toes. Similar to blister management, socks should be changed daily, and moisture in the feet should be controlled with topical foot powders, spray deodorant, and proper airing of shoes after each use. This step includes removing any sock liner or shoe insert and unlacing the shoe completely to allow the inside to dry. For athletes who have a tendency toward excessively sweaty feet, the application of 20% aluminum chloride (Drysol) for moisture control should be considered.

For athletes who develop athlete's foot, over-the-counter topical creams or solutions, such as Lamisil or Lotrimin, may be effective. Athletes suffering from athlete's foot should also consider replacing their current pair of athletic shoes. If the athlete's foot condition fails to respond to appropriate over-the-counter measures, then medical attention should be sought.

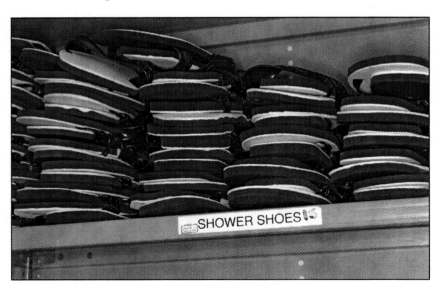

TIP/FACT #14
Strengthening and balance training are the best prevention strategies for ankle injuries.

The most commonly injured joint in most sports is the ankle. Eighty-five percent of ankle injuries are sprains; 85% are lateral ankle injuries; and 85% involve the ATFL (anterior talofibular ligament or ligament on the outside front part of the ankle). The most common mechanism of these injuries is the inversion sprain (turning the ankle in while the foot is pointing down).

The recovery and rehabilitation from an ankle injury is a staged process. The initial stage is the management of the swelling and pain, followed by the recovery of the normal range of motion in the ankle. The next step involves isometric and isotonic strengthening and, finally, proprioceptive training, with the systematic progression into sport-specific training.

Most individuals do well with the early stages of recovery and rehabilitation (managing pain and swelling). However, too many athletes do not complete the rehabilitation process. Instead, these athletes return to activity too soon after their pain and swelling has resolved. With subsequent injuries, they gradually lose strength and never develop the proprioceptive protection that can help prevent injuries in the future.

Strength training has been shown to be an effective strategy for preventing ankle injuries. Such a regimen should focus on ankle eversion (pushing the foot out) and dorsiflexion (pointing the foot toward the head) exercises. These exercises can be performed against a wall for resistance (isometrics) or with resistance tubing (theraband). Balance training is another form of training that has been found to help prevent ankle injuries. Such training focuses on proprioception. Proprioception is a joint's ability to sense where it is in space, both while in mid-air and with ground contact. Proprioceptive drills to enhance balance include assuming a single-leg stance, first on a firm floor and then with a folded towel on the floor. Proprioceptive exercises should be performed with the eyes open and closed. Hopscotch, jump rope, and the BAPS board (biomechanical ankle platform system) can also help to improve balance.

In addition to strength and balance training, ankle braces or taping may also help prevent ankle injuries. Both can play a meaningful role in the timing of return-to-play. Supportive devices function by providing additional proprioceptive input to the ankle. Numerous studies exist that demonstrate similar benefits between taping and the various ankle braces. Lace-up and other braces can be adjusted frequently during practice or competition and require no special skill to apply. Some athletes chose to use both taping and a functional brace, but no evidence exists to document any further benefit to this practice. Athletes with repetitive ankle injuries should be evaluated by a physician, physical therapist or certified athletic trainer (ATC).

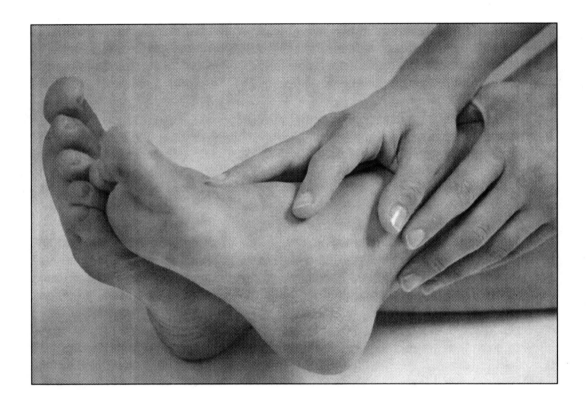

TIP/FACT #15
Maintaining adequate muscular strength and flexibility can help prevent shin splints.

"Shin splints" is a catch-all term that refers to a group of overuse injuries that manifest themselves in inflammation of muscles and tendons of the lower leg. In general, shin splints involve microscopic tears in the muscles of the legs at their points of attachment to the shin. A painful condition in the lower leg, shin splints often start out as a dull sensation that athletes experience after exercising. If left untreated, shin splints can eventually advance to an intense pain.

More often than not, shin splints result from muscular imbalances, insufficient shock absorption, or excessive pronation of the foot (a factor that can have a significant negative impact on the leg's ability to absorb shock). Increasing the strength of the lower-leg muscles enhances their ability to adequately absorb any shock (force) to which they may be exposed during physical activity. Flexibility training can help athletes maintain the correct muscular balance and avoid improper foot-plant mechanics (either of which can contribute to shin splints).

Among the treatment options for shin splints are taking anti-inflammatory medicine (aspirin), ice massage, reducing the amount of exercise, varying the training program, wearing a custom-fitted shoe orthotic, ultrasound, and electrostimulation. Whatever options athletes decide to undertake to treat their shin splint condition, they should listen to their body and use common sense at all times. If their condition persists, they should seek proper medical advice.

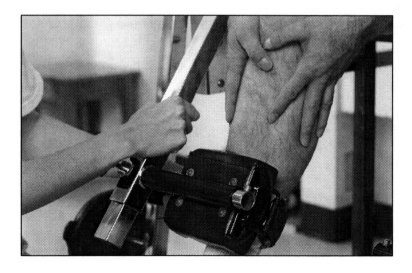

TIP/FACT #16
Hamstring flexibility and quadriceps strengthening exercises can help prevent patellofemoral pain.

Patellofemoral pain syndrome (PFPS) is the most common overuse knee condition experienced by athletes, especially young athletes. Intrinsic factors that contribute to PFPS include pronated feet (flat feet), tight hamstrings, weak quadriceps (in particular the inside or medial part of the quads), a wide pelvis, and the outward placement of the patellar tendon. Extrinsic factors include training errors (too much, too soon, too fast), worn-out or improper shoes, exercising on hard surfaces, and a history of direct trauma to the knee.

Exercises focused on treating or preventing PFPS include those that strengthen the quadriceps and that enhance hamstring flexibility. Flexibility training should be performed several times over the course of the day. Basic lower-extremity flexibility exercises include hamstring, quads, gastrocnemius and soleus, IT band, and piriformis stretching. Athletes should perform five repetitions of each exercise each stretching session and hold each position for 20 to 25 seconds.

Strengthening the quadriceps should address the medial (inside) part of the quadriceps. Quadriceps weightlifting activities include the leg extension, squat, and leg press. The squat and leg press exercises involve functional strengthening of the muscles involved in the physical demands of many different activities. Performing leg extensions is also recommended, but they may increase pressure over the patellofemoral joint and aggravate symptoms in some individuals. Several additional activities that athletes can perform to help treat or prevent PFPS do not require equipment, including wall sits, step-ups or step-downs, single leg dips, and straight leg raises.

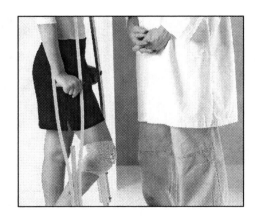

TIP/FACT #17
Lower extremity strength training and sport-specific drills can reduce the incidence of ACL injuries.

The knee is the largest joint in the body. It has a complex system of ligaments (bands of connective tissue, which connect bones together at the joints). One of the key ligaments involved in the process that helps stabilize the knee is the anterior cruciate ligament (ACL). The ACL resists forward translation or movement of the tibia on the femur.

The most common type of ACL injury is a sprain—an injury caused by tensile stress to the ligamentous fibers. Depending on the degree of damage to the fibers, sprains come in three grades of severity—first-degree (mild), second-degree (moderate), or third-degree (severe). In isolated cases, the ACL may rupture, resulting in an injury that usually requires surgery. Approximately 70 to 80% of ACL injuries occur during non-contact activities, such as landing from a jump or cutting and stopping. The majority of athletes are injured in high-risk sports (soccer, basketball, football, and volleyball).

ACL injury prevention strategies focus on performing exercises to improve hamstring strength and tone, as well as doing landing and cutting drills. Athletes who are involved in high-risk sports (those that involve pivoting and cutting) should perform these drills year-round.

Jumping drills should stress landing on two legs with the knees in a flexed (bent) position to absorb the ground contact forces of landing. Jumping drills should emphasize landing on the balls of the feet with the chest over the knees. This posture will allow more muscular absorption of ground contact and less ACL strain. Examples of specific jumping drills that could be performed in this instance include wall tucks, broad jumps, squat jumps, and cone jumps.

Cutting maneuvers should be performed with the hip and knee flexed, so that the athlete instinctively employs this position for competition. Athletes should be encouraged to do an accelerated, rounded turn for changing directions, rather than planting and cutting on a straightened knee. Stopping drills should emphasize a 3-step stop with the knee flexed, rather than a sudden 1-step stop on a single leg. In addition, proprioceptive training (balance training) may also help reduce ACL injuries.

TIP/FACT #18
Knee braces can be effective at preventing medial collateral ligament (MCL) injuries, but have limited benefit in the prevention of ACL injuries.

Prophylactic knee bracing has been the subject of many studies that have attempted to evaluate injury prevention. These studies have mostly involved football players. Unfortunately the usefulness of these investigations has been hampered by low numbers and other confounding problems.

It appears that prophylactic bracing with metal hinges on the sides of the knee can lower the incidence of MCL injuries in football linemen. However, no evidence exists that ACL injuries can be prevented with prophylactic bracing during competition. A new brace has been developed that trains athletes to maintain a flexed knee position in order to avoid dangerous positions for the knee. The clinical effectiveness of the brace has yet to be determined. On the other hand, it has been demonstrated that bracing an ACL-deficient knee will not resist further injury while engaging in high-energy (cutting) activities associated with high-risk sports.

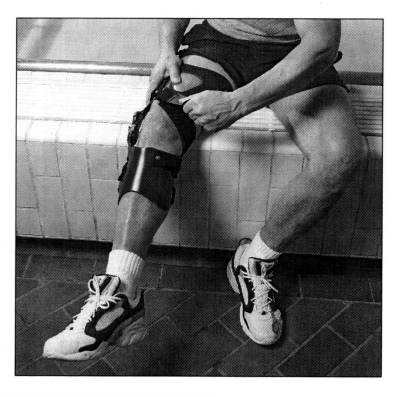

TIP/FACT #19
Avoiding overtraining can help reduce stress fractures.

Stress fractures are incomplete microscopic breaks or cracks in normal bone caused by repetitive trauma without adequate rest periods between exercise sessions. Common among basketball players, long-distance runners, aerobic dancers, and gymnasts, stress fractures usually occur as the result of the repeated impact of running or jumping. As such, stress factors emanate from the failure of bone to adequately adapt to the mechanical (force) loads experienced during exercise.

The most common stress fractures encountered are metatarsal (foot), tibia (lower leg), navicular (foot), fibula (outside of lower leg), and femur (thigh). Although most stress fractures are considered low-risk and heal uneventfully with relative rest, there are some stress fractures that can involve significant long-term disability, including the femoral neck (hip), anterior cortex of the tibia (front portion of lower leg), navicular (inside foot), sesamoid (bottom of great toe), and fifth metatarsal (outside of foot).

Causative factors for stress fractures can be divided into intrinsic factors (characteristics of the athlete) and extrinsic factors. Intrinsic factors specific to stress fractures in individuals are high-arched feet, low bone mass, menstrual disturbances, poor nutritional status, and a prior history of stress fractures. Extrinsic factors include hard exercise surfaces, worn-out or improper shoes, excessive training volume with insufficient recovery, and inadequate nutrition.

Prevention strategies should focus on minimizing the impact of the applicable intrinsic and extrinsic factors. Shoes should be properly fitted for the athlete's foot and gait. Athletes with high arches should consider placing an additional cushion in their shoes, while those with excessive pronation may benefit from wearing shoes that help correct the athlete's foot position. Some individuals may benefit from wearing custom orthotics in their running shoes. Athletes with high arches may gain additional cushion by removing the sock insert and inserting an additional cushion insole.

Two additional key considerations in preventing stress fractures are the training surface and the training regimen undertaken by the athlete. As such, to the degree possible, athletic training programs should be conducted on soft or resilient surfaces. The hardest surface to train on is concrete followed by asphalt and then natural turf or trails. Furthermore, athletes should gradually increase the intensity of their workouts. Dramatic increases (too much, too soon) should strictly be avoided.

Strength-training programs for the lower extremity, as well flexibility training, have also been shown to help enhance an athlete's resistance to multiple injuries, including stress fractures. In particular, hip abductor (side leg lifts) exercises have been shown to help decrease the risk of femoral neck stress fractures.

Another step that athletes can take to minimize their risk of stress fractures is to eat a balanced diet with adequate calcium intake. Finally, athletes should listen to their body and respond to aches and pains with appropriate adjustments in their training schedule to allow for recovery. Varying the mix of training modalities can also be a helpful measure in avoiding stress fractures. In that regard, cross training with cycling, elliptical, or mechanical stairclimbing machines can help athletes maintain their level of conditioning, with less stress on their bones than impact exercises.

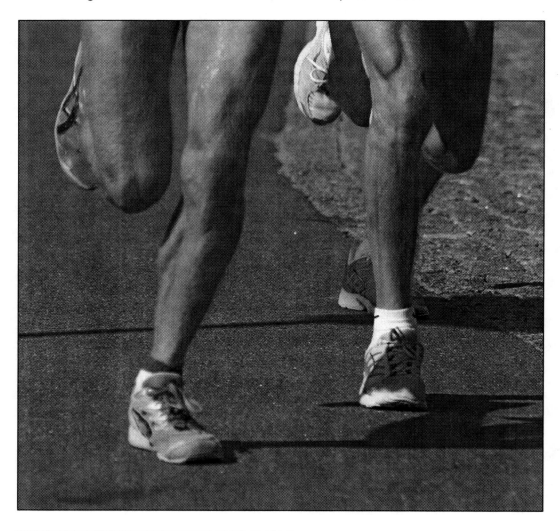

TIP/FACT #20
Stretching and avoiding overtraining can help prevent tendonitis.

Tendonitis is a generic term for a variety of overuse conditions that affect the tendons of the body (the fibrous cords that anchor muscles to bones). Athletes are particularly vulnerable to tendonitis because their tendons are exposed to the force of repetitive muscle contractions. The areas of the body most commonly affected by tendonitis are the ankle, foot, knee, shoulder, and elbow.

Engaging in a sound program of stretching and strengthening routines is the best measure that athletes can undertake to prevent tendonitis. Avoiding overstressing any part of the body can also be an essential step in minimizing the risk of tendonitis. In addition, adhering to the proper mechanics and techniques for performing sports skills can be another critical factor in preventing tendonitis. For example, an improper throwing motion or an improperly executed backhand can lead to tendonitis of the shoulder or elbow. Finally, an athlete's exposure to tendonitis can also be reduced by providing the athlete with the best equipment possible (e.g., shoes).

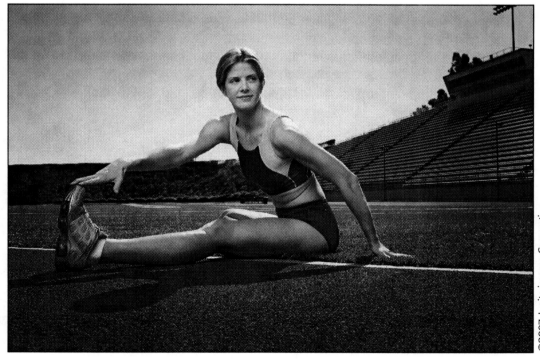

©2007 Jupiterimages Corporation

TIP/FACT #21
Adequate nutrition, hydration, and overall conditioning can help prevent exertional muscle cramps.

Muscle cramps are often debilitating and game-ending for many athletes. While they most commonly occur in the gastrocnemius (calf) or hamstring muscles, they can occur in any muscle. Their symptoms are manifested by a painful spasm of the muscle in a shortened position. Often, these cramps occur toward the end of a game or an extended period of activity (e.g., a long run or race).

Muscles require fluids and nutrients to maintain repeated contractions. Most individuals theorize that dehydrated states, electrolyte disturbances (low sodium, potassium, calcium, or magnesium), or just plain muscle fatigue are the primary causes of cramps. In team sports, athletes who engage in intense bouts of running/sprinting (e.g., running backs, defensive backs, and receivers in football; midfielders in soccer; etc.) are among the individuals who are susceptible to exertional cramps. Certain medications like asthma medications, cholesterol-lowering medications, and creatine supplementation can also precipitate exertional cramps.

Although many theories and folk remedies have been advanced for exertional muscle cramping, limited evidenced-based data exists to support many of these alternatives. Initial treatments when cramping occurs include active stretching of the muscle, hydration with a glucose-electrolyte solution, and ice massage. Some affected individuals, however, will cramp more while lying down and may benefit from slowly walking and stretching.

Three other preventive strategies for cramping that have been proposed include adequate hydration and proper nutritional intake before practice or competition (carbohydrate intake), as well as ingesting sports drinks (glucose-electrolyte solutions like Gatorade, Powerade, etc.) for exercise/activity sessions lasting > 60 minutes. Because sports that involve relatively high levels of sweating can result in a significant loss of salt (an imbalance which can lead to muscle cramping), athletes should be encouraged to liberally salt their food, although the intake of salt tablets is not recommended. On a less scientific note, some anecdotal reports have been put forth concerning the benefit of ingesting pickle juice for those individuals susceptible to cramping. In reality, however, no evidence to support this practice exists. On the other hand, proper conditioning has been shown to help reduce the incidence of exertional cramping among athletes.

Athletes who develop recurrent cramping, cramping at low levels of exertion, or in non-exercising muscles should be evaluated by a physician. Finally, athletes who resume exercising after suffering from exertional cramps should do so at a slower pace, until which time they feel reasonably comfortable extending themselves again.

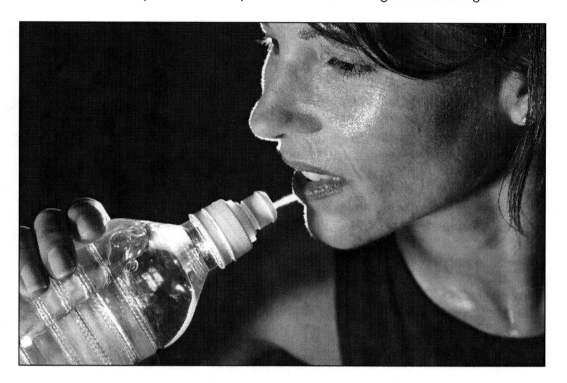

TIP/FACT #22
Warming-up and strength training can help prevent muscle strains.

A muscle strain involves overstretching the fibers within the muscle, resulting in microscopic tearing of the fibers. The greater the degree of muscle strain, the greater the degree of fiber destruction. A muscle strain typically occurs when muscles are forcefully and rapidly contracting against resistance. While any muscle can be involved, some muscles tend to be injured more frequently than others, including those in the thigh (the hamstrings and quadriceps), the lower leg (calves), and in the groin and shoulders. Each of these muscles have one key attribute in common—they're large muscles utilized for sudden, powerful movements.

The most effective way to prevent muscle strains is to warm up the entire body (e.g., jogging in place), followed by stretching the muscles involved in the activity. Another productive step for preventing muscle strains is to engage in a properly designed strength-training program that addresses any muscular imbalances that an athlete might have. The weaker muscle in any of the various pairs of antagonistic muscles that exist in the body is at a higher risk of being injured. For example, a number of athletes suffer hamstring strains because of a muscular imbalance between their quadriceps and hamstrings (i.e., their quadriceps are disproportionately too strong for their hamstrings).

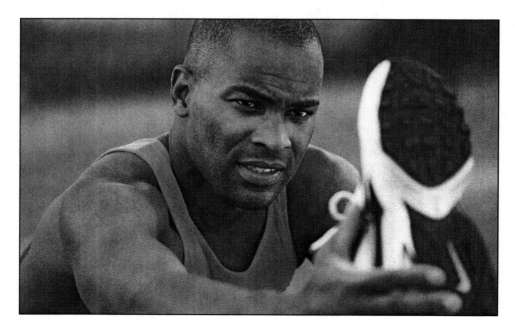

TIP/FACT #23
Strengthening of the rotator cuff muscles can reduce the occurrence of shoulder problems.

Athletes often develop shoulder problems that are related to instability (loose shoulder) and sports-induced weakness of the rotator cuff and scapular-stabilizing muscles. Because range-of-motion problems or loss of motion are relatively uncommon in athletes, stretching activities are generally not necessary, other than in the context of warming up for activity.

On the other hand, athletes who are at risk for incurring shoulder problems (e.g., those individuals who compete in throwing events or swimming) should engage in both rotator cuff-specific training and a general resistance exercise program that focuses on developing the larger muscles of the shoulders and core strengthening. Rotator cuff strengthening exercises should involve the supraspinatus and external rotators of the shoulder.

Scapular stabilizers are muscles around the shoulder blade that support and position the shoulder blade during overhead activities. These muscles include the levator scapula and trapezius (elevate the scapula), the rhomboids (retract the scapula), and the serratus anterior and posterior (retract and maintain the scapula on the chest wall with sport-specific motions). Exercises designed to develop the scapular stabilizing muscles generally involve shoulder elevation, retraction, and pinching the shoulder blades together.

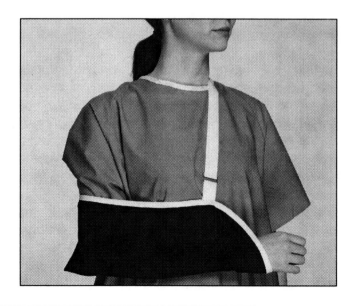

TIP/FACT #24
Proper hygiene is the most effective method to prevent skin infections.

Skin infections can be a serious concern for individual athletes, as well as for other teammates and competitors who may be infected by a particular athlete. Prevention strategies include the identification of infected athletes so they can be treated and isolated, the use of properly fitting equipment (to prevent blisters that may become infected), and the regular cleaning of equipment and uniforms. Among the problems caused by skin infections is the loss of practice and game time for athletes who participate in close-contact sports, such as wrestling, football, and martial arts.

Effective strategies for preventing skin infections in athletes should start with proper cleaning of uniforms and equipment. Practice and game uniforms should be laundered in hot water after each use. In wrestling, the mats and walls should be cleaned daily. There are multiple available disinfectants available for purchase, but a simple 1:100 strength solution of water and household bleach is adequate. If neither of the aforementioned is available, 70% Isopropyl alcohol (rubbing alcohol) or peroxide can be used. Individual equipment (shoulder pads, neoprene braces, etc.) should be wiped down after each use, not shared between athletes, and laundered regularly.

Coaches, athletic trainers, and individual athletes should be on the alert for the development of suspicious skin infections. Non-contagious skin findings include chaffing, abrasions, friction blisters, minor acne, and superficial lacerations. Contagious skin infections include herpes (zoster or shingles, cold sores, herpes gladiatorum), impetigo, tinea ("ringworm" of the head or body), moluscum, and carbuncles ("boils").

Herpetic lesions are manifested by clusters of small vesicles (blisters) on a red base. They may be crusted or oozing. Athletes with herpes should be on appropriate prescribed medications for 120 hours and have no oozing lesions prior to returning to practice or competition. Wet lesions should not be covered to allow early return to play.

Impetigo appears as a patch of crusted tissue on a red base. They may involve an ooze of pus or clear liquid. Athletes with impetigo should be on appropriate prescribed antibiotics for 72 hours, with no oozing or wet lesions prior to returning to practice or competition. Clearance to compete for an abscess or a "boil" is similar to that for impetigo. Again, wet lesions should not be covered to allow early return to play.

Ringworm appears as oval-raised or flat-red skin lesions, with some central crusting or scaling. Ringworm lesions can appear anywhere on an athlete's body. Athletes with ringworm should be on appropriate over-the-counter or prescribed medications (Lotrimin) for 72 hours prior to returning to practice or competition.

Moluscum appears like flesh-colored small dome-shaped lesions that may occur in isolation or in clusters. These lesions should be treated by a medical provider prior to the athlete returning to play. In a few instances, isolated lesions may be covered for competition.

When coaches, athletes, or parents identify suspicious skin problems, the athlete should be restricted from practice or contact until these problems have been properly diagnosed and treated. Coaches should require written notification from medical personnel as to the assessment and recommended schedule for allowing the athlete to return to competition.

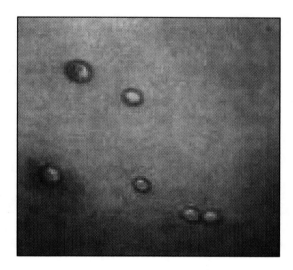

TIP/FACT #25
Water bottles should never be shared among team members, especially when an athlete is ill.

Exercising, ill athletes may pose a threat to themselves and other athletes. Strategies to prevent spread of infection begin with avoidance of the use of shared water bottles. Options include individual disposable cups for hydration or individual, personal bottles for hydration. If it is necessary to use common bottles athletes should not touch the bottle tip to their mouth. Ill athletes should be isolated from other teammates.

One well-recognized recommendation for ill athletes is the "neck check." Athletes with symptoms below-the-neck should not practice or compete. Below-the-neck symptoms include fever > 100.4°F, muscle aches, vomiting, diarrhea, or severe cough. Symptoms above-the-neck include those individuals who are ill, not with a fever, but with mild congestion and mild cough. In most cases it is safe for these individuals to compete. Ill athletes experience a decline in concentration, aerobic capacity, and a tendency to dehydrate more easily. As a rule, they are more likely to make mental mistakes and will not perform at their normal level. During recovery, athletes with symptoms below-the-neck should start exercising at 50% capacity for the first 5-10 minutes. If an athlete is fatigued at the 10-minute period, the individual should retire for the day. If the athlete experiences no fatigue, the individual can proceed with the exercise session or game.

Other prevention strategies in this regard apply to any individual concerning personal hygiene and personal safety while traveling. Mouthpieces should be cleaned, should not be placed on the ground, and should never be shared. Equipment should be cleaned with a disinfectant or bleach solution on a regular (preferably daily) basis. Traveling athletes should be aware of the source of drinking water or use bottled water.

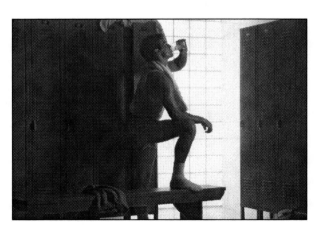

References:

Benjamin HJ, Briner WW, (2005) Little League Elbow. *Clinical Journal of Sport Medicine* **15**: 37-40.

Boden BP, Griffin LY, Garrett WE (2000) Etiology and prevention of noncontact ACL injury. *Physician and Sportsmedicine* **28**: 53-60.

Fees, M, Decker, T, Snyder-Mackler, L, Axe, MJ (1998) Upper extremity weight-training modifications for the injured athlete. *The American Journal of Sports Medicine* **26**: 732-742.

Howard TM and Butcher JB (eds) (2001) *Blackwell's Primary Care Essentials: Sports Medicine.* Blackwell Science, New York, NY.

Lyman, S, Fleisig, GS, Waterbor, JW, Funkhouser, EM, Pulley, L, Andrews, JR, Osinski, ED, Roseman, JM (2001) Longitudinal study of elbow and shoulder pain in youth baseball pitchers. *Medicine & Science in Sports & Exercise* **33**: 1803-1810.

Mellion, MB, Walsh, WM, Madden, C, Putukian, M, Shelton, GL (eds) (2002) *Team Physician Handbook,* 3rd ed. Hanley & Belfus, Inc, Philadelphia, PA.

O'Connor, FG, Wilder, RP (eds) (2001) *Textbook of Running Medicine.* McGraw-Hill, New York, NY.

Wojtys, EM, Huston, LJ, Schock, HJ, Boylan, JP, Ashton-Miller, JA (2003) Gender Differences in muscular protection of the knee in torsion in size-matched athletes. *The Journal of Bone and Joint Surgery* **85**: 782-89.

3

Direct Catastrophic Injuries in Sports

Barry P. Boden, MD

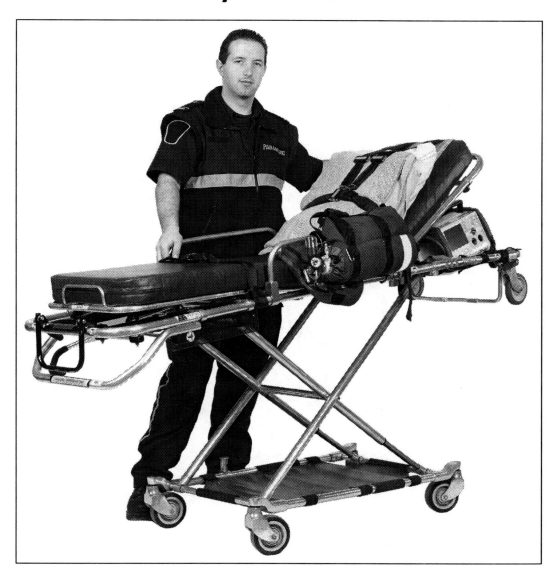

TIP/FACT #26
Catastrophic injuries are rare but tragic events.

In the United States, approximately 10% of all brain injuries and 7% of all new cases of paraplegia and quadriplegia are related to athletic activities. Information on catastrophic injuries in athletes is collected by the National Center for Catastrophic Sports Injury Research (NCCSIR), the United States Consumer Product Safety Commission (CPSC), and other organizations (Appendix 1). The NCCSIR defines a catastrophic sports injury as "any severe spinal, spinal cord, or cerebral injury incurred during participation in a school/college sponsored sport." Injuries are classified by the NCCSIR as *direct*, resulting from participating in the skills of a sport (i.e., trauma from a collision), or *indirect*, resulting from systemic failure due to exertion while participating in a sport. Indirect or nontraumatic injuries are caused by systemic failure as the result of exertion while participating in a sport and include cardiovascular conditions, heat illness, exertional hyponatremia, dehydration, and other conditions.

For all sports tracked by the NCCSIR, the total direct and indirect incidences of catastrophic injuries are 1 per 100,000 high school athletes and 4 per 100,000 college athletes. The combined fatality rate for direct and indirect injuries in high school is 0.40 for every 100,000 high school athletes and 1.42 for every 100,000 college participants.

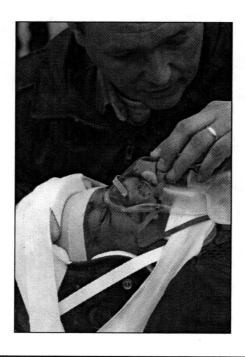

TIP/FACT #27
Football, pole vaulting, ice hockey, and cheerleading are the sports with the highest risk for a catastrophic injury.

Football is associated with the greatest number of direct catastrophic injuries for all major team sports, while pole vaulting, ice hockey, and football have the highest incidences of direct catastrophic injuries per 100,000 male participants. Cheerleading is associated with the highest number of direct catastrophic injuries for all female sports.

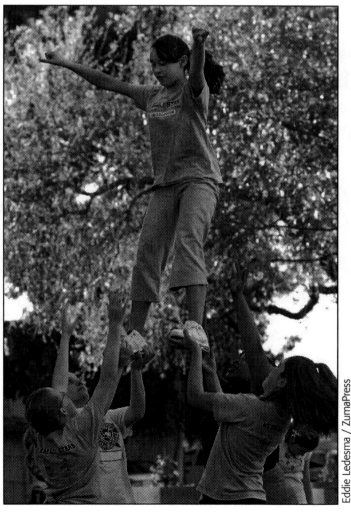

Eddie Ledesma / ZumaPress

TIP/FACT #28
Head injuries are the most common cause of fatalities in football.

Head injuries are the most common direct cause of death among football players, accounting for 69% (497 of 714 fatalities) of all football fatalities from 1945 through 1999. The majority of fatalities were associated with subdural hematomas (86%) and occurred in high school athletes (75%) during game situations (61%). A major factor in the decline of head injuries since the 1960s is improvement in the helmet design and the establishment of safety standards by the National Operating Committee on Standards for Athletic Equipment (NOCSAE). Improved medical care and technology are also likely responsible for the decline in fatalities.

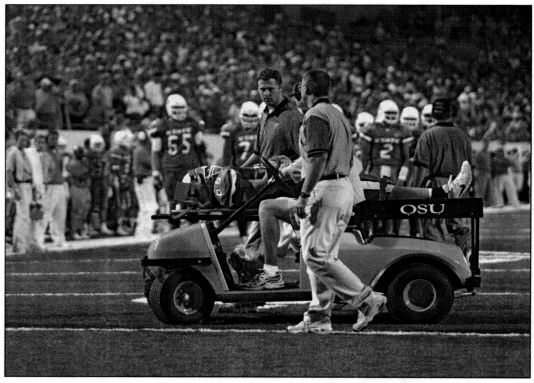

Photo by Ronald Martinez / Getty Images

TIP/FACT #29
Concussions in football typically occur to the player being tackled.

Nonfatal head injuries are extremely common in football, with nearly 900 concussions being reported in the NFL between 1996 and 2001. New data reveal that the vast majority of injuries occurred to the player being tackled. Often, the concussed player is hit from the side on the lower half of the face by the crown of an opponent's helmet. New football helmets with better padding around the ear and jaw are currently being tested.

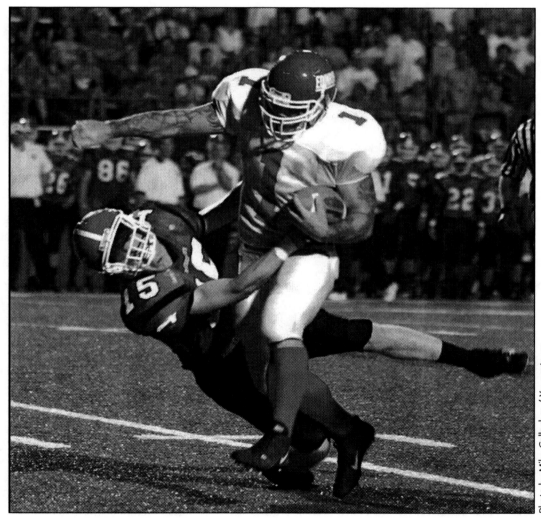

Photo by Mike Gallagher / Youngstown

TIP/FACT #30
Spear-tackling is the most common cause of cervical quadriplegia in football.

While the incidence of head-related fatalities started to decline in the early 1970s, the number of cases of permanent cervical quadriplegia continued to rise. This situation is likely due to the fact that the improved helmets allowed tacklers to strike an opponent using the crown of the head with less fear of self-induced injury. Dr. J.S. Torg was instrumental in reducing the rate of quadriplegic events by demonstrating that spearing or tackling a player with the top of the head is the major cause of permanent cervical quadriplegia. When the neck is flexed 30 degrees, the cervical spine becomes straight, and the forces are transmitted directly to the spinal structures. In 1976, spearing was banned, and the rate of catastrophic cervical injuries dramatically dropped.

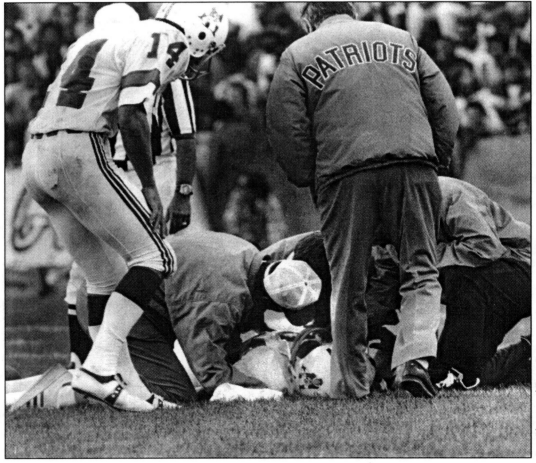

Ron Riesterer / ZumaPress

TIP/FACT #31
Most catastrophic pole-vaulting injuries occur when the athlete misses the landing pad.

Pole vaulting is a unique sport in that athletes often land from heights ranging from 10-to-20 feet. Pole vaulting has one of the highest rates of direct, catastrophic injuries per 100,000 participants for all sports monitored by the NCCSIR. The vast majority of catastrophic pole-vaulting injuries are head injuries in high school male athletes. The overall incidence of catastrophic pole vault injuries in the 1990's was 2.0 per year, while the incidence of fatalities was 1.0 per year. This number is relatively high, since there are only approximately 25,000 to 50,000 high school pole vaulters each year.

Most injuries occur when a pole vaulter either completely or partially misses the landing pad or releases the pole prematurely and lands in the vault or planting box. In response to the high catastrophic-injury rate, the landing-pad size for high school and college programs was increased in size from 16' x 12' to 19'8" x 16'5" as of January 2003. Because the majority of injuries are a result of athletes either completely or partially missing the landing pad, this rule change has the potential to significantly reduce the number of catastrophic injuries.

Any hard or unyielding surfaces, such as concrete, metal, wood, or asphalt, around the landing pad must also be padded or cushioned. In addition, a new rule has been adopted placing the crossbar farther back over the landing pad in order to reduce the chance of an athlete landing in the vault or planting box. A "coach's box" or painted square in the middle of the landing pad is also being promoted, a measure that should help train athletes to instinctively land near the center of the landing pad. Other safety measures that are under consideration by pole-vaulting authorities include marking the runway distances so athletes can better gauge their takeoff, and prohibiting the practice of tapping or assisting the vaulter at takeoff.

Pole vaulting is a complicated sport requiring extensive training and knowledgeable coaching; therefore, certification by coaches is encouraged. The value of helmets in reducing head injuries in high school pole vaulters is controversial. Without conclusive data as to their protective effect, the use of helmets is optional for pole-vaulting athletes at this time.

TIP/FACT #32
Pyramids and basket tosses are the most dangerous stunts in cheerleading.

At the college and high school levels, cheerleaders account for more than half of the catastrophic injuries that occur in female athletes. College athletes are more likely to sustain a catastrophic injury than their high-school counterparts, which is likely due to the increased complexity of stunts at the college level.

The most common stunts resulting in catastrophic injury are the pyramid, with the cheerleader at the top of the pyramid most frequently injured, and the basket toss. A basket toss is a stunt where a cheerleader is thrown into the air, often between 6 and 20 feet, by either three or four tossers. The majority of cheerleading injuries occur when an athlete lands on an indoor hard-gym surface.

The NFHS and NCAA have attempted to reduce pyramid injuries by limiting the height and complexity of a pyramid, and specifying positions for spotters. Height restrictions on pyramids are limited to two levels in high school and 2.5 body lengths in college. The top cheerleaders in a pyramid are required to be supported by one or more individuals (base) who are in direct weight-bearing contact with the performing surface. Spotters must be present for each person extended above shoulder level. The suspended person is not allowed to be inverted (head below horizontal) or to rotate on the dismount.

Safety measures have also been instituted for the basket toss, such as limiting the basket toss to four throwers, starting the toss from the ground level (no flips), and having one of the throwers behind the top person during the toss. The top person (flyer) on the pyramid is trained to maintain a vertical position and not allow the head to drop backwards out of alignment with the torso or below a horizontal plane with the body.

Cheerleading coaches need to devote equal time and attention on the technique and attentiveness of spotters in practice, compared with the athletes performing the stunts.

Coaches are encouraged to complete a safety certification, especially for any teams that perform pyramids, basket tosses, and/or tumbling. Pyramids and basket tosses should be limited to experienced cheerleaders who have mastered all other skills and should not be performed without qualified spotters or landing mats.

TIP/FACT #33
Collisions between players are the most common mechanism of catastrophic injury in baseball.

The most common mechanism of catastrophic injury in baseball is a collision either between fielders or a base runner and a fielder. Proper training is the easiest way to prevent collisions between fielders. When an outfielder and infielder are racing for a ball, the outfielder should call off the infielder. When two infielders are running for a pop-up, the pitcher should determine who catches the ball. These drills should be reinforced in practice sessions so they become instinctual in game situations.

Collisions between baserunners and fielders often involve the catcher. A typical scenario is a baserunner who dives head-first into a catcher and sustains an axial compression cervical injury similar to speartackling. Baseball rules state that the runner should avoid the fielder who has the right to the base path. Unfortunately, this rule is not always enforced when a baserunner is racing toward home plate. Since the speed of head-first sliding has been shown not to be statistically different from feet-first sliding, a strong case can be made that the head-first slide needs to be reassessed at the high school and college levels. In Little League baseball, head-first sliding is not allowed at any base.

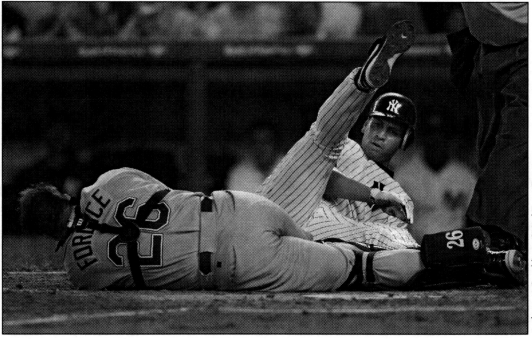

Anthony J Causi/Icon SMI / ZumaPress

TIP/FACT #34
Baseball pitchers are vulnerable from a batted ball.

After collisions, a pitcher hit by a batted ball is the next most common catastrophic injury mechanism in baseball. The pitcher is vulnerable to injury due to his proximity to the batter and from being propelled forward, often off balance, toward the batted ball. Many coaches and concerned parents perceive a problem from non-wood bats, such as aluminum bats, and have demanded that regulations be placed on non-wood bats. Due to their lighter weights, aluminum bats can be swung faster than wood bats, resulting in a higher ball-exit velocity. In response to the potential problem, the NCAA and the NFHS currently require all high school and college bats be labeled with a permanent certification mark indicating that the ball exit speed ratio (BESR) cannot exceed 97 miles per hour, as set by the Baum Hitting Machine (BHM).

Other important, new regulations designed to improve the safety factors associated with a bat are that the thickest diameter of the bat (barrel diameter) is restricted to 2 5/8 inches, and that each bat shall not weigh more than three ounces less than the length of the bat (e.g., a 34-inch-long bat cannot weigh less than 31 ounces). While these regulations show promise for reducing the number of injuries, the author is not aware of any clinical studies confirming their effectiveness.

In addition to regulating the bat, there are several other potential measures to protect pitchers. Protective screens (L-screens) are recommended at all times during practice sessions. Unfortunately, screens are not practical during game situations. Players and coaches should also be educated of the risk to pitchers and have the option of wearing protective equipment. In addition, it has been hypothesized that decreases in the ball hardness and weight may significantly reduce injury severity to players hit by a batted ball. The coefficient of restitution (COR), the measure of rebound that a ball has off a hard surface, has been adopted as the testing standard for baseballs. At the high school and collegiate levels, the COR of a baseball cannot exceed 0.555.

TIP/FACT #35
Commotio cordis may occur when a young athlete is hit in the chest by a ball.

Another area of concern in baseball is commotio cordis or arrhythmia often associated with sudden death from low-impact blunt trauma to the chest in subjects with no preexisting cardiac disease. The condition occurs most commonly in baseball, but has also been reported in hockey, softball, lacrosse, and other sports. Although the rate of rescue from commotio cordis was initially documented to be extremely low, more recent reports indicate that survival is possible with immediate resuscitative measures, such as performing a precordial thump or using automatic external defibrillators.

Preventive measures for commotio cordis have focused on chest protectors and softer-core baseballs. Unfortunately, neither has been shown to reduce the risk of arrhythmias and may actually exacerbate the force to the chest. Preventive strategies to address the risk of commotio cordis are currently limited to teaching youth baseball players to turn their chest away from a wild pitch, a batted ball, or a thrown ball. An analysis of the biomechanics of commotio cordis and the effectiveness of resuscitative measures, especially with automatic external defibrillators (AEDs), require further study.

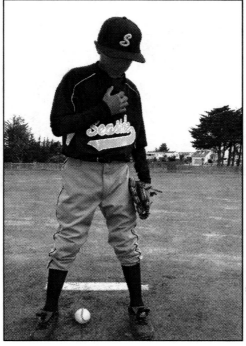

Brennan Tiffany

TIP/FACT #36
Most fatalities in soccer are caused by goalposts.

Direct fatalities in soccer are usually associated with either movable goalposts falling on a victim or player impact with the goalpost. The CPSC identified at least 21 deaths over a 16-year period associated with movable goalposts. Goalpost injuries in soccer can be prevented by never allowing children to climb on the net or goal framework. Soccer goalposts should be secured at all times. During the off-season, goals should either be disassembled or placed in a safe storage area. Goals should be moved only by trained personnel, and should be used only on flat fields. The use of padded goalposts may also reduce the incidence of impact injuries with the goalposts in soccer.

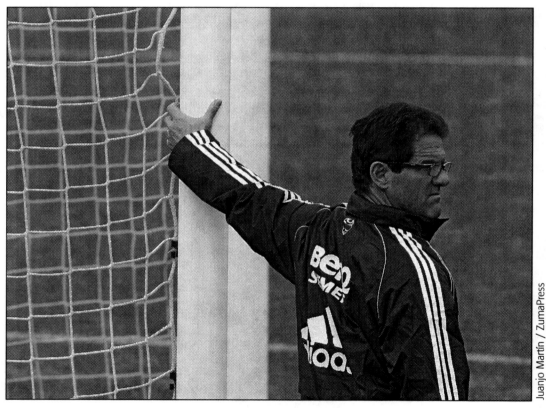

Juanjo Martín / ZumaPress

TIP/FACT #37
Children should use smaller soccer balls to reduce head impact.

No evidence exists that an isolated episode of heading a soccer ball can cause any head injury; however, there is controversy over whether repetitive soccer heading over a prolonged career can lead to neuropsychological deficits. Until conclusive data shows that repetitive heading of a soccer ball causes no long-term damage, it has been recommended that children use smaller soccer balls to reduce head impact. Leather or water-soaked soccer balls add weight to the balls and should never be used. Proper heading techniques should also be employed (i.e., contact on the forehead, with the neck muscles contracted). Soccer players should be trained to hit the ball, not to be hit by the ball. A long-term prospective study on the cumulative effects of heading a soccer ball is currently underway.

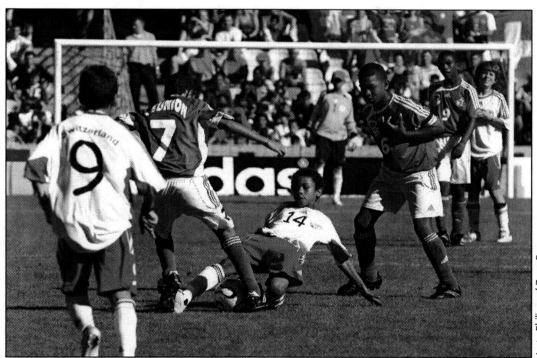

Juste Philippe / ZumaPress

TIP/FACT #38
The defensive posture during the takedown is the most common cause of catastrophic injury in wrestling.

Cervical injuries constitute the majority of direct catastrophic wrestling injuries. Most injuries occur in match competitions, where intense, competitive situations place wrestlers at a higher risk. The position most frequently associated with injury is the defensive posture during the takedown maneuver. There is no clear predominance of any one type of takedown hold that contributes to wrestling injuries.

General prevention strategies for direct catastrophic wrestling injuries rely on the referees and coaches. Referees should strictly enforce penalties for slams and should become more aware of dangerous holds. Stringent penalties for intentional slams or throws are encouraged. The referee should have a low threshold of tolerance to stop the match during potentially dangerous situations. Coaches can prevent serious injuries by emphasizing safe, legal wrestling techniques, such as teaching wrestlers to keep their head up during any takedown maneuver to prevent axial compression injuries to the cervical spine. Wrestling coaches should also emphasize adhering to proper rolling techniques, with avoidance of landing on the head, during practice sessions.

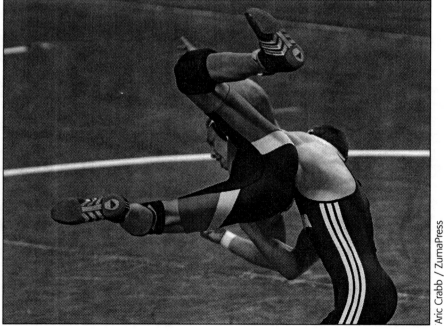

Aric Crabb / ZumaPress

TIP/FACT #39
Checking from behind is the most common cause of catastrophic neck injuries in ice hockey.

Although the number of catastrophic injuries in ice hockey is low compared with other sports, the incidence per 100,000 participants is relatively high. The majority of recent catastrophic injuries are reported to occur to the cervical spine. The most common mechanism of injury in ice hockey is checking from behind and being hurled horizontally into the boards. Contact with the boards typically occurs to the crown of the player's head, subjecting the neck to an axial load. Head and facial injuries are also common from collisions, fighting, or being hit by the puck or stick.

The frequency and severity of head and neck injuries may be reduced by enforcing current rules against pushing or checking from behind, padding the boards, and encouraging the use of helmets and face masks. In a prospective analysis of facial protection in elite, amateur ice hockey players, it was documented that players wearing no protection were injured twice as commonly as players wearing partial protection, and nearly seven times higher than those wearing full protection. Eye injuries were nearly five times greater for players with no facial protection, compared with those wearing partial protection. Aggressive play and fighting in hockey should also be discouraged and penalized appropriately. The "heads-up, don't duck" program teaches ice hockey players to avoid contact with the top of the head when taking a check, giving a check, or sliding on the ice. The Safety Toward Other Players (STOP) Program places the STOP patch on the back of the jersey of amateur athletes as a visual reminder not to hit an opponent from behind.

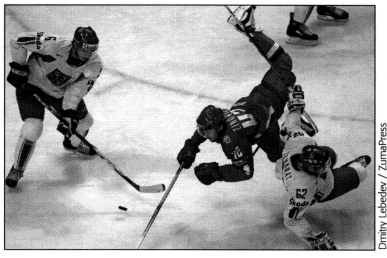

Dmitry Lebedev / ZumaPress

TIP/FACT #40
Diving into the pool is the most common cause of catastrophic injuries in swimming.

Most direct catastrophic swimming injuries are related to the racing dive into the shallow end of pools. The NFHS and NCAA have implemented rules to prevent injuries during the racing dive. At the high school level, swimmers must start the race in the water, if the water depth at the starting end is less than 3.5 ft. If the water depth is 3.5 ft. to less than 4 ft. at the starting end, the swimmer may start in the water or from the deck. If the water depth at the starting end is 4 ft. or more, the swimmer may start from a platform up to 30 in. above the water surface. The NCAA requires a minimum water depth of 4 ft. at the starting end of the pool. During practice sessions where platforms may not be available, swimmers are advised to only dive into the deep end of the pool or to jump into the water feet first.

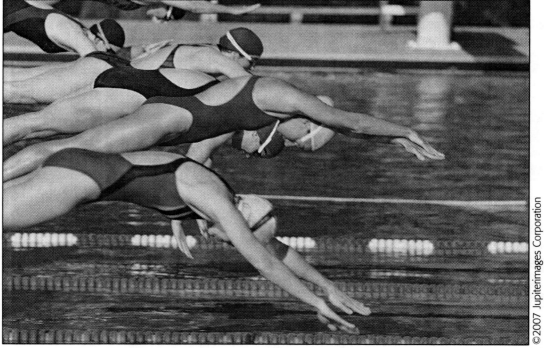

TIP/FACT #41
The cost of catastrophic injuries can be tremendous.

It has been clearly documented that physical activity has numerous health-related benefits. Nonetheless, a low risk of catastrophic injuries exists in certain organized sports, especially football, pole-vaulting, ice hockey, and cheerleading. In addition to the decreased quality of life for the patient, the lifetime cost for a complete quadriplegic individual can easily surpass $2 million dollars. Prevention is the most effective means of reducing the incidence and costs associated with catastrophic head and neck sports injuries (Appendix 2). Continued research of the epidemiology and mechanisms of catastrophic injuries is critical to prevent these injuries.

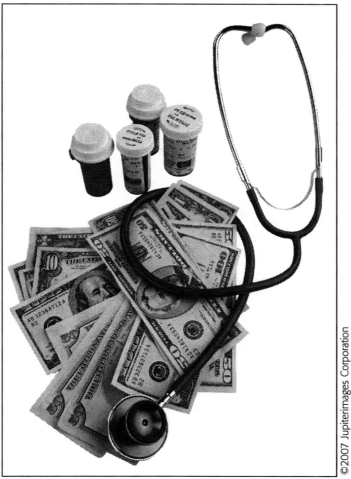

©2007 Jupiterimages Corporation

References:

Boden, BP, Kirkendall, DT, Garrett, WE (1998) Concussion incidence in elite college soccer players. *The American Journal of Sports Medicine* **26**: 238-41.

Boden, BP, Lin, W, Young, M, Mueller, FO (2002) Catastrophic injuries in wrestlers. *The American Journal of Sports Medicine* **30**: 791-795.

Boden BP, Pasquina P, Johnson J, Mueller FO (2001) Catastrophic injuries in pole-vaulters. *The American Journal of Sports Medicine* **29**: 50-54.

Boden, BP, Tacchetti, R, Mueller, FO (2003) Catastrophic cheerleading injuries. *The American Journal of Sports Medicine* **31**: 881-888.

Boden, BP, Tacchetti, R, Mueller, FO (2004) Catastrophic injuries in baseball. *The American Journal of Sports Medicine* **32**:1189-1196.

DeVivo, MJ (1997) Causes and costs of spinal cord injury in the United States. *Spinal Cord* **35**: 809-813.

Janda, DH, Bir, CA, Viano, DC, Cassatta, SJ (1998) Blunt Chest Impacts: Assessing the Relative Risk of Fatal Cardiac Injury from Various Baseballs. *Journal of Trauma-Injury Infection & Critical Care* **44**: 298-303.

Janda, DH, Bir, CA, Wild, B, Olson, S, Hensinger, RN (1995) Goal post injuries in soccer: A laboratory and field testing analysis of a preventive intervention. *The American Journal of Sports Medicine* **23**: 340-344.

Maron, BJ (2003) Sudden death in young athletes. *The New England Journal of Medicine* **349**:1064-1075.

Maron, BJ, Poliac, LC, Kaplan, JA, Mueller, FO (1995) Blunt impact to the chest leading to sudden death from cardiac arrest during sports activities. *The New England Journal of Medicine* **333**: 337-342.

Molsa, JJ, Tegner, Y, Alaranta, H, Myllynen, P, Kujala, UM (1999) Spinal cord injuries in ice hockey in Finland and Sweden from 1980 to 1996. *International Journal of Sports Medicine* **20**: 64-67.

Mueller, FO, Cantu, RC (2002) National center for catastrophic sports injury research: Twentieth annual report, Fall 1982-Spring 2002. Chapel Hill, NC. National Center for Sports Injury Research,1-25.

Pellman, EJ, Viano, DC, Tucker, AM, Casson, IR, Waeckerle, JF (2003) Concussion in professional football: Reconstruction of game impacts and injuries. *Neurosurgery* **53**: 799-814.

Stuart, MJ, Smith, AM, Malo-Ortiguera, SA, Fischer, TL, Larson, DR (2002) A comparison of facial protection and the incidence of head, neck, and facial injuries in junior A hockey players: A function of individual playing time. *The American Journal of Sports Medicine* **30**: 39-44.

Torg, JS, Guille, JT, Jaffe, S (2002) Current Concepts Review: Injuries to the cervical spine in American football players. *The Journal of Bone and Joint Surgery* **84**: 112-122.

Appendix 1. Sources of Information on Sport Safety.

AACCA   American Association of Cheerleading Coaches and Advisors
                 www.aacca.org

CPSC   Consumer Product Safety Commission
                 www.cpsc.gov

NCAA   The National Collegiate Athletic Association
                 www.ncaa.org

NCCSIR   National Catastrophic Center Sports Injury Research
                 www.unc.edu/dept/nccsi/

NCIPC   National Center of Injury Prevention and Control
                 Centers for Disease Control and Prevention
                 www.cdc.gov/ncipc

NFHS   National Federation of State High School Associations
                 www.nfhs.org

NOCSAE   National Operating Committee on Standards for Athletic Equipment
                 www.nocsae.org

PVSCB   Pole Vault Safety Certification Board
                 www.skyjumpers.com

USA Baseball www.usabaseball.com

Appendix 2. Summary of Safety Measures for Sports

Football

Helmet improvements (NOCSAE standards)
Banning spear-tackling

Pole Vault

Larger landing pad
Soft surrounding surfaces adjacent to landing pad
Moving crossbar closer to landing pad

Cheerleading

Limit height and complexity of pyramids
Maintain vertical position for flyer
Improving the skills of spotters

Baseball

Proper training to prevent collisions
Avoiding head-first sliding
Protecting pitchers (L-screens, bat and ball regulations)
External defibrillators for commotio cordis

Soccer

Goalpost safety (anchor properly, no climbing)
Proper heading technique
Smaller ball at youth level

Wrestling

Strict penalty for intentional slams
Heads-up technique

Ice Hockey

Avoid checking from behind
Helmet and face masks

Swimming

Adhere to rules on racing dive

4

Protective Sports Equipment

John P. Manta, MD

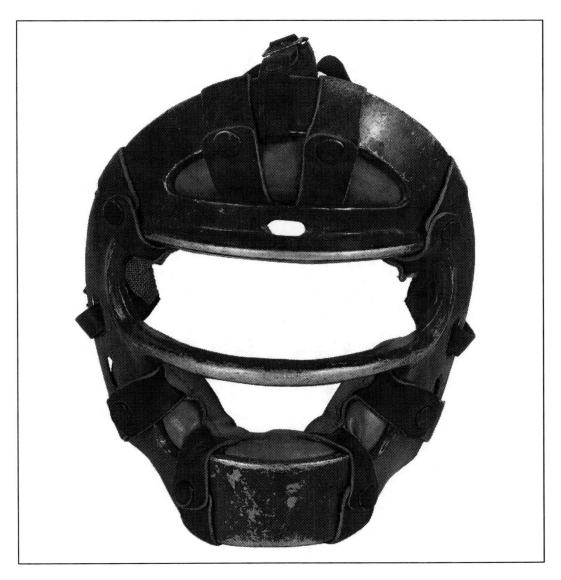

Very few instances exist when more protective gear does not ensure a safer game. It should surprise no one that American football with mandatory helmets and padding has approximately one-third the injury rate of New Zealand club rugby. Nonetheless, many sports seem slow to embrace protective equipment. For instance, girl's lacrosse only recently instituted mandatory eye protection and mouth guards.

In order to make sound decisions about protective equipment players, coaches and athletic directors need to separate the marketing hyperbole of new and improved protective equipment from the scientific studies, which often lag years behind. However certain fundamentals should always be considered. Protective equipment must be able to improve safety without hindering performance, adding liability or creating new safety concerns. Although this sounds rudimentary the mandatory hard-shelled football helmets were initially associated with an increase in head and neck injuries. This was not the result of a defective product but rather because it allowed or even encouraged the defensive player to utilize this piece of armor as a weapon. The rule change to eliminate spear-tackling with the top of the head reduced the number of fatalities and serious neck injuries in the late 1970's.

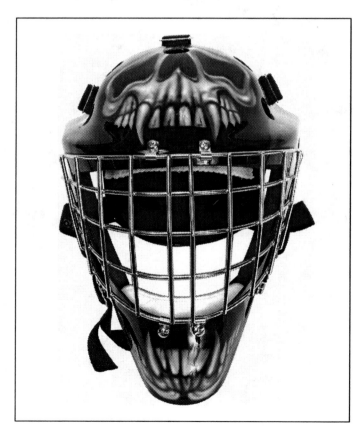

TIP/FACT #42
A proper fitting football helmet is critical for protecting the head from injury.

Collision team sports require the greatest amount of protective equipment. Protective headgear continues to evolve to protect football players from head injury. For example, over the years, American football helmets have developed from the simple leather helmet to the suspension helmet to the complex hard-shelled helmet of today. The National Operating Committee on the Safeguards of Athletic Equipment (NOCSAE) is responsible for developing the standardized game-simulating tests, as well as the standard needed to pass the test for football and many other sports helmets. The stringent criteria for helmet certification have consolidated the number of helmet manufacturers to two primary companies: Riddle and Shutt.

The NCAA has rules governing football helmets, including the helmet must have manufacturer or reconditioner certification indicating satisfaction of the NOCSAE test standard, the face mask and helmet must be secured by a four-point chin strap, and a warning label regarding risk of injury must be on the outside of the helmet. The NOCSAE warning statement is also located on a card that comes with each helmet. This statement should be read and signed by every participant and his parent.

The testing of helmets is based on the severity index (SI). The SI is an attempt to describe the significance of impact on the helmet. The SI predicts the helmet's ability to decrease forces at impact and to effectively protect the brain. A lower SI has a decreased risk of injury. In 1996, the passing SI score was decreased to 1200.

The Shutt football helmets are the Pro Air II and the Air Power. These helmets have pneumatic airliners with pads inside the helmet. These airliners do not compress like pads and have the ability to return to their original shape quickly after impact and to handle repeat impacts. These helmets have low SI values and offer good protection.

The Riddell Revolution helmet offers increased side and facial protection to potentially decrease the risk of concussions from blows to the side of the head, face, and mandible area. Emergency removal of the facemask with this helmet is a concern among Certified Athletic Trainers. This situation exists because the facemask design precludes the use of the standard removal device. Riddle does, however, provide a screwdriver for quickly removing the facemask.

The stability of the helmet on the player's head is critical to keeping the protective system in its intended place. Fitting adjustments may be necessary if the athlete's head has any irregularities. A player's head should be measured one inch above the eyebrows with helmet tape to determine proper shell size. Wetting the player's head makes the initial fit easier. The helmet should be fitted so that the ear openings are centered over the ears, the eyebrows are 1 to 1½ inches below the helmet's front edge, the faceguard is 2 to 2½ finger widths from the tip of the nose, and the jaw pads follow the contours of the cheek. Because it is relatively common for young football players to have narrow faces, the thickness of the jaw pads may need to be adjusted for a better fit. A simple test for proper fit is to rotate the helmet side-to-side, checking to make sure the forehead skin or hair moves with the helmet.

Vision should be tested peripherally, as well as up and down. The player should be able to see 180 degrees peripherally and 75 degrees in both an up and a down direction. The chinstrap should be tightened so that the cup is snug and centered on the chin. Players should not be allowed to play while wearing an unsnapped chinstrap, because the helmet can pop off on contact.

It is important to note that football helmets require maintenance. The National Athletic Equipment Reconditioners Association (NAERA) is an organization of athletic equipment reconditioners who recondition and certify helmets according to the NOCSAE standards and guidelines. NOCSAE mandates that every football helmet should be reconditioned at the conclusion of each football season. Helmets should be inspected weekly. In fact, many high schools require recertification annually. This process includes a standard drop test in which the helmet must meet the established SI value.

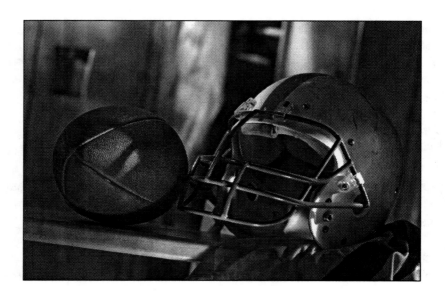

TIP/FACT #43
Football neck collars can reduce the incidence of stingers.

Stingers and burners represent a common football injury. This injury causes an intense burning pain in the shoulder often associated with tingling pain that radiates to the hand. This injury can be severe enough to cause arm weakness. Although controversy exists over the mechanism of injury, there is agreement that a stretch of the nerves appears to be fundamental to this injury. Neck rolls and collars are designed to prevent or minimize such nerve injuries.

Neck collars have three essential designs. Simple neck rolls are made from 5.08 cm open-cell foam, coated with vinyl. The Cowboy collar is a neck-roll system that combines a molded collar of polyethylene foam with a padded vest. The collar is worn under the shoulder pads and is designed to engage the side and rear of the helmet. The A-Force neck collar incorporates a molded cervical collar held in place by two straps that pass back under the axilla and fasten in the back with a plastic buckle.

All of these devices are ideally geared to reduce extreme neck motion without limiting normal motion. A laboratory evaluation of the devices revealed that all three collars limit the head and neck from bending backward. The Cowboy collar provides the greatest resistance to this type of motion. However, all three collars tested had a limited ability to restrict motion to the side. Unfortunately, this factor is likely the most common mechanism for stinger injuries.

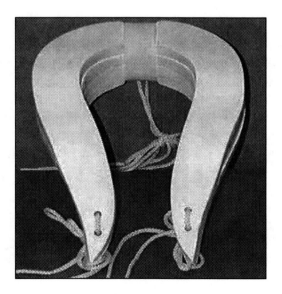

TIP/FACT #44
Facemasks and helmets can significantly reduce the incidence of head and facial injuries in ice hockey.

Facemasks and helmets are mandatory in college and most junior hockey leagues. However, the speed of play makes the weight of any protective equipment a major concern. Therefore, ice hockey helmets are not constructed in the same manner as football helmets. The Hockey Equipment Certification Council (HECC), Canadian Standards Association, and the International Standards organization (ISO) regulate ice hockey helmets.

In July 2004, NOCSAE developed specifications for newly manufactured hockey helmets. In this instance, the NOCSAE standard specifies drop tests similar to those described for football helmets. In addition, ISO also published the ISO 10256, which specifies performance requirements and test methods for head and face protection for use in ice hockey. The ISO standards address construction, shock absorption, puck-impact resistance, penetration, retention-system properties, field of vision, marking, and essential information concerning equipment that protects the head and face. Furthermore, most hockey leagues require a HECC certification.

The outer shell of the helmet is designed to deflect objects and dissipate forces over a larger area. Unlike football helmets, ice hockey helmets generally fail to restrict rotation of the head within the helmet. In that regard, a four-point chinstrap that theoretically improves the fit of the helmet and decreases the number of facial injuries is another safety feature being considered for adoption by hockey's governing bodies.

Facemasks are an extremely effective safety measure for reducing the incidence of eye and facial injuries in ice hockey. In a prospective analysis of facial protection in elite amateur ice hockey players, it was documented that players wearing no protection were injured twice as often as players wearing partial protection, and nearly seven times higher than those wearing full protection. Eye injuries were nearly five times greater for players with no facial protection, compared with those wearing partial protection.

TIP/FACT #45
Wearing helmets is mandatory in men's lacrosse.

Helmets are mandated for all men's lacrosse players and female goalies. Women lacrosse players are not required to wear a helmet, but are mandated to wear protective eyewear. The basic helmet configuration for lacrosse is similar to football and hockey, with a hard outer shell for deflective purposes. The inside layer typically has a liner or air bladder for energy absorption. Cascade is a popular manufacturer, with models that include conformity with lightweight helmets. Lacrosse helmets resemble football helmets with a facemask, four-point chinstraps, and air bladders. All men's lacrosse helmets must have the NOCSAE sticker on the outside and the NOCSAE warning statement.

Recent helmet design modifications have improved the lacrosse helmet's SI (severity index) score. Newer models are designed to be lighter, with shapes to attenuate forces when subjected to repeated impacts. Two new lacrosse helmets, the Sports Helmets Ultralite and Cascade, have the lowest rear-boss, drop-site test scores. However, all scores were within NOCSAE guidelines. Importantly, it should also be noted that a recent study found that SI values increased as the number of drops increased. Although the NOCSAE mandates football helmet reconditioning at the conclusion of each football season, the requirements are not as strict in lacrosse. Nonetheless, it is generally recommended that the lacrosse helmet be reconditioned each year and in use for only three years. Players who do not recondition their helmets and wear them for greater than three years may be at increased risk for head injury.

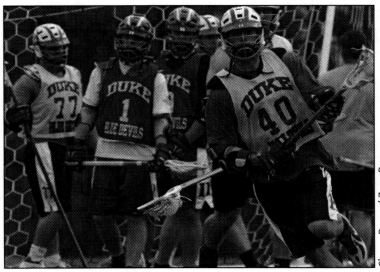

Shawn Rocco / ZumaPress

TIP/FACT # 46
Baseball helmets are mandated for batters, but not for fielders.

Although baseball is a noncontact sport, the high velocity of the ball has made double-earflap helmets mandatory. Helmets in baseball are regulated by NOCSAE, but are not subject to a drop test. In lieu of the drop test, helmets are subjected to a test where a ball, traveling at 60 mph, strikes the helmet in six different locations—one of which is random. The baseball helmet has a hard outer shell for deflection and an inner soft padding for absorption of energy. Newer models are replacing the traditional foam padding with air cells. Catcher's masks have only recently been certified, and NOCSAE has mandated built-in or attached throat guards. These helmets must also be one-piece construction, like a hockey helmet. Baseball helmets have no specifications for reconditioning, but should be inspected routinely. The paint utilized on these helmets should fulfill the NOCSAE certification requirements. Helmets are mandated for batters, but not for fielders. Due to the high incidence of pitchers and infielders being injured from a batted ball, the use of helmets for fielders should also be considered.

Although facial injuries account for less than 5% of all baseball injuries, they can have very serious consequences. Facial fractures account for 30% of all facial injuries. In youth baseball, protective faceguards are worn when the athlete is either at bat or running the bases. Polycarbonate face shields and metal cages are designed to provide minimal interference with vision. Adding the faceguard to a helmet has been found to decrease the risk of facial injuries by 35%.

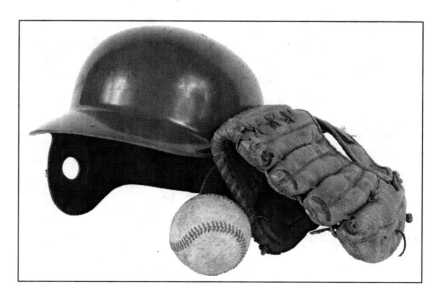

TIP/FACT #47
Safety balls, screens, and sliding bases can all reduce the incidence of injuries in baseball.

One of the most common causes of injuries in baseball is being hit by a batted ball. Although protective gear is standard for the batter, defensive players, with the exception of the catcher, have only their glove. Therefore, it is not surprising that infielders have the highest rate of ball-related injuries. In turn, being struck by a batted ball is one of the leading causes of catastrophic baseball injuries for pitchers. The use of personal protective equipment would certainly reduce these catastrophic injuries; however, helmets and faceguards are neither required nor commonly used for these positions.

Softer safety balls are commonly used at the youth baseball level to help decrease the rate of injuries to fielders. Soft-core balls usually have a polyurethane core, as opposed to the cork core in a standard baseball. The Consumer Product Safety Commission (CPSC) studied all available scientific literature on the softer-than-standard baseballs. The expert review determined that softer-than-standard baseballs reduce head injuries. In fact, a large study found soft-core balls decreased injury rates by 23%. The most significant benefit of these softer balls was with children younger than 10 years of age and less-skilled players.

The level of softness and compressibility of the baseballs are stratified for different age and skill levels. There are three main types of reduced-impact balls: reduced impact 10, reduced impact 5, and reduced impact 1. The softest ball, type 1, is recommended for children younger than 10 years old. The stiffer safety ball, type 2, is utilized until the age of 14. A recent USA baseball study showed that these balls were utilized by only 5% of leagues, 12% of which discontinued their use because of play-ability issues. The hardest safety ball, type 3, is recommended for players older than 14.

Sliding injuries account for 60% of all injuries to base runners. There are many factors that contribute to sliding injuries, including poor sliding technique and late decisions to slide by athletes. In addition to improved coaching, one way to drastically decrease injury rates involving sliding is with a detachable base. The detachable base dissipates the force being transmitted to the foot, ankle, and knee when the athlete makes contact with a standard base. Sliding bases or breakaway bases are designed in two pieces. The below-ground anchor is flush with the playing surface. The base then attaches to this mooring. Comparatively, approximately one fifth of the force is necessary to release the safety base from its mooring than the standard base.

Unlike safety balls, break-away bases have been studied in an older population. In a two-year study, 45 injuries occurred on standard bases, with only two on the break-away bases. The study also showed an 80% reduction in medical costs for players using the break-away base, compared to the standard base. The bases had to be reset an average of six times per game. The Rogers break-away system has different resistance levels for athletes of different sizes. The Rogers system includes tops, base plates, and an anchor mechanism. It is also important to note that the break-away bases are significantly more expensive than standard bases.

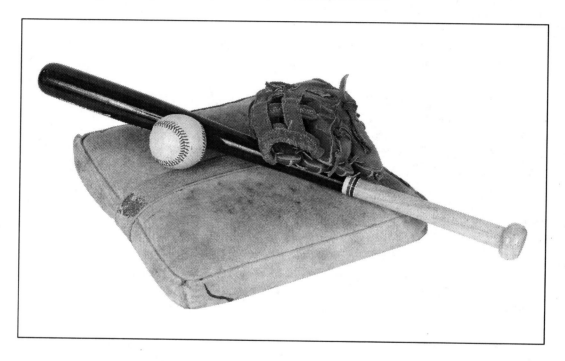

TIP/FACT #48
Mouthguards can prevent dental and orofacial injuries.

While mouthguards have the obvious benefit of preventing dental and orofacial injuries, they also may contribute to decreased concussion rates. Mouthguards are required for football, field hockey, ice hockey, and lacrosse. However, they should be utilized for every sport where a significant risk of contact exists. For example, mouthguards are not required for baseball, despite the frequency of ball-related injures to the face and teeth. Mouthguards are probably the most underutilized protective equipment available, despite the fact that they are relatively low cost, unobtrusive, and have minimal impact on performance. Mouthguards should be encouraged at an early age, so that usage becomes a habit.

Unfortunately, no standards exist for mouthguards. In addition, compliance is often low, even in sports where mouthguards are mandatory. Mouthguards should be properly fitted and of good quality in order to maximize player comfort and compliance. They should also be replaced at the first sign of wear (cracks or splits) or loss of resilience.

The role of mouthguards in concussions is theoretical. In collisions, which result in a direct blow to the chin, the mouthguard may have the ability to absorb some of the energy. The resilience of the material and the design of the mouthguard are designed to distribute the energy over a much greater surface area. In order to be effective in altering this force transmission, mouthguards must have adequate coverage and thickness over the back teeth.

Four types of mouthguards are available on the market: over-the-counter, boil-and-bite, custom-made, and heat-and-pressure laminated. Over-the-counter mouthguards offer the least protection and are considered unacceptable by most athletes. The boil-and-bite mouthguard is more customable. However, they are not very effective for concussion resistance, because they are too thin over the critical occlusal table. Fitting the boil-and-bite type of mouthguard pushes the material to the periphery and can result in a loss of up to 99% of their thickness in the posterior mouth region. The custom-fabricated mouthguard is professionally made over the dental cast of the athlete's maxillary arch. In general, they are fabricated from ethylene vinyl acetate (EVA) in single or double laminated sheets from a plaster model in a dental office or commercial laboratory. The pressures of the vacuum-forming machine can cause inconsistent and often minimal thickness across the occlusion surface. The heat-and-pressure laminated mouthguard provides a more precise fit and retains its structural integrity for longer periods of time. Upper and lower plaster models are taken of the athlete's mouth. The laminating machine has the capability of fusing multiple layers of EVA. This step enables the material thickness in the critical occlusion-surface area and allows for articulation of the aches to enhance mandibular stability during impact.

All four types of mouthguards appear to be effective at decreasing lip and mouth lacerations. The lower-cost models are more likely to interfere with speech and breathing, a feature that may decrease compliance with wearing the mouthguard.

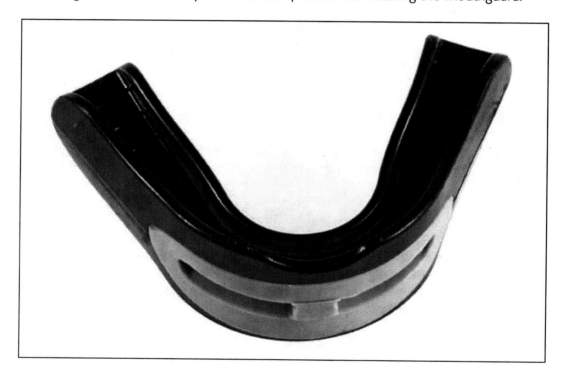

TIP/FACT #49
Protection of the head and neck in any sport involving a projectile should include eyewear.

An estimated 5.5 percent of all college varsity athletes sustain some form of eye injury each season. The U.S. consumer product safety commission estimates almost 40,000 sports-related eye injuries occur annually in the United States. For many sports with mandatory helmets, the protective eyewear is built into the helmet; however, proper fit and maintenance of the eyewear are required. The helmets mandated in football and men's lacrosse require a facemask, but this apparatus is often inadequate protection against eye injuries. Eye injures from small projectiles and fingers are not totally prevented by cage facemasks. Eye shields are available for these helmets. Most organizations require a clear, non-tinted, rigid device. This additional protection is recommended for all athletes, but is mandatory for athletes with only one functional eye (corrected vision that is less than 20/40).

Although collision sports generally require a helmet, the risk of eye injury in a particular sport is proportional to the chance for the eye being hit hard enough to cause injury and is not correlated with the classification into collision, contact, and non-contact categories. Available eye protectors can reduce the risk of eye injury at least 90 percent. On the other hand, the large number of eye-protector products available results in confusion regarding which are the most effective. The American Society for Testing Materials (ASTM) and NOCSAE are primarily responsible for sports eyewear safety standards. ASTM writes standards for sports eyewear for selected racket sports, women's lacrosse, field hockey, baseball, and basketball. Standards for hockey, youth baseball, football, and lacrosse are provided by NOCSAE.

Sports eye protection should be designed specifically for the sport. When choosing protective eyewear, the athlete's vision history is important. Only eye protectors that have been certified to national performance standards should be considered. An eye professional, such as an ophthalmologist or optometrist, can help ensure that prescription eye protection is sport-appropriate. Athletes who do not require correction lenses may use non-prescription polycarbonate eyewear. An athletic trainer can assist in selecting appropriate protective gear that fits well and is sport-appropriate for these athletes.

TIP/FACT #50
Shin guards are effective at protecting the lower leg from low-energy injuries (contusion, abrasion), but not from high-energy injuries (fractures).

During one three-year period in the early 1990s, 647,368 emergency room visits occurred from soccer injuries. Ankle and leg injuries account for 25% of these injuries. The most common mechanism of injury is a player-to-player collision from a tackle or missed kick. This encounter most commonly results in soft-tissue trauma, but can result in a serious fracture. In one surveillance study of soccer injuries, four of the 17 fractures which occurred were to the shin. The shin guard is the only mandatory protective device in soccer; however, its effectiveness in significant trauma has not been well established.

In a study of impact-load dispersion of different brand name shin guards, all were effective at reducing the peak impact force by at least 40%. The Lotto Air Italia was able to dissipate over 70% of the force. The study was performed utilizing a pendulum and a metal pipe to strike the shin of a hybrid III test dummy.

Although shin guards have obvious benefits, they are often ineffective at preventing many significant injuries. In a study of 31 tibia fractures sustained while playing soccer, the majority of fractures occurred while the athletes were wearing shin guards during game situations. The most typical mechanism was a slide tackle, often from behind, to an offensive player's planted leg. In over half of these incidents, the fracture was within the portion of the bone protected by the shin guard.

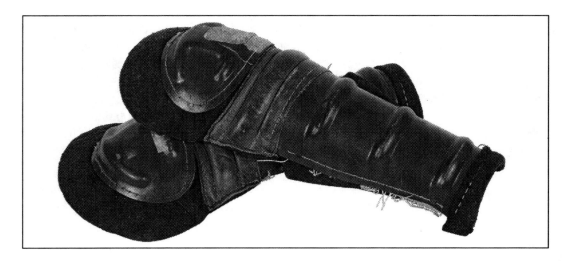

TIP/FACT #51
Soccer headgear has yet to be proven effective.

Soccer headgear has recently been added to the armamentarium of personal protective equipment. In soccer, head contact can have devastating consequences. Injuries from head-to-head, head-to-knee, and head-to-goalpost collisions can be catastrophic. However, severe head injury from head-to-ball contact is rare. The current generation of soccer headgear is designed only for impact with a ball and not for these other serious, yet unintentional, impacts.

The incidence of concussions in collegiate soccer, where there is significantly more contact than youth soccer, was shown to be approximately one concussion per team per season. Head-to-head and head-to-ground collisions were the major causes of concussion. No concussions occurred as a result of intentionally heading the soccer ball. Despite this, repetitive heading has been criticized for subjecting the athlete to impact forces that may cause long-term harm to the athlete's brain. Although no definitive evidence exists, arguments have been made that repetitive heading may lead to neurocognitive deterioration. It should be noted that other sports that involve direct head trauma, such as boxing, have already mandated some type of headgear.

In a study utilizing a JUGS Soccer Machine that projected soccer balls at a force platform, all three headbands tested had a decrease in force transmission. The three headbands tested were of similar design. This headgear is not similar in construction to the hard-shelled football helmet, but rather is a band of closed-cell foam. Some headgear also contain a hard-plastic insert. All types circle the head like a headband. The type with the hard-plastic insert was the most effective.

In another study, soccer headgear was noted to have limited benefit. A decrease in force transmission was only noted at low velocities and was not of a significant magnitude. According to the author of this study, a soccer ball and soccer headgear are approximately equal in terms of softness. As a result, no significant change occurred in soccer-ball force and acceleration when the ball hit the headgear.

The debate over soccer headgear demonstrates the problem in determining the efficacy of personal protective equipment. Although the headgear is actively marketed as a safety device, its indication and effectiveness is unproven. It may make heading the ball more comfortable. On the other hand, it may provide a false sense of security and provide little real protection to substantial injury. Further clinical trials are necessary before recommending headgear in soccer.

References:

Biasca, N (2002) The avoidability of head and neck injuries in ice hockey: an historical review. *British Journal of Sports Medicine* **36**: 410-427.

Cross, K (2003) Training and equipment to prevent athletic head and neck injuries. *Clinics in Sports Medicine* **22**: 639-67.

Halstead, PD (2001) Performance-Testing Updates in Head, Face, and Eye Protection. *Journal of Athletic Training* **36**: 322-327.

Hawn, K (2002) Enforcement of mouthguard use and athlete compliance in national collegiate athletic association men's collegiate ice hockey competition. *Journal of Athletic Training* **37**: 204-208.

LaPrade, R (1995) The effect of the mandatory use of face masks on facial lacerations and head and neck injuries in ice hockey. *The American Journal of Sports Medicine* **23**: 773-775.

Powell, J (2001) Cerebral concussion: causes, effects, and risks in sports. *Journal of Athletic Training* **36**: 307-311.

Vinger, P (2000) A practical guide for sports eye protection. *The Physician and Sportsmedicine* **28**: 49-58.

Washington, R (2001) Risk of injury from baseball and softball in children. *Pediatrics* **107**: 782-784.

5

Environmental Issues in Sports

Brian V. Reamy, MD, Colonel, USAF, MC

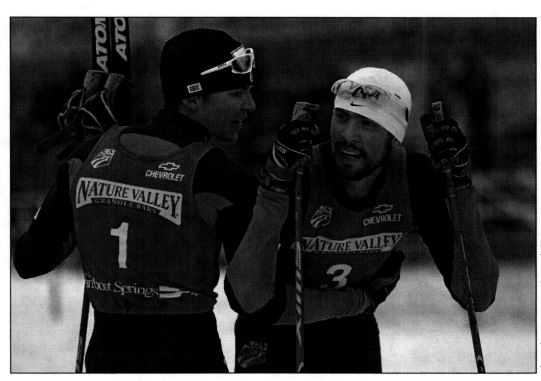

Photo by Doug Pensinger / Getty Images

TIP/FACT #52
The athlete with hypothermia may demonstrate symptoms that mimic mild alcohol intoxication.

Hypothermia occurs when the body's core temperature drops below 95°F. The athlete with hypothermia will show very nonspecific symptoms, such as confusion (forgetting plays, rules, or how to put on equipment), memory problems (inability to find proper ski lifts or skiing off course, forgetting the score), poor judgment (fighting, causing penalties, screaming at teammates), slurred speech, sleepiness, and eventually loss of consciousness. The overall appearance is similar to someone who is mildly intoxicated.

Extremes of age, use of alcohol, psychiatric illness, dehydration, injury, and improper clothing all increase the risk for hypothermia. Hypothermia is not restricted to days where temperatures are below freezing. It can occur even when outdoor temperatures are in the 50's (°F), especially if the athlete is wet and fatigued for an extended period of time. Endurance events are a particular risk, due to prolonged evaporative heat loss, exhaustion, and clothing dampened by sweat.

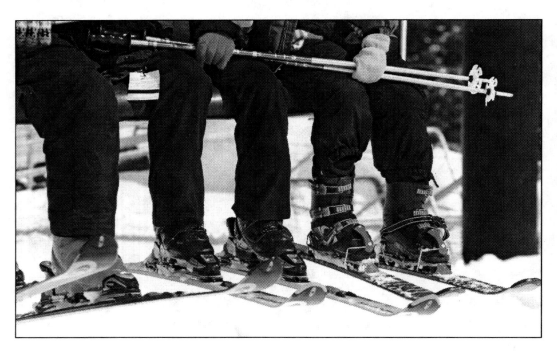

TIP/FACT #53
Field treatment of hypothermia should focus on the "3 W's" and transport to a hospital.

Hypothermia causes the heart to be unstable. Jostling or rough handling can trigger heart rhythm disturbances that can lead to death. It is important to move and treat the athlete with hypothermia very gently. The field treatment of someone with hypothermia should focus on the "3 W's." **W**et clothing should be removed and dry clothing or a blanket applied. **W**arm, non-caffeinated beverages should be provided to help reverse dehydration, and to begin core rewarming. **W**ind protection should be provided by placement in a shelter, vehicle, or behind a windscreen. Transport for definitive rewarming should be arranged as soon as possible to a hospital or medical-aid station.

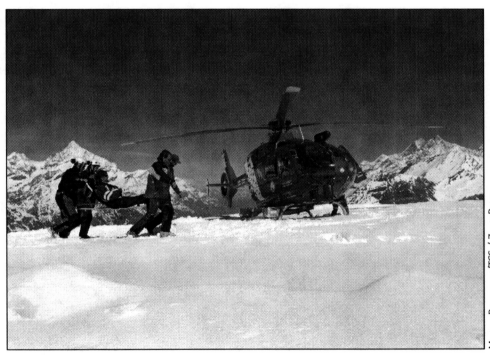

Menno Boermans/TCS / ZumaPress

TIP/FACT #54
The prevention of hypothermia revolves around the "3 L's" of proper clothing.

The prevention of hypothermia is possible through good conditioning, proper nutrition, experienced leadership and coaching, normal hydration, avoidance of alcohol or smoking, and habituation to a cold environment. Deciding what clothing to wear to avoid undue risk of hypothermia should adhere to the "3 L's." It should be **L**ayered, **L**oose, and **L**ightweight. Layering permits removal of layers as the athlete begins to warm with exertion. It is important to limit sweating, which can wet the clothing and increase the risk of hypothermia. The minimum number of layers is three—a silk or a wicking synthetic near the skin (e.g., Capilene®), a thick fluffy, insulating middle layer (e.g., Thinsulate®), and a water-resistant outer layer (e.g., Gortex®).

Clothing should be loose, to provide lots of air space between the layers—warming the air within fabrics and between layers creates optimum insulation and warmth. Finally, clothing should be lightweight to reduce sweating and optimize athletic performance. Not only can sweating dampen clothing, which increases the hypothermia risk, it can also cause dehydration, because the thirst drive is impaired in the cold.

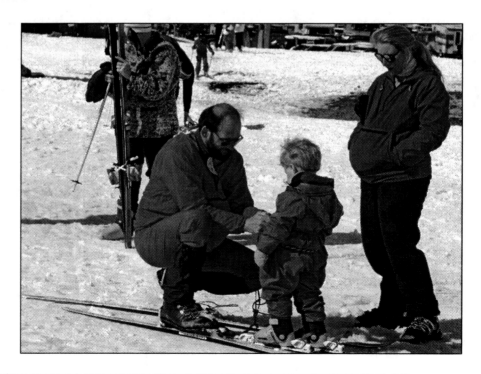

TIP/FACT #55
Prolonged exposure to cold is more dangerous than brief exposure to very cold temperatures.

Frostbite requires prolonged freezing of skin to occur. The feet and hands are most at risk and account for 90% of all injuries. But, the ears, nose, cheeks, and the penis (a particular concern for runners) are also at risk. The severity of injury is linked to prolonged exposure to cold, much more than to brief exposure to severe cold. It is most common in athletes from 30 to 49 years of age who engage in high-risk sports in inclement environments (back-country skiing, base jumping, expedition racing). Runners, who prefer to have unrestricted movement during races, present a particular problem. They may not wear sufficient clothing—especially if wind chill is severe. The 3 L's still apply (refer to tip/fact #54).

Superficial frostbite (1st degree) is characterized by skin that is normal-to-red in color, maintains sensation, and can be indented with pressure. Milky blisters are features of a 2nd-degree injury. Deep frostbite (3rd and 4th degree) is characterized by purple skin that contains small blood-filled dark blisters, is wooden to the touch, and does not indent with pressure. Healing from frostbite is hard to predict. Because the survival of skin is not determined until three weeks after injury, all frostbite should be treated the same in the early stages.

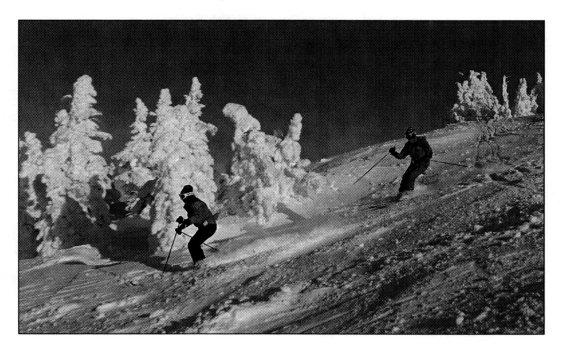

TIP/FACT #56
Field warming of frozen parts should not be instituted until refreezing can be prevented.

The peak period of damage to body parts from frostbite *occurs during the rewarming* of a frozen part. Therefore, rewarming should be done only once, and recurrent cycles of freezing and rewarming should be avoided. It is far more important to spend time on transport to a fixed medical facility than on rewarming. A useful mnemonic is, "it is better to walk out on a frozen part then to stop to rewarm it." The injured part should be protected with a loose, bulky insulated splint during transport. During treatment of hypothermia smoking, alcohol, and massage of the frozen part should be avoided.

Many homespun remedies are harmful if applied to fragile frostbitten skin, (brandy, bag balm, Vaseline, vegetable oil, rubbing alcohol, tar, snow) and should be avoided. Definitive treatment requires rewarming in temperature-controlled water at 104-108°F, and should be left to physicians working in a fixed medical facility. Pure aloe vera (Dermaide Aloe®), a topical medication, and oral ibuprofen (Motrin®) can help to treat frostbite if definitive treatment is delayed.

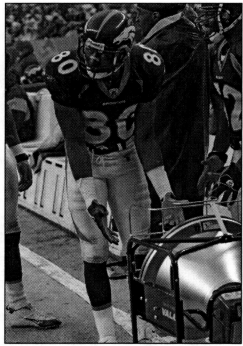

Byron Hetzler / ZumaPress

TIP/FACT #57
Field-side treatment for heat illness should be started early to prevent further damage.

Heat illness is best thought of as a spectrum that progresses from the mild (heat cramps) through the moderate (heat exhaustion) to the life threatening (heatstroke) if treatment is not provided. Heat cramps are painful contractions of muscles that typically occur after prolonged exercise. Heat exhaustion is a sign of impending body-wide system collapse. Athletes may have headaches, dizziness, fatigue, irritability, chills, nausea, vomiting, and fainting. Heatstroke can have similar symptoms, plus confusion and seizures. It represents a complete failure of the body's cooling system and requires emergency medical treatment with cold water immersion (partial or complete). Although athletes in the end stages of heatstroke may stop sweating, athletes with early heatstroke may sweat profusely.

The field-side treatment of heat illness revolves around immediate cooling. Athletes should stop activity, move to a shaded, cool environment, and drink cool water or sports beverages. Fanning after spraying the athlete with a cool mist is also helpful. Stretching and massage can treat heat cramps. If altered consciousness is present, heatstroke should be presumed, and emergency evacuation should be arranged.

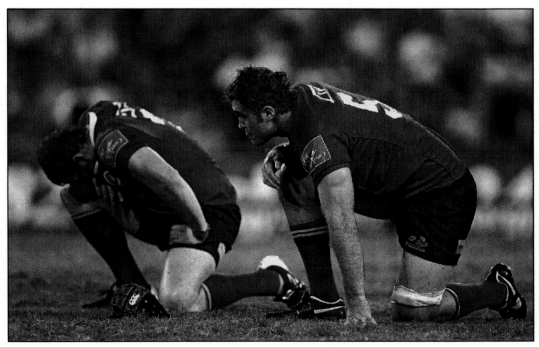

Photo by Krystle Wright / Getty Images

TIP/FACT #58
Prevention of heat illness is optimized by proper hydration and clothing, acclimatization, and modification of activity, based on the heat index (WBGT).

Preventing heat illness involves focusing on five key factors. First, *acclimatization* to high heat and humidity for 10-14 days prior to competition is ideal. The first four-to-five days are when the body improves its ability to cool itself. Second, *clothing* should be light colored, lightweight, and offer sun protection. Third, *medications* that impair heat loss by reducing sweating and increasing the metabolic rate should be stopped. Two examples of such medications are antihistamines (change to nasal steroid sprays to treat nasal allergies) and weight-loss supplements that contain caffeine, ephedra, or related compounds. Fourth, *prehydration and hydration* should adhere to the American College of Sports Medicine (ACSM) recommendations. Athletes should drink 16 oz. of water or sports beverage two hours before exercise. If this step does not induce urination, an additional 16 oz .should be consumed 15 minutes before exercise. During exercise, athletes should drink 20 to 40 oz. every hour. Fifth, *activity planning or reduction* should be based on the heat index or Wet Bulb Globe Temperature scale (WBGT). This scale incorporates humidity and radiant heat, along with temperature, to predict risk for heat injury at different climatic levels. Commercially available portable meters measure WBGT, and some communities broadcast the WBGT over the airways or telephone.

When the heat index is above 90, the risk of heat exhaustion or heatstroke is very high and consideration should be given to canceling and rescheduling practices or games. Table 5-1 summarizes the WBGT recommendations for athletes.

WBGT	Risk	Recommendations
>90	Extremely High	All activities should stop.
85-90	Very High	Unacclimated athletes should not participate.
75– 85	High	Take frequent rest breaks. Focus on hydration.
65-75	Moderate	Proceed with event and monitor conditions.
< 65	Low	Proceed with event.

Table 5-1. Activity modification for athletes, based on WBGT

TIP/FACT #59
An athlete who has suffered a heat injury is at greater risk for a recurrent and more severe injury for 24-48 hours and should be held out from practice and competition.

A risk factor for severe heat illness is a prior heat injury 24 to 48 hours earlier. If an athlete responds to field treatment of heat exhaustion, that individual should be held out of practice and avoid exertion for 24 to 48 hours before resuming full activity. Cases of death in athletes due to heatstroke have been preceded by a milder heat injury on the previous day. Kory Stringer, a professional football player, is a recent example of such a catastrophic occurrence.

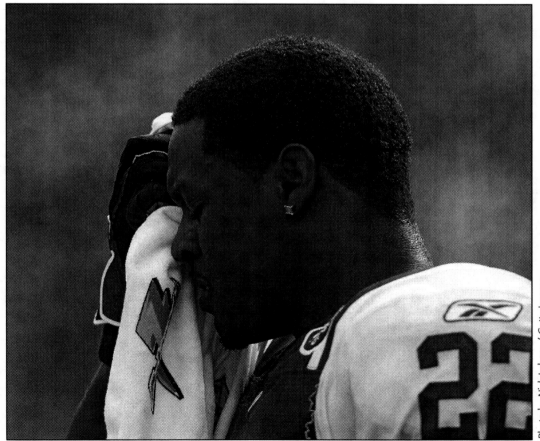

Photo by Nick Laham / Getty Images

TIP/FACT #60
Altitude illness can occur unpredictably in even the most well-conditioned athletes with ascent past 8,000 feet.

Rapid ascent past 8,000 ft. leads to decreased oxygen in the bloodstream. This situation can affect any individual, including the most highly conditioned, in an unpredictable fashion. The mildest symptom is a high-altitude headache (HAH). This condition may or may not progress to the syndrome of acute mountain sickness (AMS). AMS includes HAH and at least one of four symptoms: nausea/vomiting, fatigue, dizziness, or insomnia. Untreated AMS will progress to high-altitude cerebral edema (HACE—stumbling, decreased consciousness, confusion, or coma) or high-altitude pulmonary edema (HAPE—wet cough, shortness of breath at rest, and weakness).

The key to treatment is to stop the ascent and rest. A lack of improvement in 12 hours should lead to a descent in altitude of 1000 to 3000 feet. Ibuprofen or aspirin can be used for headache, and, if available, acetazolamide (Diamox® – prescription only) should be given. Any symptoms of HACE or HAPE should trigger immediate descent and evacuation. These are life-threatening conditions.

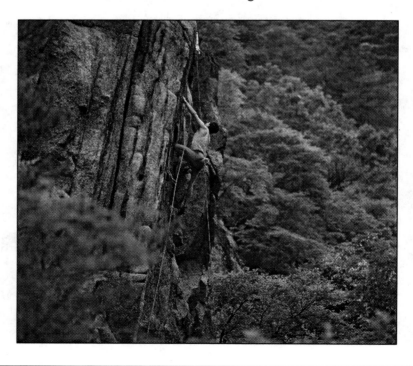

TIP/FACT #61
Altitude illness is preventable.

Altitude illness is entirely preventable by proper acclimatization. It takes several days for the body to fully adapt to altitude changes. Exertion should begin below 8,000 feet. Two to three nights should be slept at 8,000 to 10,000 feet before continuing with the ascent. A limit of 1,500 feet per day may be climbed above 10,000 feet. A summary of prevention recommendations is listed in Table 5-2.

1. Begin exertion below 8,000 ft. Spend two-to-three nights sleeping between 8,000 and 10,000 ft. before ascending above 10,000 ft.
2. Sleep no more than 1,500 ft higher each day above 10,000 ft.
3. Avoid alcohol or sedatives.
4. Avoid dehydration or hypothermia.
5. Consider getting a prescription for Diamox®, 250 mg twice a day, beginning the day before ascent as a preventive treatment. This step is especially important for anyone with a history of AMS, when climbing past 11,400 ft., or when acclimatization is not possible. The Rx should be continued until after 48 hrs. at peak altitude. (Diamox® causes carbonated beverages to taste foul and increases the need to urinate.)
6. In the face of symptoms of AMS, do not go higher. Descend if symptoms do not improve in 12 hours.

Table 5-2. Prevention of altitude illness

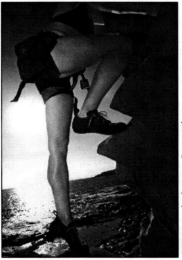

©2007 Jupiterimages Corporation

References:

Armstrong, LE, Epstein, Y, Greenleaf, JE, Haymes, EM, Hubbard, RW, Roberts, WO, Thompson, PD (1996) American College of Sports Medicine Position Stand. The female athlete triad: Heat and cold illnesses during distance running. *Medicine & Science in Sports & Exercise* **28**: 139-148.

Convertino, VA, Armstrong, LE, Coyle, EF, Mack, GW, Sawka, MN, Senay Jr., LC, Sherman, WM (1996) American College of Sports Medicine Position Stand. Exercise and fluid replacement. *Medicine & Science in Sports & Exercise* **28**: i-ix.

Danzl, DF (2001) Accidental hypothermia, in Auerbach, PS (ed) *Wilderness Medicine,* 4th ed. Mosby, St. Louis, MO. pp 135-177.

Hackett, PH, Roach, RC (2001) High-altitude medicine, in Auerbach, PS (ed) *Wilderness Medicine,* 4th ed. St. Louis, MO, Mosby, pp 2-43.

Moran, DS, Gaffan, SL (2001) Clinical management of heat-related illnesses, in Auerbach, PS (ed) *Wilderness Medicine,* 4th ed. Mosby, St. Louis, MO, pp 290-316.

Reamy, BV (1998) Frostbite: Review and current concepts. *Journal of American Board of Family Practice* **11**: 34-40.

6

Sports Nutrition

Patricia A. Deuster, PhD, MPH
Jamie A. Cooper, MS

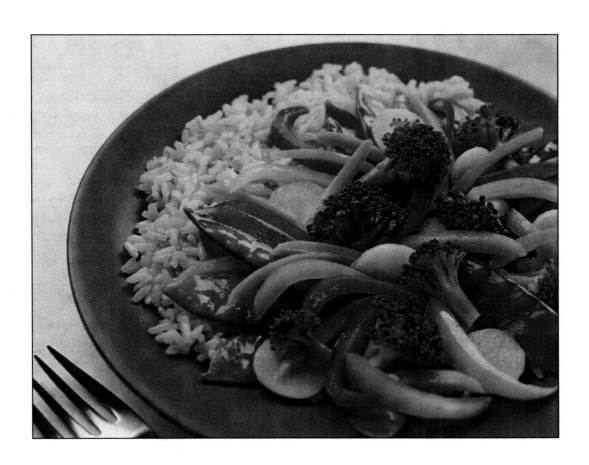

TIP/FACT #62
All athletes can meet their protein requirements by eating a balanced diet with adequate energy intakes.

An individual is comprised of water (40 to 60%), protein (12 to 15%), adipose tissue (8 to 50%), and minerals (2 to 8%). Most of the body's protein is in skeletal muscle, which is approximately 20% protein; the remainder of muscle is made up of water (75%) and other organic material (5%). The protein in skeletal muscle and other tissues is not a primary source of energy, but rather serves other important functions, such as the maintenance and repair of cell functions, energy production, muscle contractions, and delivery of oxygen and other nutrients to tissues. Therefore, protein is essential for all aspects of function and is important for all athletes, regardless of the sport.

The recommended dietary allowance (RDA) for protein intake for normal, healthy people (0.8g/kg of body weight per day) is not adequate for athletes. Strength-trained athletes may need 1.6 to 1.7 grams of protein per kg of body weight, whereas endurance athletes may require 1.2 to 1.4 grams per kg body weight each day. This amount would equate to 0.5 to 0.8 grams of protein per pound of body weight, or 75 to 120 grams for a 150-pound athlete. Many athletes consume four times the RDA each day in an effort to increase strength, muscle mass, and size. However, consuming more protein than recommended has not been shown to increase muscle mass. In fact, excess protein, which is broken down into amino acids, is stored as fat in the body. Further, excessive intake of protein increases fluid needs and may compromise kidney function.

The need for dietary protein also depends on total energy intake and protein quality. For example, female endurance athletes may need more protein than men because their energy intakes are usually lower. However, protein needs can and should be met by eating good foods, rather than by taking protein supplements.

TIP/FACT #63
Vitamin, mineral, and other supplements are not needed, if a healthy, well-balanced diet is consumed.

Vitamins, minerals, and other cofactors are essential for good health, growth, and development. These essential nutrients do not provide energy for muscular contraction, but rather participate in energy-providing reactions and muscle growth and repair. Despite the availability of vitamins and minerals in the foods athletes eat, many athletes take a vitamin and/or mineral supplement because they think it will improve their performance. No study has ever shown a benefit from vitamin and mineral supplements on performance, unless there was already an existing vitamin or mineral deficiency. Eating a well-balanced diet that includes vegetables, fruits, grains, dairy products, and meats should ensure adequate amounts of vitamins, minerals, and other cofactors in their natural forms. However, taking a well-balanced supplement that provides only the recommended amounts of vitamin and/or minerals should not cause any problems.

Any athlete who is not eating a balanced diet may consume inadequate amounts of certain vitamins and minerals. Dietary intakes of calcium, iron, and zinc may be low, but this can be avoided by making appropriate food choices. Dairy products and other foods, such as sardines, canned salmon, broccoli, tofu, turnip greens, milk, cheese, yogurt, and kale, are high in calcium and should be consumed daily. Meat, fish, and poultry provide iron that is highly available, whereas vegetables (spinach, kidney beans, and others) and grains provide iron that is not absorbed as readily. Blackstrap molasses and many fortified foods (pastas and cereals) are also good sources of iron.

Lean red meats and seafood, in particular oysters, are the best sources of zinc, but cereals and rice, beans, cheese, and nuts, including peanut butter, also provide zinc. Zinc from meat and seafood is more readily available than zinc from grains and vegetables, because the fiber in such foods can bind the zinc. Vegetarians should plan their diet so they take in adequate amounts of zinc and iron.

In addition to calcium, iron, and zinc, young, growing athletes should consume sufficient amounts of folate, vitamin B_6, and vitamin B_{12}. Additional folate, vitamin B_6, and vitamin B_{12}, which serve important roles in growth, energy metabolism, and development, may be needed during high periods of growth. Eating a well-balanced diet by choosing a wide variety of foods should provide the necessary vitamins, minerals, and other cofactors required by young athletes.

TIP/FACT #64
Maintaining hydration status is the most critical nutritional concern for athletes.

The human body is approximately 60% water, and as such, water is the most important "nutrient" of all. Proper hydration is critical for athletes, because dehydration, or loss of body fluids, will compromise performance. Water in the body serves many functions as a primary component of blood, where water is essential for maintaining circulation, body temperature, and blood pressure, and delivering nutrients and oxygen to tissues. In particular, it is the loss of water, or sweating, which dissipates the excess body heat produced during exercise.

During exercise, the body's fluid volume decreases due to water lost through sweat and respiration. Athletes who exercise for extended periods of time, especially when training in hot and humid weather, are at high risk for dehydration. If an athlete trains or competes more than once a day, the risk of dehydration is high. Fluid losses amounting to only 2% of body weight can cause decrements in performance. Symptoms of dehydration (other than loss of body weight) include feeling thirsty, dry mouth, nausea, headache, and difficulty concentrating. One good indicator of dehydration is urine color. When fluid levels are adequate, urine will be pale yellow, whereas urine will be dark when fluid status is compromised.

Although dehydration is a vital issue, it is also important not to over-hydrate when exercising for a long period of time. Drinking too much water can lead to a condition called hyponatremia, or a low-blood sodium level. This situation involves a very serious health condition and can result in death. Although the general population has been advised to restrict their sodium intake, athletes should not. Athletes require sodium due to the large amounts lost in sweat, and those losses must be replaced. The American College of Sports Medicine and the National Athletics Trainers Association recommend that athletes liberally salt their food and drink sports drinks, particularly when exercising in the heat, to maintain sodium balance and to help in rehydration.

Water, juice, and sports drinks are good choices for replacing fluid. In general, athletes should drink 16 ounces of water or a sports drink two hours before exercise. During exercise, athletes should begin to drink early and at regular intervals so fluids are ingested at a rate sufficient to replace the water lost through sweating. At least four-to-eight ounces should be ingested every 15 to 20 minutes during exercise, and the fluid should be cool (between 59° and 72°F), rather than warm, because cool fluids are absorbed more rapidly than warm ones. Finally, it is important that the taste and flavor of the beverage are appealing, since more fluid will be ingested if the taste and flavor are suitable.

After exercise, the fluids lost during exercise should be replaced as soon as possible. The appropriate amount of fluids to be replaced can be calculated from body weight, urine losses, and fluid ingested during exercise. Specifically, athletes should measure their weight before and after exercise to determine weight loss during exercise (in ounces) and then add how much fluid they consumed during exercise (in fluid ounces). This total is the amount of fluid they should drink to replace sweat losses and ensure adequate rehydration. Thus, optimal hydration status is based on the individual needs of the athlete, and all athletes should be instructed to pay attention to their fluid needs by "weighing in" before and after training.

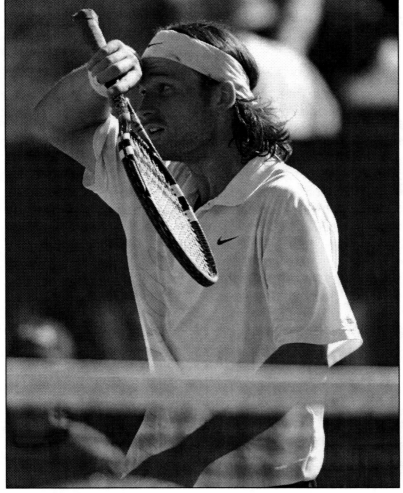

Photo by Brian Bahr / Getty Images

TIP/FACT #65
Athletes should select a fluid replacement beverage, based on the duration and intensity of the exercise and their preferences.

Both water and sports beverages are important for athletes, but several issues should be considered when selecting a sports beverage. The usual beverage of choice for maintaining hydration status during exercise is water, because it is both readily absorbed and inexpensive. A general rule is that water is preferred when the duration of the exercise is 60 minutes or less.

In contrast to water, sports drinks typically provide both carbohydrates (CHO) and electrolytes. However, the athlete should be aware that two types of beverages are marketed to athletes: sports and energy beverages. Although fundamentally similar, sports and energy beverages serve two different purposes. Both typically contain energy-rich CHO and other performance-enhancing ingredients, but a sports beverage is intended to maintain hydration.

Carbohydrate and electrolyte replacement is important for exercise of long duration (i.e., greater than one hour), which can deplete energy stores and compromise electrolyte balance. As discussed in tip/fact #64, sodium and chloride are lost through sweat, and need to be replaced. Energy in the form of CHO can extend performance and delay fatigue. Although sports drinks do not necessarily promote rehydration more rapidly than water, people are more likely to drink sports drinks because they taste better. The optimum CHO content for a sports drink is between 4-and-8% or 9.5-to-19 g of CHO per 8-oz. serving, which equates to ≤ 96 kcal/8oz. Also, the drink should have a sodium content between 40 to 240 mg/8oz., be non-carbonated, and contain no substances other than CHO electrolytes. If it contains protein, the CHO-to-protein ratio should be less than 4.

The type of CHO in the sports drink is important as well. Glucose and maltodextrin empty more rapidly from the digestive tract than fructose, and fructose can cause gastrointestinal problems. Like water, 4 to 8 oz. of a 4 to 8% sports drink should be ingested every 15 to 20 minutes, during exercise lasting longer than one hour, to reduce the risk of dehydration. Drinking this amount should also provide enough CHO (30 to 60 g per hour) to maintain blood glucose and delay fatigue. Sports beverages can be useful for athletes who must spend the day at athletic events, such as track or swimming meets, basketball, volleyball or wrestling tournaments, or gymnastic competitions, where nutritious foods and beverages may be difficult to find. Table 6-1 provides the names and composition of sports beverages that are available and appropriate during and after exercise.

Unlike sports drinks, energy drinks should NOT be used for fluid replacement, and if used, should be used with caution. Most energy drinks contain too much CHO to allow for rapid fluid replacement. The CHO content may be as high as 52 grams per 8 oz., and although this amount of CHO may be useful after exercise, it would be detrimental during exercise. In addition, many energy drinks contain amino acids, caffeine, vitamins, herbs, and other factors, which are not needed during exercise, and which can be very expensive. Because there are so many energy and sports beverages on the market, it is very important to read the labels and have the athletes try the beverage during training before using it during a competition.

PRODUCTS	Energy kcal/8oz	CHO g/8 oz	CHO:Pro $\geq$ 4:1	Sodium mg/8 oz
Cerasport	76	13	-	102
Gatorade Original	50	14	-	110
Gookinade	86	10	-	64
GU2O	50	13	-	120
MetRx ORS	75	19	-	125
Powerade	72	19	-	53
Power Bar Endurance Sports Drink	70	17	-	160

Table 6-1. Recommended fluid replacement beverages

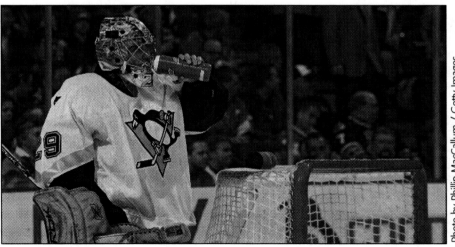

Photo by Phillip MacCallum / Getty Images

TIP/FACT #66
The glycemic index of foods should be used for selecting the foods consumed prior to and after training and competitions.

Carbohydrates (CHO), the body's primary source of energy during exercise, are found primarily in grains, fruits, and vegetables. CHO can be categorized into two main groups: simple and complex. Simple CHO is found in fruits, candy, and table sugar, whereas complex CHO is found in breads, cereals, vegetables, and foods high in starch. All foods promote changes in blood glucose after they are ingested. Comparisons of blood glucose responses to foods gave rise to the term, glycemic index (GI), which signifies how rapidly blood glucose increases in response to the ingestion of the food. The GI is now recognized throughout international communities as a reliable and scientific way to rate and classify foods, based on how they affect blood glucose. This measure is important for young athletes.

Foods are classified as having either a low, moderate, or high GI. The GI of a specific amount of a particular food is expressed relative to the glycemic response after ingestion of 50 g of glucose or white bread. The division between a low, moderate, and high GI depends on the reference used (glucose or white bread). The higher the GI, the greater the change in blood glucose that will occur and the greater the amount of glucose delivered to the body. The GI allows for specific foods or combinations of food to be compared.

Although GI values are usually consistent across the world, some foods are highly variable. Two notable foods in this regard include rice and carrots. The GI for rice has been reported to range from a low of 27 to a high of 104, depending on differences in rice across countries. Carrots are highly variable, with a low GI of 32 to a high GI of 92, and these differences may reflect the nutrient content and/or the methods of preparation. Otherwise, GI values are fairly consistent, and whenever possible, should be used to make food choices before and after training and competition.

Athletes should try to use the GI index when planning meals and snacks to optimize performance. Eating foods that have a moderate or low GI is important for endurance athletes prior to long training sessions and competition. Consuming high GI foods prior to exercise can result in hypoglycemia when an individual starts to exercise, a condition where blood sugar levels drop rapidly and symptoms such as dizziness, sweating, palpitations, and the like may occur. This situation happens because the rapid rise in glucose will cause insulin to be released, which, in turn, results in glucose uptake by tissues and lowers blood glucose. In contrast, foods with a high GI will cause the most rapid repletion of liver and muscle glycogen, because first blood glucose and then the insulin response will be high. Thus, consuming high GI foods is most beneficial immediately after a long and/or intense workout when glycogen depletion may have occurred. Table 6-2 (pg. 109) presents the GI of various foods. Appealing foods from both groups should be identified and made available before, during, and after exercise.

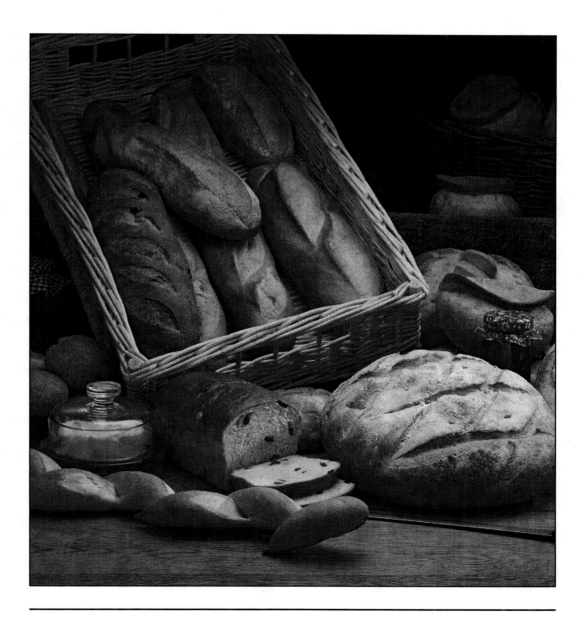

TIP/FACT #67
The precompetition meal is very important, and foods must be chosen and timed appropriately.

Many athletes are unsure about what to eat or even if they should eat before competing. *Under no circumstance should an athlete try to eat something new on a competition day.* One way to approach the precompetition meal is to try different foods before training and/or practice to see what works best. Because eating certain foods can cause gastrointestinal distress in some people, athletes need to find out during training what foods cause them problems.

In general, an athlete should consume some form of CHO two-to-four hours before a competition to avoid low blood glucose levels, which can cause symptoms of lightheadedness, fatigue, and indecisiveness. The CHO consumed prior to the event will help fuel the brain and muscles during the competition. If the competition is in the morning, a small, low GI CHO food should be eaten, since blood glucose levels decline during the night. If the competition is later in the day, it is important to consume CHO foods throughout the day, but allow at least two hours without eating any solid food before the actual competition begins.

How much an athlete eats before competition depends on the time of the competition. A big meal (1,200 calories or 4 to 5 grams of CHO/kg) will require at least four hours and a lighter meal (about 600 calories) around three hours for digestion. A light snack (about 200 to 300 calories or 0.8 to 1.0 grams of CHO/kg body weight) may require about two hours for digestion.

Whenever the meal is eaten, it should contain primarily CHO and be easy to digest. In this regard, foods such as breads, cereals, pasta, rice, fruits, and vegetables, are good choices, since they are predominantly CHO. Alternatively, some athletes will select a sports beverage or liquid fuel, rather than solid foods, as a light snack, in order to minimize gastrointestinal problems. Foods with a high GI should be restricted when there is less than one hour before the competition in order to avoid hypoglycemia. Fried and high-fat foods should be avoided for all precompetition meals, because these foods take a long time to digest. Table 6-3 (pg. 109) provides a list of healthy precompetition foods that supply about 50 grams of CHO. The GI of the food selected will depend on when the meal is eaten relative to the competition.

The intensity of the sporting event may also impact decisions on precompetition meals. If the activity is very low intensity, the body can digest light foods during exercise, so eating less than four hours prior to a competition should not hinder performance.

On the other hand, intense activities will divert blood flow from the stomach and intestines to the working muscles. As a result, adequate time prior to the competition is needed for digestion. To prevent discomfort and possibly nausea, eating four hours prior to intense competition is typically safe. Under all circumstances, athletes should be well nourished and have consumed some form of CHO prior to a competition.

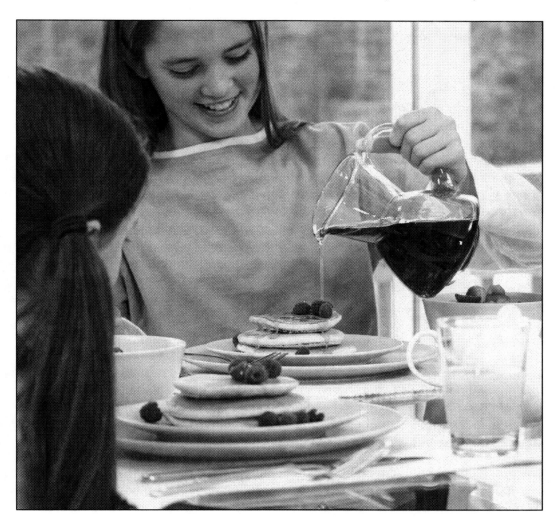

TIP/FACT #68
A diet low in carbohydrates will not provide enough energy for optimal athletic performance, whatever the sport.

Carbohydrates (CHO), the body's primary source of energy for muscular contraction, are stored as glycogen in the muscles and liver. CHO is important for maintaining blood glucose levels during exercise and preventing premature fatigue. During exercise of moderate intensity, blood glucose is readily taken up by skeletal muscles for energy, whereas with high intensity exercise, glucose for energy is obtained from the breakdown of glycogen. One hour of high-intensity exercise can reduce glycogen levels by about 55%, whereas two-to-three hours of strenuous exercise can deplete glycogen stores. Thus, a diet low in CHO will rapidly deplete both muscle and liver glycogen and will negatively affect both short-term intense and prolonged high- and low-intensity exercise performance. Moreover, mood appears to be better when a high CHO, as compared to a low or moderate CHO, diet is consumed. Maintaining a high CHO intake may also prevent, or at least reduce, symptoms associated with overreaching and, possibly overtraining. Finally, persons who ingest low CHO diets (20 to 100 grams per day) typically have reduced exercise tolerance and are unable to improve their performance through training.

Given that dietary CHO is essential for maintaining and repleting muscle and liver glycogen to support continued high levels of activity, athletes should be careful to consume sufficient amounts for their sport. Athletes undergoing regular high intensity endurance sessions should consume between 6-and-12 grams of CHO/kg of body weight daily, whereas an athlete participating in low to moderate intensity exercise may require only 4 to 7 grams of CHO/g body weight. Stated differently, approximately 55 to 70% of the total daily energy should come from CHO, with serious endurance athletes being at the upper end of the recommendation. Other athletes (weightlifters, basketball players, and other "short burst" athletes) may find that 55% of the total energy from CHO is adequate. That translates into a daily intake of approximately 6-to-12 g of CHO/kg of body weight.

Any athlete who is not eating enough CHO should be educated and encouraged to consume healthy, CHO rich foods, such as pastas, whole grains, cereals, beans, fruits, and vegetables. This step will also help ensure that they are receiving other essential nutrients. As discussed previously, sports drinks also provide CHO, but should not be relied upon as a good source of other essential nutrients. These beverages can supplement the diet, but should not dominate the energy needs of an athlete. In summary, daily CHO intake is directly related to an athlete's ability to sustain performance and recover from intense exercise, whether the activity is aerobic or resistance training.

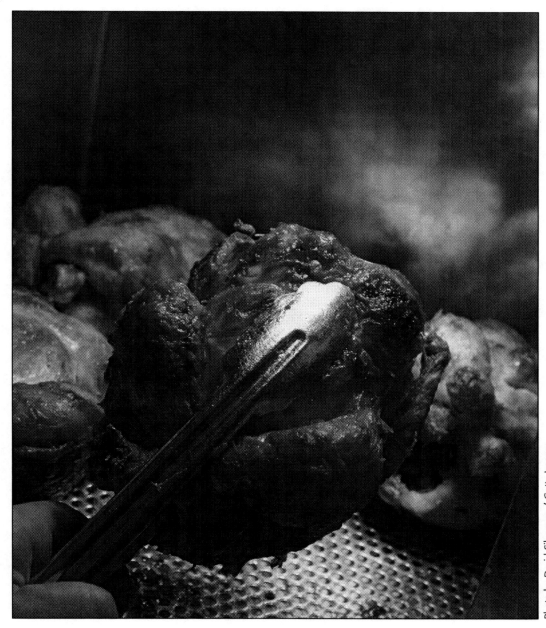

TIP/FACT #69
Female athletes should ensure they obtain adequate amounts of energy, calcium, iron, and zinc.

Female athletes are at risk for what is known as the "female athlete triad." The female athlete triad comprises (1) cessation of menses, (2) eating disorders, and (3) premature osteoporosis. Nutrition is a primary component of this triad, which is particularly common among ballet dancers, runners, and gymnasts, where an intense desire and/or pressure to be thin may exist. This quest for thinness results in energy intakes that are much lower than what is currently recommended for inactive females of the same age. Adequate energy intake is very important, because recovery from intense training requires energy for regeneration and repair of muscle tissue and is a requisite for normal functioning. An inadequate energy intake is also associated with low intakes of all nutrients (CHO, protein, and fat), but in particular with the minerals calcium, iron, and zinc.

Calcium is important for bone growth and strength, and when an athlete consumes a diet low in calcium-rich foods, she may be at risk for stress fractures and premature osteoporosis. This issue is a great concern if the female athlete is not having regular menstrual cycles. Female athletes should consume at least 800 to 1,200 mg of calcium daily, whereas females who do not have regular menses (amenorrhea) should consume up to 1,500 mg of calcium per day.

Female endurance athletes often have low iron stores and may be at risk for iron deficiency anemia due to menstrual losses of iron and inadequate intake of iron-containing foods. Iron deficiency limits oxygen transport in the blood and may decrease physical performance. Most female athletes take in less than 10 mg of iron each day, even though the RDA is 15 mg/day.

Athletes seeking to increase their iron stores should select foods that are rich in iron, such as green leafy vegetables and red meat. Consuming a combination of animal and vegetable iron sources at the same time will increase iron absorption from vegetables. In addition, an adequate intake of Vitamin C is important for iron status, because it enhances iron absorption. If a female athlete is anemic or has symptoms of anemia, to include fatigue, difficulty sleeping and/or concentrating, lethargy, headaches, and/or rapid heart rate, a physician should be consulted. Iron supplements should only be taken under the direction of a physician, since large doses can be toxic. Blood tests are the best way for assessing iron status and anemia.

Finally, zinc status may be compromised in female athletes because of poor dietary patterns and depletion of zinc due to exercise. Most female athletes take in around 7 mg or less of zinc, substantially lower than the RDA of 12 mg for females. As stated previously, zinc is essential for tissue repair, reproductive function, protein synthesis, immunity, and many other essential actions. Female athletes should be encouraged to take in foods that are high in zinc, to include seafood, meats, tofu, miso, chick peas, milk, and eggs.

Overall, female athletes should be educated about the importance of nutrition for optimal performance and evaluated or monitored to ensure they are consuming a balanced diet with adequate energy and micronutrients to meet their energy demands. If any athlete is not having her menses, then care should be taken to develop nutritionally sound dietary practices for the athlete and monitor her progress and menstrual patterns.

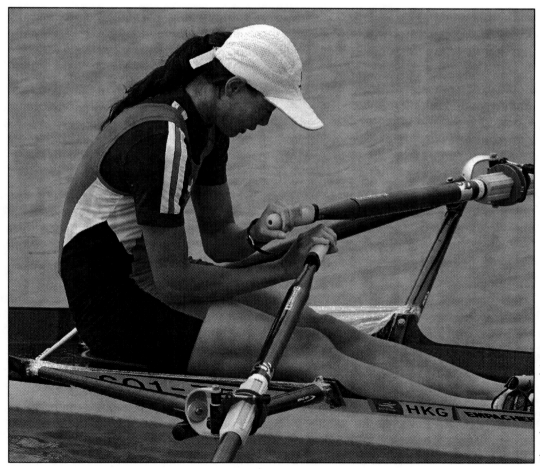

Photo by Ross Land / Getty Images

TIP/FACT #70
Dietary supplements should be carefully researched, since many lack adequate scientific evidence and could be dangerous and/or contain banned additives.

The supplement market is teeming with pills, powders, and sports foods designed and marketed to athletes who are seeking the extra edge on athletic performance or physique. Millions of dollars are spent annually on protein powders and other products, yet scientific evidence demonstrating beneficial effects is lacking. In fact, most studies indicate that more protein is NOT better. Every month, new products emerge, but one supplement that has been around for a relatively long time is creatine.

Creatine is one of the most common supplements taken for improving muscular strength and mass. It is well established that creatine supplementation will cause water retention and weight gain, which may benefit an individual who is trying to gain weight. In addition, some research indicates that creatine can help sprint and power athletes, although creatine is not effective for endurance sports. Examples of other common and routinely used supplements that do not have sufficient evidence for any use include carnitine, chromium, coenzyme Q10, Gamma-oryzanol, ginseng, lecithin, medium chain triglycerides (MCT), omega-3 fatty acids, and hydroxy-methyl butyrate. More evidence may emerge over the next few years, but at this time, such supplements should not be used.

Another problem with taking supplements is that many people are not aware of the actual product ingredients. Many products have ingredients or additives that consumers are unfamiliar with, and many have labels that do not match the actual contents. In addition, when several compounds are mixed together, the combination may produce effects that do not occur when taken alone. One example is Hydroxycut, which contains chromium, hydroxagen, garcinia cambogia, glucomannan, alpha lipoic acid, willow bark extract, L-Carnitine, green tea leaf extract, caffeine, and guarana extract, to name a few. Hydroxagen alone may be fine, but untoward interactions have and can predispose athletes to heat injuries, muscle damage, and other adverse events when combined with caffeine or other compounds.

In addition, understanding what is in the supplement becomes vital when the issue of drug testing arises. Some products contain agents that could yield positive drug testing results. Finally, some additives, such as those in bee pollen, Ma Huang, and Jin Bu Huan, for example, have been proven dangerous to individuals. Bee pollen may contain proteins that can trigger serious allergic reactions, while Ma Huang is an amphetamine-like substance that when combined with caffeine has been implicated in more than 100 adverse events and several deaths. Similarly, Jin Bu Huan has been known to cause life-threatening respiratory problems. In summary, because many supplements do not have a scientific basis and contain additives, some of which are banned or can be harmful, eating a healthy, balanced diet that meets the athletes' needs is the best option. Supplements should be used only with extreme caution.

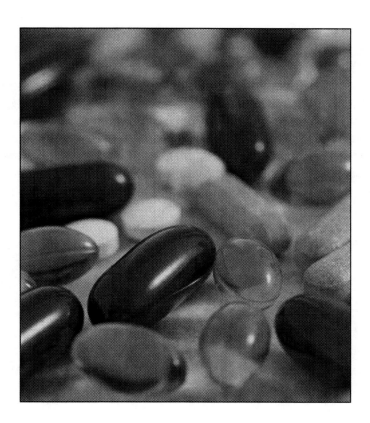

TIP/FACT #71
Recovery from training and competition can be accelerated by ingesting a combination of carbohydrates and protein within 30 minutes after completing the activity.

Accelerating recovery after training is important for replenishing muscle and liver glycogen and providing amino acids to the muscles for repair. Endurance and resistance exercise can deplete muscle glycogen, which must be replaced. In addition, exercise breaks down muscle proteins, and amino acids are needed to repair them. Thus, what and when an athlete eats following physical exertion becomes very important. Optimal recovery is accomplished by consuming the appropriate foods at the appropriate time.

Most people would agree that consuming a healthy meal or snack containing CHO and some protein is the best choice after training or competing. Strength and power athletes should consume a mixture of CHO (0.5 to 1 gram CHO/kg body weight) with some protein (up to 0.2 grams/kg body weight) within 30 minutes to one hour after a workout to replete glycogen and enhance muscle protein synthesis. This timing appears critical for providing nutrients to the muscles and helping the athlete to recover faster in preparation for the next workout. This dietary practice may also reduce injuries.

For endurance athletes or athletes exercising for long periods of time, consuming a form of CHO right after exercise that is readily digested and absorbed is important. These athletes should consume high GI liquids or solid foods providing 0.5 to 1.5 grams of CHO/kg body weight within one hour after exercise and every two hours for the first four hours. Stated in a more simplistic way, 50 to 100 g (or 200 to 400 kcal) of high GI CHO should be ingested by athletes immediately after extended exercise-training bouts. This step will help ensure that liver and muscle glycogen levels are restored and recovery from exercise occurs quickly.

Ingesting some protein with CHO during recovery will accelerate glycogen repletion and enhance protein synthesis. The amount of protein depends on the amount of CHO, but a good rule of thumb is that no more than one gram of protein should be eaten for every four grams of CHO. This step can easily be achieved by eating mostly CHO. The most important point is to eat healthy foods right after a training session and focus on CHO rich foods. Table 6-2 provides a selection of foods that are good after intense-training sessions.

GI < 60	60 < GI < 85	GI > 85
Apples	Banana	Angel Food Cake
Apricots (dried)	Corn Tortilla	Corn Chips
Beans	Cracked Barley	Cornflakes
Brown Rice	Green Peas	Doughnut
Cashews	Linguine	English Muffins
Grapefruit/Oranges	Oatmeal, Cooked	Hard Candy
Milk (whole/skim)	Orange/Grapefruit Juice	Ice Cream
Peanuts	Soy Yogurt	Raisin Bran Cereal
Pears (fresh)	Sponge Cake	Raisins
Plums	Sweet Corn	Rice Cakes
Rye bread	Sweet Potato	Shredded Wheat
Soybeans	White Rice (long-grain)	Sports Drinks
Yogurt	100% Whole wheat bread	White Bagel

Table 6-2. Glycemic index for various foods

Sport Drinks (check label)
1 Sports Bar (check label)
Baked/Mashed Potato
Medium Bagel
Soft Pretzel (small)
1 cup Macaroni and Cheese
1.5 cups Couscous
2 English Muffins, plain
1 cup Whole Wheat Crackers
1.5 cups Corn Puffs Cereal with Milk
1 cup Raison Bran Cereal
2 cups Pineapple (fresh) with 1/2 cup Walnuts
Banana and 2 Tbsp. Peanut Butter
1 cup canned Apricots in heavy syrup and 4 oz. Cottage Cheese
1/2 cup Figs and 1 oz. Peanuts
1 cup Kidney Beans and 1/4 cup White Rice
Turkey burger on Whole-grain Roll with Vegetables

Table 6-3. High GI foods that supply at least 50 grams of CHO in a 4:1 ratio of CHO and protein

References:

Foster-Powell K, Holt SH, Brand-Miller JC (2002) International table of glycemic index and glycemic load values. *The American Journal of Clinical Nutrition* **76**: 5-56.

Kern, M (2005) CRC Desk Reference on Sports Nutrition. CRC Press, San Diego State University, San Diego, CA.

Deuster PA, Singh A, Pelletier, PA (2004) The Navy SEAL Nutrition Guide: 1994. Gatorade Sports Science Institute. http://www.gssiweb.com/.

Driskell, JA, Wolinsky, I (eds) (2005) *Sports Nutrition: Vitamins and Trace Elements,* 2nd ed. CRC Press, Boca Raton, FL.

7

Common Ergogenic Aids in Sports
Donald T. Kirkendall, PhD

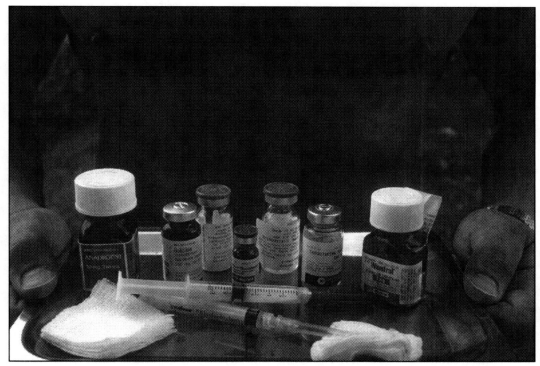

Photo by Karen Levy / Allsport

For many individuals, sports are about performance and outperforming an opponent. The problem is that athletes sometime think that training is not enough…that they might need something else for 'an edge' to perform better. It's an attitude that has been around since the dawn of competition and will continue despite the best medical and ethical oversight. In groups, most athletes would deny that they would take something illegal if it would help them win, but if asked individually, many athletes would admit that they would. The BALCO scandal of 2004 demonstrated that the 'crooks' are still trying to stay one step ahead of the 'cops' by using a steroid that was effective, yet undetectable.

Many athletes probably know more about supplements than most coaches and sports-medicine professionals. When a doctor says something doesn't work, chances are the athletes will know if the doctor is being truthful or just overly righteous. Ergogenic aids improve performance. If something increases muscle mass but doesn't improve strength performance, it is not ergogenic. Ronald Maughan, the prolific sports performance researcher from the UK, once made the following observation about supplements and ergogenic aids: "If it works, it's probably banned. If it isn't banned, it probably doesn't work."

One flaw with many research studies is that the methodology is 'below' the gold standard of research—the randomized clinical trial. There are only four outcomes of research: true positive (it works and studies show it works); true negative (it doesn't work and studies show it doesn't work); false positive (it doesn't work, but studies show it does work); and false negative (it works, but studies show it doesn't work).

Using inadequate research designs and small numbers of subjects increases the chance of false positive or false negative findings. False negatives were a common problem of early research on anabolic steroids. Athletes knew steroids worked, but research methods failed to show their effectiveness. The results of most supplement research must be considered as potential false positives or false negatives because of the designs, subject type, and subject numbers in the study. The placebo effect also always needs to be considered in any well-designed study.

Given the aforementioned discussion, the remainder of this chapter provides an overview of ten of the most commonly utilized ergogenic aids in sports. For each item, a general summary of the ergogenic aid is detailed, including a review of what the substance is, why it should work, what the research says about it, what safety concerns are attendant to its use, what organizations (if any) have banned its use, and an abridged compendium of comments about it.

TIP/FACT #72
Caffeine

☐ *What is it?* Caffeine is a commonly found product in many non-pharmaceutical items and in numerous prescription medicines. It is considered both a drug and a supplement. Caffeine's most obvious effect is as a mild central nervous system (CNS) stimulant. Chemically, caffeine is a stimulant in the dimethylxanthine class, a class of compounds that stimulates the release of adrenaline and other transmitters in the brain.

☐ *Why should it work?* Its CNS actions should place the athlete at a higher level of arousal and alertness. A more important effect is that its class of compounds stimulates the release of free fatty acids for use as a fuel. When free fatty acids are available during aerobic exercise, muscle will use the fats as a fuel, sparing the use of stored muscle carbohydrates (glycogen). This factor will allow the athlete to go farther into the contest before running low on muscle glycogen (a common reason for fatigue in aerobic sports).

☐ *What does the research say?* Caffeine has been effective at improving performance (by 1 to 3%) in endurance events like one-hour cycling time trials and 2000m rowing races. These are small improvements, but could be the difference between winning and losing. There does not seem to be a dose-response effect (taking more doesn't make one perform better). Single sprint performance, but not multiple sprints, might be improved.

☐ *Safety concerns:* People can develop a dependence on caffeine and experience withdrawal symptoms. Caffeine is a mild diuretic, but this feature seems to be blunted by exercise.

☐ *Banned by:* IOC, FIFA at urine levels >12µg/ml, NCAA at urine levels >15µg/ml

☐ *Comments:* Caffeine is most effective taken as a pill rather than a liquid (as in coffee or high energy drinks). The doses used in the published research (250 to 700mg or 2 to 9mg/kg) of caffeine within an hour of performance did not trigger a positive drug test. However, urine tests for caffeine are notoriously inaccurate. Caffeine in coffee is quite variable. For example, an 8 oz. cup of Maxwell House® has 110mg, while 8 oz. of coffee from Starbucks® has 250mg.

TIP/FACT #73
Ephedrine and Pseudoephedrine

☐ *What is it?* Ephedrine and pseudoephedrine are both called sympathomimetic amines, because their actions mimic the action of the sympathetic nervous system. Ephedra is also marketed as an herbal supplement called ma huang. Athletes who use these substances believe they will increase energy supply and delay fatigue. Ephedrine is an ingredient in over-the-counter, weight-loss supplements and energy pills that can still be found in convenience stores, gas stations, and truck stops.

☐ *Why should it work?* It has been suggested that compounds like these spare glycogen and delay fatigue, because running out of glycogen occurs later. Ephedrine (and its metabolite, phenylpropanolamine) dilate bronchioles and are used as a nasal decongestant. In combination with caffeine, ephedrine is effective at burning fat and promoting muscle growth. As a mimic of the central nervous system, these compounds also stimulate arousal.

☐ *What does the research say?* Ephedrine has been shown to improve performance in a 30s maximal cycling task (called the Wingate Test), due to what the authors called an arousal effect, and in a 10K run time, suggesting an ergogenic effect. There are no studies on single-sprint performance. Pseudoephedrine's ergogenic effect is unproven. No effects have been shown for such events as one hour of cycling or 5,000m running performance. Some improvements in strength (isokinetic torque output of knee extensors) have been shown. Overall, pseudoephedrine is effective in endurance activities. As with ephedrine, there are no studies on single-sprint performance. There does not appear to be a dose-response effect.

☐ *Safety concerns:* Ephedrine side effects may involve major cardiovascular events, hypertension, hypotension, adverse drug interactions, and psychoses. Ephedrine has been linked with nearly 1,000 incidents and 50 deaths. Frequently, adverse effects are related to excessive dosages, but many of the reported adverse effects of ephedrine were within the recommended dosage. Pseudoephedrine has been implicated in nervousness, restlessness, and insomnia, plus some infrequent side effects, like headaches, palpitations, sweating, and others.

☐ *Banned by:* IOC, NCAA, NFL

☐ *Comments:* About 1/3 of the positive drug tests at the Olympics are for ephedrine, pseudoephedrine, or phenylpropanolamine. Ephedra was headline news when it was implicated in the 2003 death of Steven Bechler of the Baltimore Orioles. Nearly 2/3 of all complaints about herbal supplements are related to ephedrine despite being <1% of all sales. Many states have removed ephedra products from their shelves, and the FDA has recommended that ephedra should be avoided. Several years ago, *Sports Illustrated* had an article on the use of Sudafed® (pseudoephedrine) in the NHL.

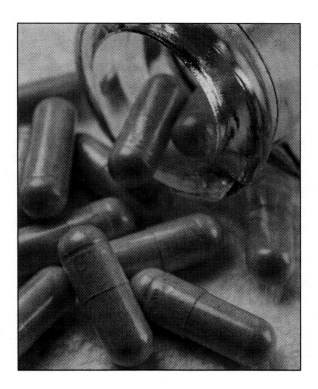

TIP/FACT #74
Bicarbonate

□ *What is it?* Normally, this substance is found as sodium bicarbonate—ordinary baking soda. Another option is sodium citrate.

□ *Why should it work?* The body's chemistry exists within a narrow acid-base range. Lactic acid lowers the body's pH, making the body more acidic. When lactic acid is enough, as from very high-intensity exercise like a 400m sprint (maximum exercise of up to around two minutes in length), power output is reduced, causing the athlete to slow down. If the body's pH can be raised with a base compound, then it will take longer for lactic acid's role in fatigue to take effect. Bicarbonate is a base compound readily available from any grocery store.

□ *What does the research say?* Bicarbonate is ineffective in exercise that is not limited by lactic acid, so athletes participating in events in the 30 second to two-to-four minute range (e.g., 200m-to-mile running and swimming, cycling races of similar duration) may benefit using bicarbonate (.3 to .5g/kg). In a study evaluating an 800m run, athletes using bicarbonate effectively improved their finish by around 20m, which would drastically improve their placement. Other laboratory studies on performance demonstrate its effectiveness in high power-output exercise. However, there are almost as many studies that show no effectiveness of bicarbonate. Because most of these studies used times to exhaustion outside of the one-to-four minute duration that is limited by lactic acid, consuming bicarbonate would not be expected to be beneficial.

□ *Safety concerns:* There are numerous reports of gastrointestinal (GI) problems (cramps, bloating, vomiting, and diarrhea) in up to half the subjects studied. These problems seem to occur one to two hours after ingestion. In some cases the athlete is unable to compete due to severe GI side effects. The GI problems are unpredictable and may not occur with each ingestion. There is no way to predict when the GI issues will occur. As a result, bicarbonate is rarely used.

□ *Banned by:* none

□ *Comments:* Some people have minimized GI problems by increasing their water intake and extending the time to ingest that bicarbonate or using sodium citrate as an alternative. A 70kg athlete at .5g/kg would need 35g of bicarbonate, which is a hefty amount of baking soda. Simple practicality restricts its use.

TIP/FACT #75
Anabolic Steroids

☐ *What is it?* Anabolic-androgenic steroids ('steroids') are oral or injectable synthetic versions of testosterone that usually are more potent than testosterone. These drugs are a class III controlled drug in the U.S. and allegedly are still available over-the-counter in Mexico (although purchasing them will get you arrested at the border)! The scientific research now supports what athletes have known for decades; steroids work…but not without substantial risks.

☐ *Why should it work?* Steroids increase muscle mass by increasing protein synthesis, similar to the increase in muscle mass that occurs with puberty. Steroids have been shown recently to increase erythropoiesis (red blood cell production). Increased muscle mass improves very high power-output activities (weightlifting, sprints, etc). The disclosure in 2004 that some MLB baseball players used steroids provides some anecdotal evidence that steroids might also be beneficial for the highly skilled activity of hitting a baseball.

☐ *What does the research say?* Early research showed little effect of steroids in most sporting activities, mostly due to inadequacies of research design or dosage. Little effect was shown, because the dosages were too small or the investigations used an inadequate subject population. Strength, muscle mass, and high power-output performance all improve with steroid use. More recent evidence reveals a benefit to endurance performance.

☐ *Safety concerns:* Steroids users pay a price. Among the consequences of taking steroids are documented liver problems, increased risk of cardiovascular disease (documented heart attacks, stroke, bypass surgery, very low HDL-cholesterol levels), selected cancers, and premature death. Other steroid-related issues involve acne, aggressive behavior ('road rage'), testicular atrophy, and gynecomastia (in males), as well as coarsening of the voice, menstrual irregularities, virilization, and male-pattern baldness and facial hair (females). Social issues are also a concern. It's not just athletes who use steroids. Non-athletic individuals also use steroids to bulk up (i.e., increase their level of muscle mass).

☐ *Banned by:* IOC, NCAA, NFL, NBA, FIFA, MLB

☐ *Comments:* Athletes will stop listening as soon as someone says that steroids don't work. A trip to almost any weight-lifting facility can expose the reality of the easy access that exists to steroids. I recently asked my exercise physiology classes how many people could locate someone who uses steroids with one or two phone calls and over half the class raised their hand. There are many different dosing regimens that come from trial and error. It's not unusual to hear people refer to steroids, not as performance enhancing drugs, but as recovery-enhancing drugs. Many users claim they can perform high-intensity workouts with less recovery between workouts (employing semantics in an attempt to rationalize the use of anabolic steroids). There have been a number of recent positive drug tests for a steroid called nandrolone®. The IOC has shown that up to 15 to 20% of over-the-counter supplements are contaminated, many with steroids or their precursors, some with nandrolone®, and innocent use of a contaminated supplement will trigger a positive drug test. No athlete has ever beaten a positive drug test by claiming ignorance. People sometimes confuse anabolic steroids with corticosteroids, which are potent anti-inflammatory compounds. Corticosteroids are substances that are injected into joints to promote healing or are used as inhalants for patients with respiratory problems. Corticosteroids have wide use in medicine.

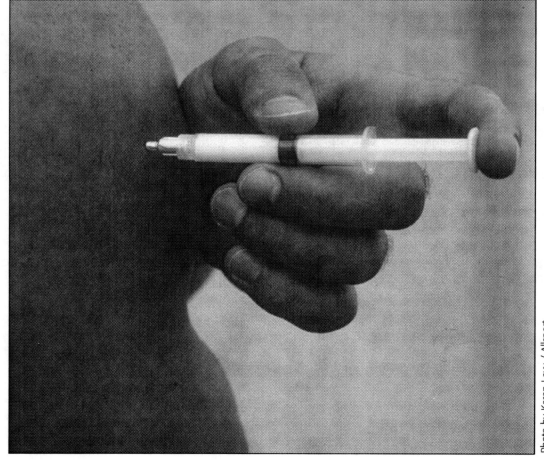

Photo by Karen Levy / Allsport

TIP/FACT #76
Steroid Precursors

☐ *What is it?* To make testosterone, the body goes through an extensive, complicated chemical process. Some individuals believe that if selected building blocks (precursors) are ingested, more testosterone will be made. The most visible of this class of compounds are dehydroepiandrosterone (DHEA) and androstenedione ('andro'). Neither of these is classified as a drug, but as supplements.

☐ *Why should it work?* Because each is involved in the production of testosterone, it is assumed that more of the building blocks will lead to more testosterone and the resulting responses from increased testosterone. Steroids are actually anabolic-androgenic drugs. Anabolic refers to the muscle-building aspects, while androgenic refers to its masculine-producing effects (voice, hair growth, etc.). It's the anabolic aspects that are ergogenic, performance-enhancing. Androstenedione is androgenic in its action, so it's unlikely to have much performance-enhancing effects. DHEA is more likely to have some anabolic effects.

☐ *What does the research say?* Before Mark McGuire's run on the homerun record in 1998, little attention was paid to androstenedione, and no performance studies were reported in the medical literature. After 1998, a few clinical trials were performed. No study demonstrated any ergogenic effect, muscle mass increase, or protein synthesis, and only one revealed a transient, short-term, elevation of testosterone. Similar results have been shown with DHEA.

☐ *Safety concerns:* Similar to anabolic steroids, these compounds reduce the good cholesterol, HDL, placing the athlete at increased risk for cardiovascular disease. There are reports of irreversible androgenic effects (e.g., hair growth, male-pattern baldness, gynecomastia).

☐ *Banned by:* IOC, NCAA, FIFA, NFL, NBA

☐ *Comments:* Both types of steroid precursors can trigger a positive drug test. While there might be animal studies that show conflicting results, the only projects discussed in this chapter are those looking at sports performance in humans. An ingested precursor is not likely to arrive intact to the cells involved in making the compound. When the compounds pass through the liver, they are disassembled, and the pieces are transported to wherever they might be needed. Since neither DHEA nor andro seem to be effective (keep in mind, however, the caveat about false positive and false negative findings), and both can trigger a positive drug test, this class of compounds should be avoided. Why take the chance of a positive drug test, using a drug that doesn't seem to work?

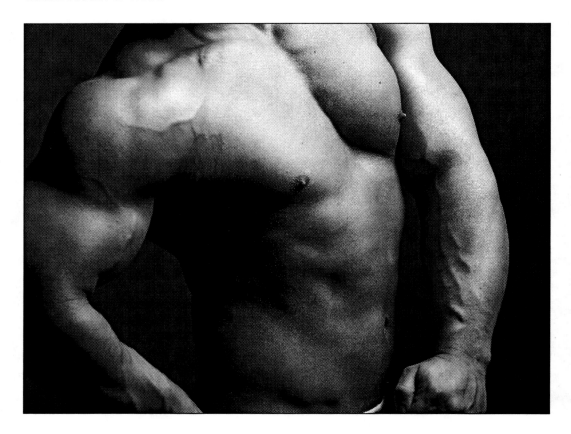

TIP/FACT #77
Erythropoietin

☐ *What is it?* Erythropoietin is the hormone produced by the kidneys that stimulates the production of red blood cells that carry oxygen to the cells. Once erythropoietin was synthesized in a test tube, it was possible to produce longer-acting replicas of the hormone that could be injected. There are a number of definite medical uses for erythropoietin. The sporting slang for erythropoietin is EPO.

☐ *Why should it work?* There are three ways to enhance oxygenation: deliver oxygen-rich blood to the tissues (increase the cardiac output), increase the amount of oxygen used by the muscles (increased oxygen extraction by the muscles), or increase the amount of oxygen carried by the blood. While all three can be improved with training, the latter factor is what can be influenced by EPO, because more oxygen-rich red blood cells can send substantially more oxygen to the muscles. The earliest method of increasing red blood cells was through blood doping—this process involves removing blood, training until the blood had been naturally replaced, and then re-infusing the withdrawn blood. With the advent of recombinant EPO, the need to follow the blood-doping procedure was unnecessary.

☐ *What does the research say?* Unquestionably, an increase in red blood cells and subsequently the oxygen-carrying capacity of the blood will improve endurance performance. Early work with blood doping showed substantial improvements in endurance performance, and subsequent studies on EPO found similar results. Endurance performance is consistently improved with EPO.

☐ *Safety concerns:* EPO increases the number of red blood cells—the solid portion of the blood. As a result, more blood exists in the limited space of the cardiovascular system, leading to reports of hypertension and thromboembolism. Seizures have also been reported. The 'thicker' blood means the heart has to work harder to pump blood. Most medical professionals are convinced that the unfortunate deaths of several cyclists were due to EPO administration.

☐ *Banned by:* IOC, NCAA, FIFA, NFL, UCI, FIS

☐ *Comments:* There is no doubt that the indiscriminant use of EPO to improve performance is a very dangerous proposition. EPO is very expensive, as is the testing necessary to detect EPO use. All injectable compounds carry the risk of needle contamination, because most athletes aren't likely to be as antiseptic as a medical facility. If steroids are *the* drug for strength sports, EPO is *the* drug for endurance sports.

EPO use in endurance sports is reported to be widespread and can only be detected with very expensive blood tests, not the typical urine tests.

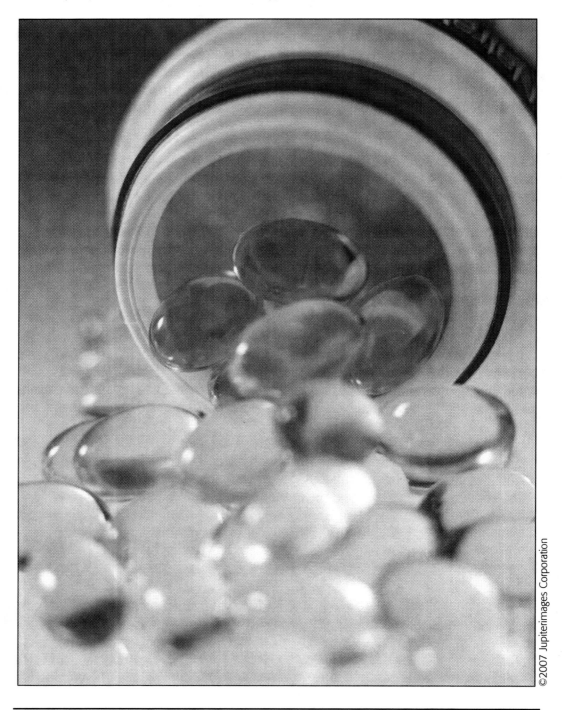

TIP/FACT #78
Human Growth Hormone

☐ *What is it?* Human growth hormone (HGH) is produced by the human pituitary gland and has numerous actions, not the least of which are soft tissue (including muscle) growth and fat loss. Recombinant HGH is currently the medication of choice in the medical community.

☐ *Why should it work?* The purported ergogenic effects of HGH relate to its ability to enhance protein and glucose uptake by cells, as well as releasing fatty acids from fat to serve as an energy source. HGH gained strong support among the athletic community from an endorsement in the out-of-print book, *"The Underground Steroid Handbook."*

☐ *What does the research say?* Most of the research on HGH is in the clinical, medical literature. The only paper to show some muscle mass effects was from injectable HGH given to 60+ year-old men. Other reports on HGH failed to show an ergogenic effect.

☐ *Safety concerns:* Hypoglycemia, weight gain, breathing difficulties, rapid pulse rate, and increased risk of lung and colon cancer. Underground HGH may be reported to be of pituitary origin, but the risk of transmitting disease is a serious concern.

☐ *Banned by:* IOC, NCAA, FIFA, NFL

☐ *Comments:* HGH is available only as an injectable. HGH is too large a molecule to be handled by the GI system, so it gets broken down to individual amino-acid building blocks. Anything marketed as an oral source is inaccurate. Anything marketed as a precursor of a stimulant of HGH release is also inaccurate, although the amino-acid arginine does stimulate pituitary release of HGH if given intravenously. Most marketed HGH products are not the recombinant drug. The chance that an athlete is injecting actual HGH is highly unlikely.

TIP/FACT #79
Proteins and Amino Acids

☐ *What is it?* Powdered forms of amino acids or proteins used to increase protein intake.

☐ *Why should it work?* Amino acids are the building blocks of protein, and muscle is protein. If more amino acids are supplied, more muscle should be built.

☐ *What does the research say?* Dietary recalls of athletes show that they receive sufficient protein in their diet without protein supplementation. The normal RDA for protein is .8g/kg/day, and most athletes are in the 1.2 to 1.8g/kg/day range, with many strength-trained athletes ingesting 2g/kg/day. Most well-controlled studies in untrained and strength-trained athletes show no effect after a few months of protein supplementation. A subgroup of amino acids, the branched-chain amino acids, has received special attention. This particular group of amino acids can serve as a fuel for energy when muscle glycogen levels are very low. They have also been reported to reduce muscle damage (as suggested by low CPK levels), but there hasn't been any evidence that performance is improved. Good evidence does exist that the post-exercise replenishment of muscle glycogen is faster if the post-exercise meal includes some protein (a 4:1 cholesterol:protein ratio is suggested). This approach is reported to improve performance in the next bout of exercise, because more glycogen was stored when protein accompanied the post-exercise carbohydrate.

☐ *Safety concerns:* Conceptual concerns exist over renal damage. Excess, unused protein is likely stored as fat.

☐ *Banned by:* none

☐ *Comments:* There is no more heavily marketed corner of the supplement business than protein and amino-acid supplementation. Nutritional stores (e.g., GNC, etc) have entire sections of protein supplements, and some industries (e.g., the Joe Wieder fitness empire) are based on protein supplements. Athletes who believe in protein supplementation typically claim that research studies disallowing the "benefits" of comsuming extra protein were too brief.

TIP/FACT #80
Creatine

☐ *What is it?* Creatine is a naturally occurring nitrogenous compound that is a backbone for the high-energy molecule phosphocreatine (also called creatinephosphate or PCR). Creatine is ingested from meat or fish.

☐ *Why should it work?* Energy turnover during high-intensity, short-term exercise uses a chemical exchange of energy from phosphocreatine to ADP (adenosine and two phosphates), leading to creatine and ATP (adenosine and three phosphates). Although this pathway is very fast, there is only a small amount of each chemical. As a result, energy transfer using this pathway is limited. The thought is that if there is more creatine, then more energy can be held as phosphocreatine. If so, then the ATP-PC system can exchange energy for a longer time. Some individuals believe that the combination of water and creatine also stimulates protein synthesis, leading to increased muscle mass.

☐ *What does the research say?* Creatine has been shown consistently to improve activities where energy turnover using the ATP-PC system is paramount in performance. Thus, short-term, high-power activities, like weightlifting, cycling (e.g., Wingate Test, repetitive cycling), and repeated sprints (typically six to ten 30-60m sprints) all benefit. Non-responders are rare (i.e., most people get some benefit). Creatine has no effect on endurance performance. The only study to demonstrate a benefit in a 'field' setting (soccer) showed a benefit in running performance. However, only eight players were studied, and it's difficult to blind subjects to creatine use (the weight gain is obvious, and most athletes 'know' that creatine works), leading to research design questions that raise the issue of false positives. Finally, creatine, when compared to carbohydrate loading, lost in a performance contest.

☐ *Safety concerns:* There are anecdotal reports of kidney failure occurring (on rare occasions) in athletes taking creatine. In addition, there are increasing reports that creatine is implicated in muscle cramping, but this finding has not been scientifically verified. The main side effect is a substantial weight gain from water retention. Increases in body mass of 4kg (10 lbs.) or more in the first week of use are common.

☐ *Banned by:* Creatine is not banned by any governing body or the World Anti-Doping Agency (WADA). However, the NCAA prohibits Division 1 universities from supplying creatine to its athletes.

☐ *Comments:* Despite its ergogenic effects, women are reluctant to use creatine because of the weight-gain side effect. Surveys of users in colleges show that baseball, wrestlers, and football players are the most frequent creatine users. Plenty of athletes think of creatine as a 'safe' ergogenic aid. The typical dosing is a loading phase (20g/d for five days), followed by a maintenance phase (5g/d). Research, however, shows that 2g/d is a sufficient maintenance dose. Until more is known about creatine, athletes take this supplement at their own risk.

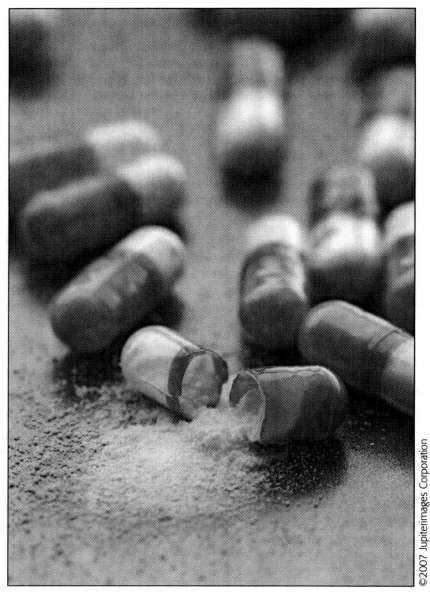

©2007 Jupiterimages Corporation

TIP/FACT #81
Energy Bars

☐ *What is it?* Energy bars are commercially marketed nutritional supplements. These bars are high in calories (200 to 300 cal/bar, similar to most candy bars), high in carbohydrate (30 to 50gm/bar), and contain some protein. Energy bars are much lower in fat and substantially more expensive than a traditional candy bar.

☐ *How should it work?* The carbohydrate in energy bars is rapidly absorbed by the GI system, thereby elevating blood sugar and supplying blood-borne energy to skeletal muscle. Energy bars are also used after exercise to jump-start the replenishment of muscle glycogen exhausted during exercise.

☐ *What does the research say?* While a number of master's theses and undergraduate research projects have looked into the effectiveness of energy bars, there is little in the published, peer-reviewed, literature on 'energy bars.' Most reviews of ergogenic aids state that good reasons might exist for athletes to supplement their diet with energy bars, especially when athletes make poor food choices and need to increase their carbohydrate intake.

☐ *Safety concerns:* It is unlikely that these products have much in the way of adverse effects.

☐ *Banned by:* None. But as newer bars come on the market, they may contain compounds that the NCAA might not want its members to supply to their athletes.

☐ *Comments:* Energy bars are commonly called "Power Bars," which is a specific product that has become the generic term for most bars. There are dozens of competitors that can be found in most supermarkets, drug, nutrition, and specialty sports stores. If an athlete has an inadequate carbohydrate intake, energy bars (as well as some high-carbohydrate drinks) are viable options for increasing carbohydrate intake.

Abbreviations

IOC   International Olympic Committee

USOC   U.S. Olympic Committee

FIFA   Federation Internationale du Football Associations

UCI   Union Cycliste Internationale

FIS   Federation Internationale du Ski

WADA   World Anti-Doping Agency

NFL   National Football League

NBA   National Basketball Association

MLB   Major League Baseball

NHL   National Hockey League (As of 2003, the NHL does not keep a banned substances list, preferring to be in accordance with local laws.)

References:

Find the WADA list of banned substances at:
   www.wada-ama.org/rtecontent/document/list_2005.pdf

For information on the extent of supplement contamination (in German), go to:
   www.dopinginfo.de

NCAA bylaw 16.5.2.2 states the following concerning what members can supply to their athletes:

"An institution may provide only nonmuscle-building nutritional supplements to a student-athlete at any time for the purpose of providing additional calories and electrolytes, provided the supplements do not contain any NCAA banned substances. Permissible nonmuscle-building nutritional supplements are identified according to the following classes: Carbohydrate/electrolyte drinks, energy bars, carbohydrate boosters, and vitamins and minerals."

The NCAA's website on drugs and sports is www.drugfreesport.com. College athletes have to consult their athletic trainer for the most up-to-date list of NCAA banned substances. Amateur and professional athletes need to do the same with their team or governing body.

8

Sports Conditioning and Training

Robert P. Wilder, MD, FACSM

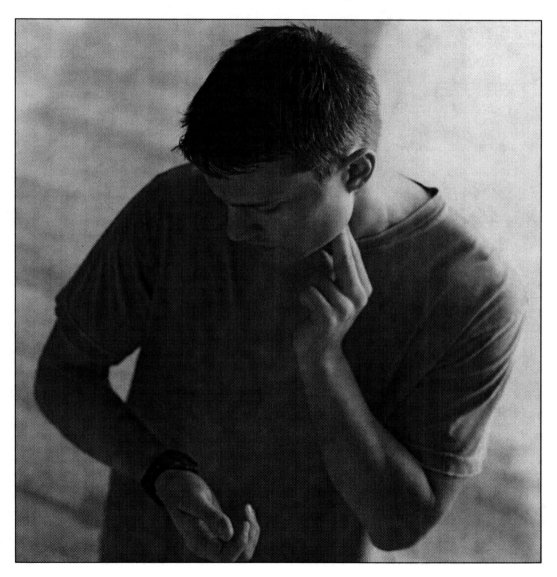

Whether it is better to exercise or train *this way* or *that way* has been debated for years. Unfortunately, much of the dialogue concerning what constitutes the proper way for athletes to condition themselves has been based on unfounded superstitions and institutions. What is not in dispute, however, is whether the benefits of a sound sports-conditioning program outweigh its risks. The answer to this issue is a resounding "yes." Not only can proper conditioning enhance sports performance, it can also minimize an athlete's risk of being injured. The ten tips/facts presented in this chapter address selected elements of sound conditioning.

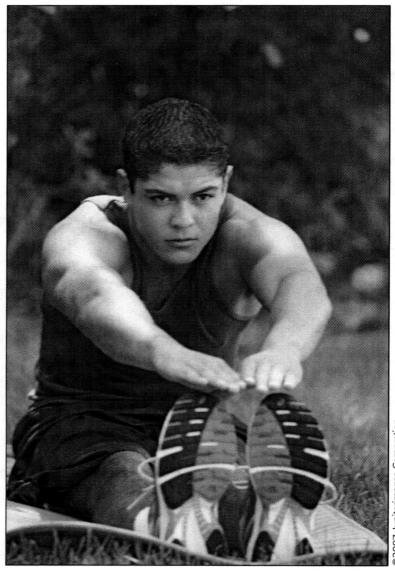

©2007 Jupiterimages Corporation

TIP/FACT #82
Athletes should adhere to certain common-sense precautions while training.

The following common-sense guidelines can help enhance the level of safety and effectiveness of an athlete's training efforts:

☐ *Be smart.* While it appears that no worthwhile human endeavor is totally risk free, the risks of training can be minimized. For example, every athlete should complete a preparticipation examination. Furthermore, an athlete should avoid doing too much, too soon in their training regimen.

☐ *Keep the muscles in balance.* Aerobic exercise should be combined with a sound strength-training program. When muscles are proportionately strong to each other, they are less likely to be injured.

☐ *Take care of your feet.* Proper foot care starts with the selection of shoes that will provide adequate support and cushioning. Respond quickly and accordingly to any exercise-related problem that plagues your feet (e.g., blisters, bone bruises, blackened toenails, etc.).

☐ *Train by stressing the body to its limits and then just a little bit more.* Allowing the body to adapt to a relatively small increase in stress is the safe, common-sense way to train. The main cause of musculoskeletal injuries is overstress—especially from a sudden increase in how much exercise an individual does or how the athlete trains.

☐ *Use proper techniques while exercising.* By keeping the body biomechanically aligned when exercising, an athlete reduces the orthopedic trauma to the body and decreases the likelihood of being injured.

☐ *Respect signals from the body that something may be wrong.* An athlete should stop exercising if any of the common termination signals are experienced, including abnormal heartbeats, pain or pressure in the chest, dizziness, light-headedness, nausea during or after exercise, prolonged fatigue, or insomnia.

☐ *Get adequate rest.* The importance of obtaining proper rest in conjunction with an exercise program cannot be overemphasized. An inadequate amount of rest can prevent athletes from achieving the maximum benefits from their exercise regimen.

☐ *Keep a training diary.* If an individual is injured, a training diary may help determine how and why an injury occurred (a sudden increase in the intensity of the athlete's efforts, a change from one (safe) exercise modality to another (unsafe) mode, etc.). Having essential background data can help in the diagnosis and specification of treatment by the athlete's healthcare provider.

☐ *Keep in mind that conditioning in isolation cannot produce the level of fitness that athletes need to perform their best.* Although extremely beneficial, exercise is only one factor in a sound, training program and must be combined with others if athletes are to be truly fit (sound nutrition, adequate rest, no smoking or recreational drugs, etc.).

☐ *Minimize the constant stress on the joints.* Keep the pounding on the body's joints to a minimum. If the athlete prefers to engage in high-impact exercise, try to also include low- or non-impact forms of exercising in the training regimen on a regular basis (preferably on an alternating basis).

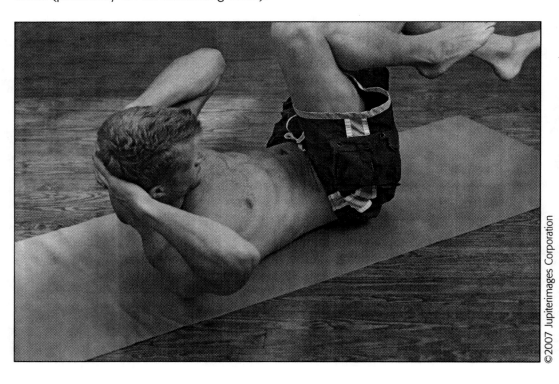

TIP/FACT #83
Athletes should avoid the common mistakes that often occur while strength training.

Athletes should abstain from making the following common mistakes while strength training:

☐ *Focus on demonstrating, rather than developing strength.* When athletes engage in a strength-training program, their primary goal should be to build strength, not show other people how much they can lift. More often than not, such a misplaced focal point will compromise training efforts by its natural tendency to lessen adherence to proper exercise technique.

☐ *Not strengthening what the athletes think they're strengthening.* Specific exercises develop specific muscles. When designing a strength-training program, it is important that athletes select the exercises that will enable them to achieve their particular training goals.

☐ *Not controlling the speed of the exercise.* When performing strength exercises, athletes should raise and lower the weight under control; otherwise, they're "throwing" the weight, as opposed to lifting it. As such, they should avoid all ballistic movements (e.g., dropping, jerking, and bouncing) while lifting.

☐ *Not exercising through a full range of motion.* To ensure that their musculature retains its natural elasticity and is developed to its fullest, athletes must perform every exercise in their strength-training regimen through its full range of motion. Otherwise, their muscles will tighten up, resulting in a condition commonly referred to as being "muscle bound."

☐ *Not exercising opposing muscles.* The human body has muscles that oppose each other (e.g., the quadriceps muscles are "opposed" by the hamstring muscles). These pairs of muscles have a proportionate strength relationship that must be maintained in relative balance. If one muscle becomes too strong for the other, an athlete risks injury to the weaker muscle.

☐ *Holding your breath while exercising.* Some individuals occasionally hold their breath while lifting to "gut-out" an extra repetition. Such a practice will lead to a substantial rise in pressure in the chest that may result in either dizziness or (in extreme instances) unconsciousness. The basic rule of thumb is that individuals should never hold their breath while strength training.

☐ *Not exercising at the right level of intensity.* A muscle becomes stronger when a demand is placed on it. If athletes place less demand than their muscles can handle, they'll get less improvement than they are capable of achieving. On the other hand, too much demand will either expose an individual to an undue risk of injury or make the exercise too difficult to perform properly.

☐ *Not giving the muscles an appropriate amount of time between workouts to recover from the demands placed upon them.* When a muscle is stressed beyond what it can normally handle, some rest is needed for the muscle tissues, tendons, and ligaments to recover. If the recovery time is too brief, the muscle may be unable to make the needed physiologic adaptations before being stressed again. Conversely, if athletes take too much time between workouts, their muscles will gradually return to their untrained level.

☐ *Trying to do too much too soon.* An athlete's strength-training program should be progressive in nature. As such, athletes should gradually increase the stress they place on their muscles as they are able to meet the imposed demand. Keep in mind that lifting too much too soon can lead to failure and injury.

☐ *Not performing the exercise properly.* Only one proper way exists to perform a specific exercise. As such, athletes should always adhere to the correct technique when strength training. If athletes compromise the recommended mechanics for doing an exercise, they will compromise their results.

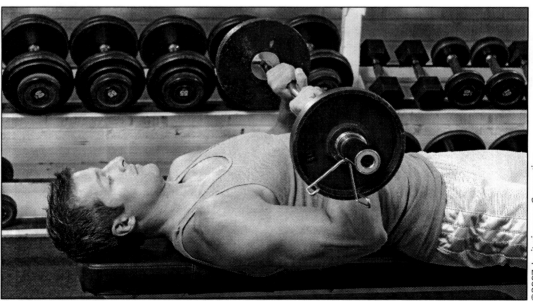

©2007 Jupiterimages Corporation

TIP/FACT #84
Athletes should avoid common mistakes that often occur while performing aerobic exercise.

Athletes should abstain from making the following common mistakes while engaged in aerobic-type training:

☐ *Rely upon "muscle burn" as an accurate indicator of exercise intensity.* For an aerobic training effect to occur, individuals must exercise at or above a specific intensity of exercise (e.g., 60 to 90% of their maximum heart rate). In reality, the heart's response to the demands of exercise is not related to how much your muscles "burn" during physical activity. It is more important for athletes to focus upon their overall perception of effort (rating of perceived exertion, or RPE), which is closely linked to their training heart rate.

☐ *Mistake neuromuscular difficulty as a meaningful barometer of training intensity.* Some exercise activities require a greater degree of motor skills (including coordination, agility, balance, and power) than others. Even though individuals may find it relatively difficult to perform whatever combination of limb and trunk movements are involved in a particular activity (e.g., exercising on a cross-country skiing machine), it does not necessarily mean that they are achieving the desired training effect.

☐ *Work out at an inappropriate level of intensity.* Getting the most our of aerobic-exercise efforts requires that athletes exercise within a particular training zone. If individuals fail to work out hard enough, they won't achieve the desired training effect. On the other hand, if they work out too hard, they may incur other negative consequences (e.g., be unable to exercise sufficiently or simply injure themselves).

☐ *Engage in activities that place too much stress on the lower extremities.* Some aerobic activities involve a greater degree of impact forces on the lower body of the exerciser than others. By the same token, some individuals can withstand greater loads on their lower extremities than others. As such, it is critical that athletes select their aerobic-exercise modality wisely.

☐ *Worry more about the clothes on their body than the footwear on their feet.* How athletes look while working out has no impact whatsoever on the nonsocial benefits they might otherwise achieve from their exercise efforts. As a rule, the most important personal wear item while exercising is proper footwear.

☐ *Lean on the exercise machine while working out.* Many individuals compromise the safety and quality of their aerobic workouts by excessively leaning on the handrails of whatever aerobic equipment device they are using while exercising (e.g., treadmills, elliptical cross-trainers, or stair climbers). Such a practice reduces the overall quality and safety level of the workout.

☐ *Fail to warm up before exercising.* To diminish the likelihood of overdoing things with their heart and to help make their exercise efforts orthopaedically safer, athletes need to warm up before they work out.

☐ *Fail to get enough rest.* Even though they may feel passionate about exercising, athletes need to give their body an occasional day off (or two) from working out to provide their body with the opportunity to recover from the physical demands they have placed upon it.

☐ *Wear weighted items (such as vests, wristbands, or ankle weights) while exercising.* In addition to offering limited training benefits, the practice of wearing weighted items while exercising increases an athlete's risk of changing the proper exercise mechanics during the activity. Such a change may expose the individual's musculoskeletal system to a heightened level of undue stress.

☐ *Rely upon aerobic exercise gimmicks marketed on television and the Internet.* Geared to individuals who are wishfully looking for a quick, easy, and painless way to achieve the innumerable benefits of proper exercise, most of these items look too good to be true…and they are.

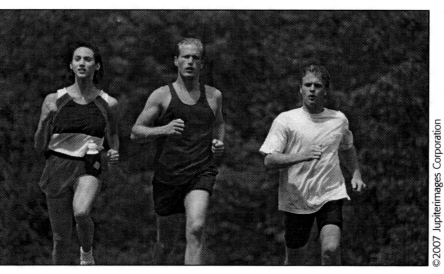

©2007 Jupiterimages Corporation

TIP/FACT #85
All exercise-conditioning equipment is not equal.

Athletes should be aware of the basic features that make some exercise equipment more appropriate for their training efforts than others. In that regard, the following factors can be used to differentiate between the various exercise-equipment options:

☐ *Safety*. Some exercise equipment is much safer than other equipment. One of the primary selection criteria is that equipment does not place undue load force on the joints of the body. Another criterion is that the equipment has instructions for use that are both clearly defined and easy to follow.

☐ *Functional effectiveness*. Some exercise equipment enables users to achieve more meaningful results (i.e., improvements that enhance the ability to perform the activities of daily living). All other factors being equal, the more productive an athlete's exercise efforts, the more well spent the time and the more likely individuals will stick to their exercise program.

☐ *Size.* With regard to size, exercise equipment has two dimensions. On one hand, the actual physical size of the equipment (i.e., its footprint) may give rise to a space issue. On the other hand, some equipment may be better designed to accommodate exercisers of different sizes. To exercise without compromising the possible results, athletes should use equipment that is relatively compatible with their body type and size.

☐ *Time efficiency.* Some exercise equipment is engineered so as to enable the users to achieve their exercise goals in less time. To a point, the time-efficiency level of a particular machine is a by-product of several factors, including at what intensity level the machine allows a person to exercise and how many components of fitness are being developed simultaneously by the exercise session.

☐ *Performance feedback.* The format and extent of performance-related feedback tends to vary from one exercise machine type and manufacturer to another. To provide maximum benefit to the user, such feedback should be both meaningful (i.e., relevant to the exerciser's needs and interests) and accurate (i.e., it is precisely what it says).

☐ *Sweet spot.* Exercise machines, similar to sports equipment, such as golf clubs and tennis racquets, have a "sweet spot." The sweet spot of some machines is larger than that of others. The larger a machine's sweet spot, the greater the likelihood that athletes will be able to exercise in their comfort zone—the area of mechanical efficiency that allows individuals to challenge themselves safely.

☐ *User-friendliness.* Some exercise equipment has a greater level of ease-of-use than others. The user-friendliness of a machine can have an impact on an individual's exercise experience in several positive ways, particularly the degree to which the exercise session is perceived as enjoyable. Of course, it is also true that unduly complicated-to-use machines can have an adverse impact on a person's exercise experience.

☐ *Serviceability.* Some exercise devices require more attention and effort to properly maintain than others. Not surprisingly, in our time-constrained society, most individuals would prefer exercise equipment that places the fewest demands on their time for service and maintenance.

☐ *Cost.* Exercise machines vary in cost. Unfortunately, efforts to decrease the cost of a product often result in a substantial loss of quality. Although not a hard-and-fast rule, the general guideline is that if something seems too good to be true (i.e., an exceptionally low price), it probably is.

☐ *Total fitness-orientation.* Some exercise equipment is designed to develop more than one basic component of fitness at a time. To a point, the more the better.

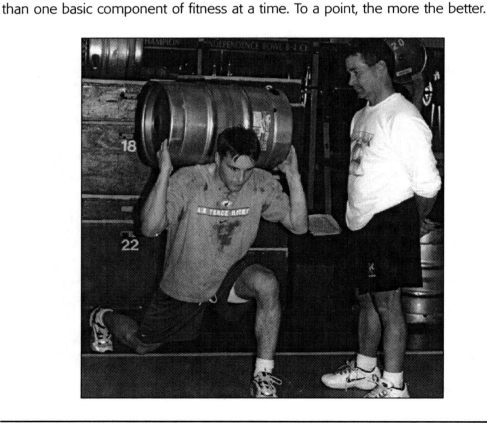

TIP/FACT #86
Athletes should design their exercise-training program in a systematic, sound manner.

Developing an effective conditioning program requires that an athlete answer three fundamental questions: "What is my existing level of fitness? What level of fitness do I want to achieve? and How can I more effectively achieve my fitness goals?" Providing honest, accurate responses to these questions is essential if athletes are to identify a productive conditioning regimen.

As a rule, athletes can evaluate their existing level of fitness by determining how fit they are on each of the basic components of physical fitness: cardiovascular fitness, muscular fitness (strength and endurance), flexibility, and body composition. Fortunately, each aspect of physical fitness can be evaluated by means of simple, non-laboratory tests.

Once athletes have evaluated their level of physical fitness, the next step is to establish realistic goals for their conditioning and training program. The objectives of the program should be based on at least three key factors, an accurate assessment of the athlete's level of fitness; a reasonable determination of what degree to which improvement can be achieved in the athlete's level of fitness within existing time, equipment, and environmental considerations; and the fitness requirements of the athlete's sport.

Based on the aforementioned factors, athletes should design their conditioning regimen in a systematic, sound manner. Whatever training program is eventually adopted, athletes should periodically reevaluate their level of progress in order to determine whether program goals/objectives are being met and whatever adjustments in their conditioning efforts are required.

TIP/FACT #87
Athletes should base their conditioning efforts on five key principles.

Athletes should incorporate the following five general guidelines into their training regimen in order to maximize their conditioning efforts:

☐ *Individual differences principle.* Athletes should understand that because of such factors as genetics and the initial level of fitness, individuals may respond to the same training stimulus in different ways.

☐ *Overload principle.* Athletes should know that in order for substantial improvement to occur in a particular system of the body (or in a component of physical fitness), the system must be stressed beyond its normal limits.

☐ *Reversibility principle.* Athletes should be aware of the fact that once they terminate their exercise programs, any adaptations that might have occurred as a result of their conditioning regimen will be reversed—a process that is often referred to as detraining. Furthermore, the effects of detraining occur more rapidly than training gains.

☐ *SAID principle.* Athletes should be cognizant of the SAID principle (specific adaptations to imposed demands), which states that a muscle will adapt to a specific demand imposed on it, making it better able to handle the greater load.

☐ *S.E.E. principle.* Athletes who want to make a meaningful comparison between various elements of a training regimen (e.g., exercise prescription, exercise modalities, available time, etc.) should employ the S.E.E. principle as the basis for distinguishing between the utility of the options under consideration. The S.E.E. principle is based on the concept that the effectiveness of a training regimen should involve three primary factors: safety, effectiveness, and efficiency. In other words, how safe is the program, how productive will the program be, and how much time will the program take?

☐ *Specificity principle.* Athletes should be aware of the fact that training for specific movements should be undertaken in the exact manner and position in which the movements will be performed. In other words, for athletes who want to improve a specific skill, the best approach is to practice that activity. Nothing totally replaces the activity itself in this instance.

TIP/FACT #88
Training efforts should be personalized to target the appropriate energy system.

Given the principle of specificity, which states that training should mimic the physiologic and biomechanical demands of competition, athletes should engage in a training regimen that produces improvements in the specific energy-delivery systems critical to obtain optimal success. Energy for exercising muscles ultimately comes from ATP (adenosine tri-phosphate), which is provided by four major energy sources. The first source is stored ATP, which is limited, only providing energy for brief (5 to 10 seconds) high-intensity work. The second source, the creatine phosphate system, can be used to replenish ATP for an additional 25 seconds, providing energy for activities such as sprinting and weightlifting. The third source, glycolysis, uses carbohydrate as a fuel source. This process results in lactic acid production, which ultimately leads to muscle fatigue. This system provides energy for activities lasting one to two minutes in length. Finally, the fourth source, the aerobic oxidation system, utilizes oxygen as an energy source and fuels activities lasting longer than two minutes.

Most programs will include some training that target each of the four energy systems. The majority of training time, however, will emphasize the energy system most used for that sport or event. For example, a long-distance runner will participate in longer endurance runs, whereas the training of a sprinter will involve a greater emphasis on repetitive higher-intensity bouts, lasting 5 to 30 seconds each.

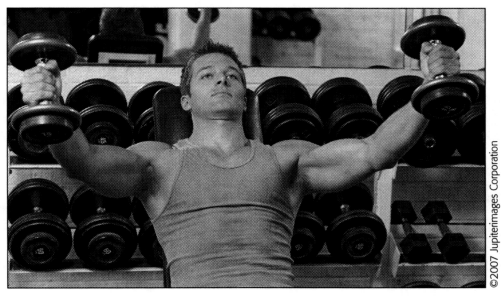

©2007 Jupiterimages Corporation

TIP/FACT #89
Excessive training can lead to the overtraining-fatigue syndrome.

Overtraining-fatigue syndrome presents itself as a prolonged decreased sport-specific performance, usually lasting greater than two weeks. It is characterized by premature fatigability, emotional and mood changes, lack of motivation, infections, and overuse injuries. Recovery is markedly longer and variable among affected athletes, sometimes taking months before the athlete returns to baseline performance.

The symptoms of overtraining can include:

• Sudden decline in quality of work or exercise performance

• Extreme fatigue

• Elevated resting heart rate

• Early onset of blood lactate accumulation

• Altered mood states

• Unexplained weight loss

• Insomnia

• Injuries related to overuse

Overtraining affects 5 to 15% of elite athletes at any one time and may be more common in amateur athletes. It is most common in endurance athletes, affecting up to 2/3 of all runners at some point. Most susceptible athletes are highly motivated and self-coached.

The exact physiologic contributors to chronic-fatigue syndrome are unknown. Potential causes include the following:

• Chronic glycogen depletion leading to peripheral muscle fatigue

- Prolonged sympathetic activity and chronically increased catecholamine levels leading to receptor down regulation and fatigue

- Excessive breakdown of branched-chain amino acids leading to central fatigue

- Depressed glutamine production from stressed muscles may depress the immune system leading to repeated minor infections

- Incomplete recovery of tissue damage can cause a systemic inflammatory response, increased cytokines, and CNS fatigue

A useful marker is to monitor baseline resting heart rest upon awakening. An elevation > 10bpm may indicate a need for training modification. Chronic elevation may indicate the chronic-fatigue syndrome.

Recovery requires rest, a period that may take up to several weeks in some athletes. Prevention measures may be considered the best "treatment," and include individualized training programs with proper periodization, reasonable goal setting, appropriate rest between hard bouts of training, cross-training, and relaxation and visualization techniques.

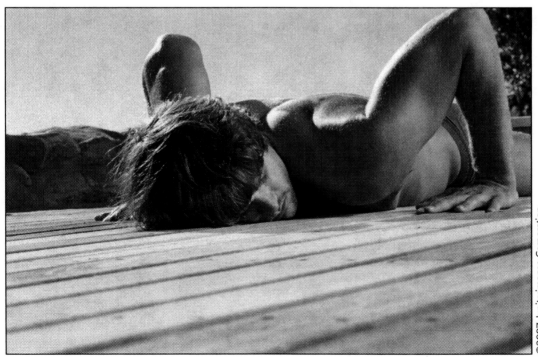

©2007 Jupiterimages Corporation

TIP/FACT #90
Peaking for competition includes tapering of training.

Training provides the basis for improved performance in competition. Peaking represents the result of physiologic and psychological training designed to produce optimal results on a given day. Peaking occurs when fitness and emotional arousal is high and fatigue is low. Peaking results not just from a reduction in training volume for a few days prior to competition, but also from a culmination of physiologic and psychologic forces leading to optimal fitness, self-confidence, motivation, and an ability to tolerate frustration. Peaking culminates with a performance at the highest level of the athlete's mental and physical powers.

Tapering, one of the last aspects of a peaking program, is a gradual reduction in training volume leading to an important competition. Most commonly, a gradual reduction in training volume begins two-to-three weeks prior to the main competition. Intensity remains high throughout the unloading process. The gradual reduction in volume allows fitness to remain at high levels.

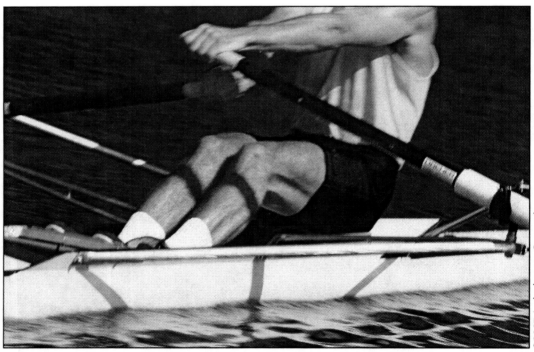

©2007 Jupiterimages Corporation

TIP/FACT #91
Athletes should be aware of the more common exercise and conditioning myths and train accordingly.

The seemingly endless array of myths, misinformation, and inappropriate practices that are incorporated into many conditioning programs have at least one trait in common— they are counterproductive to achieving the maximum results from a training regimen. The following diet, fitness, and exercise myths are examples of the more commonly held perceptions that are without foundation.

☐ *More is better.* In some things, yes; in training, no. An individual's body will respond in a positive manner to an appropriate amount of stress (demand) placed upon it. Exceeding that amount is usually a waste of time (depending on the reasons for exercising), and quite possibly may be counterproductive.

☐ *The more a person sweats, the more fat an individual will lose.* If athletes exercise in extreme heat and/or humidity or in "rubberized" clothing, they certainly will sweat and lose weight. Any weight lost in this manner, however, represents lost water—not fat. When they replenish their body fluid stores by eating and drinking, those lost pounds will return.

☐ *Muscle will turn to fat when an athlete stops lifting weights.* Absolutely not possible. When individuals stop strength training, their muscles may lose some of their girth, but will not be transformed into fat.

☐ *Performing aerobic-type exercise at a low—rather than a high—level of intensity promotes a greater loss of body fat.* While it is true that the lower a person's exercise-intensity level, the more the individual's body prefers to use fats, rather than carbohydrates, as fuel, the absolute amount of fat calories burned during high-intensity exercise tends to be equal or greater than the number expended during low-intensity activity. Athletes lose weight and body fat when they expend more calories than they consume, not because they burn fat (or anything else) when they exercise.

☐ *During exercise, individuals will become thirsty when their body needs water.* Not true. An athlete's thirst mechanism almost always tends to underestimate the body's fluid needs during exercise. As a result, an individual should consume a small amount of fluid at least every 15 to 20 minutes while exercising.

☐ *Exercise is a contest.* The word "contest" usually connotes a natural dichotomy of "winners" and "losers." Exercise, however, should not be viewed as a contest, for several reasons, not the least of which is the fact that if athletes exercise properly, there are no losers—only winners.

☐ *No pain, no gain.* Not true. Exercise should not be painful. A feeling of *discomfort* (e.g., a "burning" sensation in your muscles, muscular soreness, etc.) is generally a sign that athletes are asking their body to do something that it is not used to doing. Pain, on the other hand, is the body's signal to an athlete that they are exercising to the point where they may be harming themselves. Keep in mind that the individual who first coined the popular phrase, "no pain equals no gain" probably meant to say, "no pain equals no gain equals no sense."

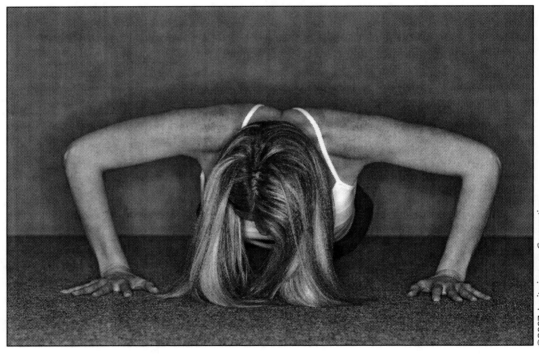

References:

Fields, K (2005) Exercise and Chronic Disease in O' Connor, F, Sallis, R, Wilder, R, St. Pierre, P (eds) *Sports Medicine: Just the Facts.* McGraw-Hill, New York, NY.

Franklin, B, Whaley, M, Howley, E (eds) (2000) ACSM's Guidelines for Exercise Testing and Prescription. Lippincott, Williams, and Wilkins, Philadelphia, PA.

Hill, J, Trowbridge, F (1998) Childhood obesity: Future directions and research priorities. *Pediatrics* **101**: 570-574.

Howard, T (2005) Overtraining Syndrome/Chronic Fatigue in O'Connor, F, Sallis, R, Wilder, R, St. Pierre, P (eds) *Sports Medicine: Just the Facts.* McGraw-Hill, New York, NY.

O'Connor, F, Wilder, R, Nirschl, R (2001) Basic Treatment Concepts in O'Connor, F, Wilder, R, (eds) *Textbook of Running Medicine.* McGraw-Hill, New York, NY.

Seto, CK (2005) Basic Principles of Exercise Training and Conditioning in O'Connor, F, Sallis, R, Wilder, R, St. Pierre, P (eds) *Sports Medicine: Just the Facts.* McGraw-Hill, New York, NY.

Vaughan, R (2001) Principles of Training in O'Connor, F, Wilder, R (eds) *Textbook of Running Medicine.* McGraw-Hill, New York, NY.

Wilder, R, Jenkins, J, Seto, C (2007) Therapeutic Exercise in Braddom, R (ed) *Physical Medicine and Rehabilitation,* 3rd ed. Elsevier, London.

9

Musculoskeletal Training (Stretching and Strengthening)

Robert P. Wilder, MD, FACSM

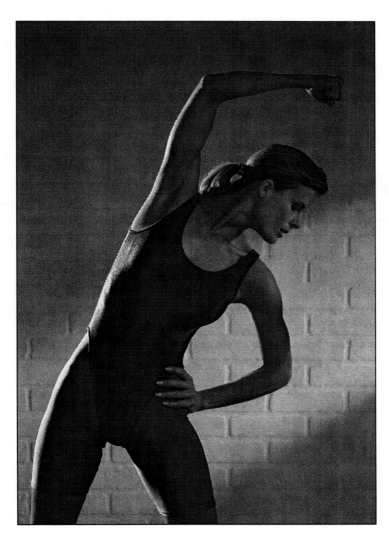

TIP/FACT #92
Appropriate amounts of stretching may help enhance performance and minimize injury.

Controversy exists concerning two of the most important proposed benefits of flexibility training: prevention of injury and performance enhancement. In athletics, flexibility has been extensively studied and applied. Among the proposed benefits of flexibility training are injury prevention, reduced muscle soreness, skill enhancement, and muscle relaxation.

With regard to injury prevention, muscles possessing greater extensibility are less likely to be overstretched during athletic activity, thereby lessening the likelihood of injury. Although the literature remains inconclusive regarding these specific benefits, a number of studies have documented a positive effect of stretching. For example, studies involving soccer players have correlated a proportion of injuries to poor flexibility, as well as demonstrated an improved range of motion and a reduction in muscle tears. There is some evidence that delayed-onset muscle soreness (DOMS) can be prevented and treated by static stretching.

On the other hand, it has also been proposed that a certain degree of tightness might protect against injury by allowing load sharing when the joints are stressed. Accordingly, hypermobility or excessive stretching could theoretically result in increased stress on the ligaments, bone, and cartilage at the joint, resulting in injury or arthritis. A major predictive factor for joint injury includes a previous joint injury resulting in excessive flexibility, rather than inadequate flexibility.

Flexibility has also been hypothesized to improve athletic performance through skill enhancement. For example, the tennis serve requires sufficient shoulder flexibility. Golf requires flexibility of the hips, trunk, and shoulders. Studies of runners have demonstrated a lower level of oxygen consumption among less flexible individuals. On the biomechanical level, pre-stretching a muscle has been shown in several studies to enhance the force of muscle contraction.

TIP/FACT #93
Static Stretching is the safest and easiest form of stretching.

Numerous stretching techniques exist. Superiority of any one method has not, however, been demonstrated. Stretching techniques are divided into four basic categories: static, passive, ballistic, and neuromuscular facilitation.

Static stretching applies a steady force for a period of 10 to 60 seconds. This method is the easiest and probably the safest type of stretching. Static stretching seems to be particularly helpful as a warm-up to other exercise, including athletic activity. Static stretching has the added advantage of being associated with decreased muscle soreness after exercise.

Passive stretching involves the employment of a partner who applies a stretch to a relaxed joint or extremity. This method requires communication and the slow and sensitive application of force. This method is most appropriately and safely used in the athletic training room or in physical therapy. Otherwise, passive stretching can be dangerous for recreational or competitive athletes due to increased risk of an injury.

Ballistic stretching employs the repetitive, rapid application of force in a bouncing or jerking maneuver. Momentum carries the body part through the range of motion until the muscles are stretched to the limits. This method is less efficient than other methods, due to the fact that muscles will contract under these stresses to protect from overstretching. The rapid increase in force can also cause injury.

The efficacy of stretching afforded by neuromuscular facilitation techniques has been well-documented. This approach involves both hold-relax and contract-relax techniques, characterized by an isometric or concentric contraction of the musculotendinous unit, followed by a passive or static stretch. The pre-stretch contraction is thought to facilitate relaxation and, therefore, flexibility. This method typically requires a trained therapist, aide, or athletic trainer.

TIP/FACT #94
Athletes should warm up before stretching.

Stretching cold muscles expose athletes to an undue risk of injuring themselves. At cooler muscle temperatures, it takes less force and stretch to tear the fibers. "Warming up" literally means increasing the individual's body temperature. Activities that can warm an athlete enough to safely begin exercise are large-muscle exercises, like pedaling a bicycle, slow jogging (in place), or doing jumping jacks. Stretching doesn't raise the body's temperature, so it's not a warm-up. Athletes should wait to stretch until after they've warmed up. When they've exercised enough to get sweaty, they've warmed up enough to stretch.

With regard to warming up before stretching, the following factors apply:

• Stretching is not a warm-up.

• Stretching before warm-up can lead to muscle tears, cramps, and other injuries.

• Athletes should warm up at least 5 to 10 minutes before stretching.

• Athletes are warmed up when they begin to break a sweat.

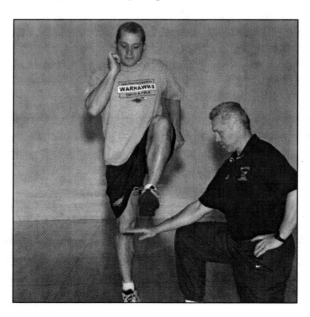

TIP/FACT #95
Athletes should stretch their muscles, not their ligaments.

Ligaments are fibrous bands that hold the body's bones together. Ligaments normally are not supposed to stretch much. They retain their length, within a range, to hold the bones in position, so the bones glide past each other along anatomically healthy paths.

The body's joints need to be flexible, but not too loose either. When injury or chronic improper stretching forces ligaments to lengthen, they do not readily go back to their former length. Technically speaking, they are *plastic*, but not *elastic*. Stretched ligaments may become irreversibly loose, like worn-out underwear waistbands.

Stretched ligaments can be a problem, because they don't hold the bones in line, allowing them to rub and grind at unhealthy angles. The friction contributes to degenerative changes over time and all the pain and disability that accompany it. Ligament instability predisposes athletes to sprains and dislocations. For example, too much looseness on the sides of the athlete's ankle increases the chance of ankle sprains. Lax shoulder capsules may slip out of place from forces that healthier joint capsules tolerate. Athletes with overly lax joints need strengthening exercises for the supporting musculature, to offset the potential for injury.

Everyone has different amounts of natural ligament looseness. Men generally have less natural flexibility than women, but can attain healthy flexibility with regular stretching. It should also be noted that some individuals have too much flexibility. Extreme ligament laxity is a common problem among dancers, and sometimes swimmers who overdo shoulder stretching. Although dancers need extreme flexibility for their art, and swimmers get better reach and range, it is not always healthy for them.

There are several steps that athletes can do to avoid stretching their ligaments when they are trying to stretch their muscles, including keeping the limb that they're stretching in line with the joint (i.e., avoid holding the joint at an angle that puts too much weight and pressure on ligaments) and not placing constant pressure on joints over extended periods of time. With regard to stretching the muscles, rather than the ligaments, the following factors apply:

- Ligaments normally are not supposed to stretch much.

- Stretched ligaments don't hold the bones in line, allowing them to rub and grind at unhealthy angles.

- Athletes should avoid putting weight and pressure on ligaments, such as in the "hurdler's stretch" and pulling their arms high up behind them.

- Athletes should avoid positions that place constant pressure on joints over extended periods of time, such as slouching, which weakens muscles and joints and puts pressure on the spine.

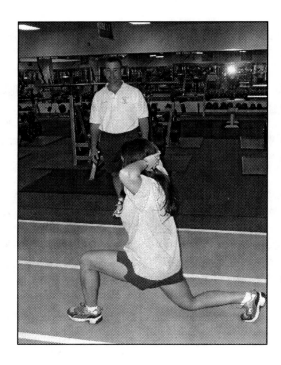

TIP/FACT #96
Athletes should strengthen, as well as stretch, the musculature surrounding the joints.

Being highly flexible, by itself, does not make an athlete fit. It can even create problems. A joint must be able to move, but not so much that it moves out of place, rubs adjacent structures, or shifts loosely during daily movement. Joints that are too loose and not strong can become unstable and not seat well. Like any two surfaces in a car or other machinery that don't seat well, an athlete's joints suffer wear and tear. As such, a difference exists between flexibility and instability. It is important to keep the musculature surrounding the joints strong, to support the joints, and to keep joint angles and movement in healthy directions and ranges. Accordingly, athletes should strengthen the musculature surrounding of a joint, as well as stretch it. In that regard, the following factors apply:

• By itself, being flexible is not synonymous with being fit.

• Stretching a joint without exercising it to be strong may allow it to stretch too far, injuring it, or to become so weak and overstretched that the joints rub and don't seat well.

• Athletes should combine strengthening exercises with their stretching exercises.

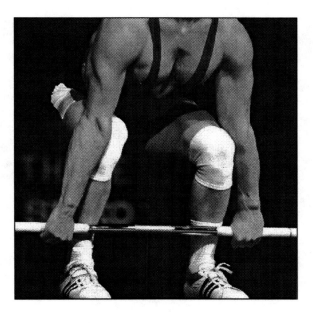

TIP/FACT #97
Muscles do matter.

When attempting to consider whether the numerous benefits of strength training make the effort involved worthwhile, it would be helpful for athletes to view their body as a car. The fuel pump for that car is their heart, while their muscles are the engine of the car. In order to function at its best, the car needs *both* a well-adjusted fuel pump and a finely-tuned engine. Sound exercise is the means for achieving both attributes.

In reality, a strong argument can be made for the need of athletes to engage in a sound strength-training regimen on a regular basis. First and foremost, improved muscular fitness has a well-documented positive impact on the performance of a variety of sports-related skills. Few athletic endeavors (if any) would not be enhanced by an improved level of strength. In addition, a higher level of muscular fitness can greatly reduce an athlete's chances of suffering muscle and skeletal injuries. It's estimated that about half of the various injuries that occur in physical activity (particularly sports) could be prevented through greater muscular fitness. As such, strength training should be viewed as an effective (and relatively inexpensive) form of health insurance for athletes. Strength training performed over an extended period also increases bone density, which helps to lower an individual's risk of osteoporosis (a concern for both female and male athletes). Finally, strength training seems to play a valuable role in preventing and treating lower back pain.

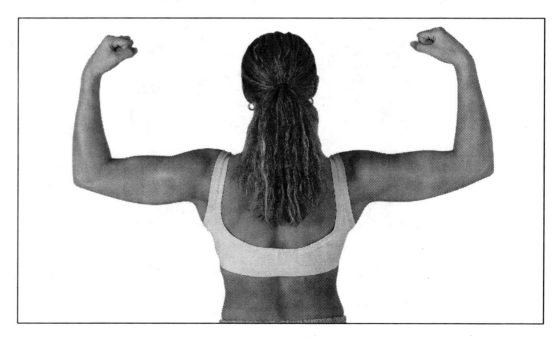

TIP/FACT #98
Athletes should select and use the type of strength-training equipment that addresses their needs and situation.

A variety of equipment is available to help athletes reach their strength-training goals. Some are more expensive. Some are more complex. Some require more skill to use. Some are more time-efficient. Some are safer. Almost all of this equipment can enable individuals to meet their personal-training goals.

Like most people, athletes might not have access to all the commonly used types of strength-training equipment. If they do, they may be uncertain about what equipment is best for them. The basic guideline to follow when selecting equipment is to choose what will best meet the athlete's interests and needs. At the minimum, equipment should be selected that is readily accessible and is consistent with the athlete's personal preference.

If an athlete has a choice of strength-training equipment, one approach is to list the advantages and disadvantages of each type and then make a subjective decision. Table 9-1 compares the three most common types of equipment on selected criteria.

	Free Weights	Multistation Machines	Variable Resistance Machines
Cost	Relatively low	Somewhat high	High
Functionality	Excellent	Limited	Limited
Learning curve	Limited	Excellent	Excellent
Muscle isolation	Variable	Excellent	Excellent
Rehabilitation	Excellent	Excellent	Excellent
Safety	Relatively safe	Very safe	Very safe
Space efficiency	Variable	Excellent	Variable
Time efficiency	Variable	Excellent	Excellent
Variety	Excellent	Limited	Limited
Versatility	Excellent	Limited	Limited

Table 9-1.

TIP/FACT #99

Adhering to the specific guidelines that have been established for strength training can enhance both the results achieved by the exercise regimen and the athlete's level of adherence to the program.

Considerable controversy exists over what constitutes the proper "recipe" for strength training. In that regard, a number of protocols and approaches exist concerning how to best structure the design of a strength program (e.g., DeLorme, Oxford, DAPRE), single-set, pyramid, periodization, etc.). In reality, all of these techniques work—some better than others. Truth be known, to a point, strength training is part art, part science. The art aspect involves subjectively injecting personal opinions and feelings into the program design project, while the scientific element is based on the documented findings of well-controlled studies. As such, athletes should base their strength-training efforts as much as possible on science, rather than art.

In an attempt to lend credibility to the issue of how to properly design a strength-exercise program, The American College of Sports Medicine developed the following prescription guidelines:

- Mode: Perform a minimum of 8 to 10 exercises that train the major muscle groups.

- Intensity: One set of 8 to 12 repetitions resulting in volitional fatigue for each exercise

- Duration: The entire program should last no more than one hour. Programs lasting greater than one hour are associated with a higher dropout rate.

- Frequency: At least two days per week

While more frequent training with additional sets or repetitions might elicit additional strength gains, a review of the literature indicates that any additional improvement would be considered relatively small (if at all) for most individuals. Furthermore, increasing the volume of work performed may have a negative impact on both the risk of injury and the level of exercise adherence (i.e., the willingness of the athletes to stick with their strength-training program).

TIP/FACT #100
Delayed onset muscle soreness may occur following initiation or a change in a strength-training program.

Delayed muscle soreness is defined as skeletal muscle pain 24 to 72 hours after unaccustomed physical activity. The pain lasts approximately five-to-seven days and can range from mild soreness to severe discomfort. Loss of muscle strength, loss of joint range of motion, tenderness, and elevated muscle enzymes are also present. Delayed muscle soreness occurs most commonly in muscle-performing eccentric activity and is related to both the intensity and duration of activity. Strength loss results from pain and a decrease in the inherent force-producing capacity of the muscle fibers. No permanent muscle injury occurs and complete muscle recovery is seen within 7 to 14 days. During eccentric-muscle activity, high tension can result in cellular damage, inflammation, and pain.

The most effective method of diminishing symptoms associated with delayed onset muscle soreness appears to be further low level exercise. This feature may be due to the production of endorphins or stimulating other neural pathways. Non-steroidal anti-inflammatory drugs may be useful in especially painful cases, because they provide an early benefit by limiting inflammation, however, their negative effects on maximal muscle function preclude their routine use.

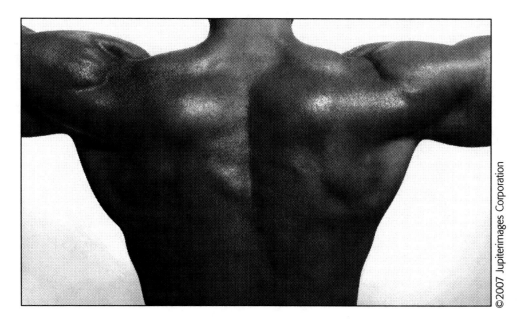

©2007 Jupiterimages Corporation

TIP/FACT #101
Athletes should know what strength will—and will not—do to their bodies.

Considerable misinformation exists concerning what individuals who strength train can expect from their exercise efforts. The more athletes are aware of the actual consequences of strength training, the better able they will be to assess the ability of their strength-training regimen to meet their needs and interests. In that regard, the following claims are among the most commonly held myths about strength training:

- *Strength training makes an individual muscle-bound.* Muscle-bound is a term that connotes a lack of flexibility. Proper strength training doesn't make athletes less flexible; it can make them *more* flexible.

- *Lifting weights results in bulky muscles.* Not true. In fact, most people don't have the genetic potential to develop large muscles. As such, over 75% of men and 90% of women can't develop substantial muscle hypertrophy without artificial means (e.g., hormonal drugs).

- *The muscles that athletes develop will turn to fat when they stop training.* Not true. Muscles cannot turn to fat. They don't have the physiological ability to change from one type of tissue to another.

- *Proper strength training has to be complex.* Not true. All factors considered, the simpler an athlete's approach to strength training, the more likely the individual's efforts will be successful. Making an endeavor too complicated can lead to a heightened level of confusion and frustration—either of which can compromise the results of engaging in a strength-training program.

- *Proper strength training is expensive.* Not true. Muscles respond to the stress applied to them, not to the cost of the equipment an athlete trains on or the money spent to join a health/fitness facility or to hire a personal trainer.

References:

American Academy of Pediatrics (2001) Strength training by children and adolescents. *Pediatrics* **6**:1470-1472.

Bookspan, J (2002) *Health & fitness in plain english.* Healthy Learning, Monterey, CA.

Franklin, B, Whaley, M, Howley (eds) (2000) ACSM's *Guidelines for exercise testing and prescription,* 6th ed. Lippincott, Williams, & Wilkins, Philadelphia, PA.

Hart, J, Ingersoll, C (2005) Weightlifting, in O'Connor, F, Sallis, R, Wilder, R, St Pierre, P (eds) *Sports medicine: Just the facts.* McGraw-Hill, New York, NY.

Nelson, B, Taylor, D (2005) Muscle and tendon injury and repair in O'Connor, F, Sallis, R, Wilder, R, St Pierre, P (eds) *Sports Medicine: Just the Facts.* McGraw-Hill, New York, NY.

Wilder R, Jenkins J, Seto C (2007) Therapeutic Exercise, in Braddom, R (ed) *Physical Medicine & Rehabilitation.* Elsevier, London.

About the Contributors

Barry P. Boden, MD, is an associate professor at the Uniformed Services University of the Health Sciences School of Medicine in Bethesda, MD, and a practicing orthopedist at The Orthopedic Center in Rockville, MD.

Jamie Cooper, MS, is a doctoral student in nutritional sciences at the University of Wisconsin—Madison.

Patricia A. Deuster, PhD, MPH, is a professor at the Uniformed Services University of the Health Sciences School of Medicine in Bethesda, MD, and director of their Human Performance Laboratory.

Thomas M. Howard, MD, is the program director of the VCU-Fairfax Family Practice Sports Medicine Fellowship in Fairfax, VA.

Donald T. Kirkendall, PhD, is an adjunct assistant professor in the Department of Exercise and Sport Sciences at the University of North Carolina-Chapel Hill. He is also a member of the sports medicine committee of US Soccer and a corresponding member of the FIFA Medical Assessment and Research Centre (F-MARC).

John Manta, MD, is an orthopedic consultant for the Downingtown Area School District and team physician for Bishop Shanahan High School in Exton, PA.

Francis G. O'Connor, MD, MPH, is an associate professor at the Uniformed Services University and medical director for the Consortium on Health and Military Performance.

Brian V. Reamy, MD, is the chair of the Department of Family Medicine of the Uniformed Services University in Bethesda, MD.

Robert P. Wilder, MD, is an associate professor of physical medicine and rehabilitation at the University of Virginia.

About the Editors

Barry P. Boden, MD, is a board-certified orthopaedic surgeon with fellowship training in sports medicine and arthroscopic knee and shoulder surgery. He participated on the varsity soccer and track and field teams at Haverford College and then completed medical school and both his general surgery internship and an orthopaedic residency at Temple University in Philadelphia. Dr. Boden continued his training with a fellowship in sports medicine at Duke University, where he served as the assistant team physician for the varsity athletes. Since returning to the Washington, DC area, Dr. Boden has been active in advancing the study of sports medicine. He enjoys teaching and has lectured at local hospitals, national conferences, and as an instructor for the Orthopaedic Academy. He is a consultant at the National Institutes of Health (NIH) and an adjunct associate professor at the Uniformed Services University of the Health Sciences (USUHS). He is currently involved in several multi-center funded studies, including one evaluating head injuries in athletes and another studying the etiology of ACL injuries.

Francis G. O'Connor, MD, MPH, associate professor at the Uniformed Services University and medical director for the Consortium on Health and Military Performance, has been a leader in sports medicine education and research for the military for over 15 years. Dr. O'Connor has authored over 30 articles in scientific journals and numerous book chapters/technical reports/health promotion resources for the military. In addition, Dr. O'Connor is the editor of four texts on sports medicine, including the *Textbook of Running Medicine* and *Sports Medicine for the Primary Care Physician, 3rd Edition*. He is on the board of several leading organizations in sports medicine, including the American College of Sports Medicine, the American Medical Society of Sports Medicine, and the American Medical Athletic Association. A colonel in the United States Army, Dr. O'Connor is a 1981 graduate of the United States Military Academy at West Point. Prior to his recent posting at Uniformed Services University in the Department of Military Medicine, he served one year as a command surgeon with Special Operations in the Middle East.

Robert P. Wilder, MD, is an associate professor of physical medicine and rehabilitation at the University of Virginia. He received his undergraduate degree from the University of Dayton, where he ran cross-country for the Flyers, serving as team captain in 1983. He received his medical degree from the University of Virginia. Following a residency in physical medicine and rehabilitation at the Baylor College of

Medicine in Houston, he completed a fellowship in primary care sportsmedicine at the Nirschl Orthopaedic Sportsmedicine Clinic and the Virginia Sportsmedicine Institute. He practiced in Dallas from 1993-1998, during which time he served as medical director of the Runner's Clinic at the Tom Landry Sportsmedicine and Research Center and as head team physician for the Dallas Burn of Major League Soccer. Since 1998, he has been on faculty at the University of Virginia, where he serves as medical director of the Runner's Clinic at UVa and as a team physician for University of Virginia Athletics. He lives in Charlottesville with his wife, Susan, and their four children, Lauren, Stephen, Ryan, and Caroline.

CALL-SIGN KLUSO

An American Fighter Pilot in
Mr. Reagan's Air Force

RICK TOLLINI

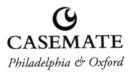

CASEMATE
Philadelphia & Oxford

Published in the United States of America and Great Britain in 2021 by
CASEMATE PUBLISHERS
1950 Lawrence Road, Havertown, PA 19083, USA
and
The Old Music Hall, 106–108 Cowley Road, Oxford OX4 1JE, UK

Hardback Edition: ISBN 978-1-61200-981-0
Digital Edition: ISBN 978-1-61200-982-7

A CIP record for this book is available from the British Library

Printed and bound in the United Kingdom by TJ Books

Typeset by Versatile PreMedia Services (P) Ltd.

For a complete list of Casemate titles, please contact:

CASEMATE PUBLISHERS (US)
Telephone (610) 853-9131
Fax (610) 853-9146
Email: casemate@casematepublishers.com
www.casematepublishers.com

CASEMATE PUBLISHERS (UK)
Telephone (01865) 241249
Email: casemate-uk@casematepublishers.co.uk
www.casematepublishers.co.uk

Contents

Introduction

I really had no desire to write a book about my combat exploits in the USAF, for many reasons. First, the narrative had already been repeated many times in my own accounts to those who wanted to hear the stories. It has been published in other books (even if by other people) and infamously (if somewhat inaccurately) chronicled in the History Channel's *Dogfight* series of TV shows.

Over the years I have also tried to extricate myself slowly from a single series of events during Operation DESERT STORM, because to many people it is how they know me, the prism through which they characterize my life and whatever success I have had. In actuality, I have come to view it as just one small episode in my life (and even of my Air Force career) compared to the many other events that have not only defined my life, but brought me to where I am today.

One day, at work I believe, I was sitting at my computer when I started re-running some of the events, both mundane and pivotal, that formed the map of my life. I quickly opened a word-processing document (as I have come to do when an idea for a song strikes me nowadays) and I jotted down some notes that to a casual observer might have seemed trivial or completely unconnected. But to me they started painting a picture of a life, one that at first appeared to have no coherent destiny, but then somehow flowed into multiple streams and rivers of events, eventually combined into raging rapids before settling into a calm ocean. Maybe another way of thinking of it is as an impressionist piece of art. At first glance, it may not be apparent what the artist is depicting, but after greater observation it suddenly becomes clear to the witness. Thereafter it's less about the physical image and more about the sense of being within the work.

The point at which I had arrived—its how, when, and where—suddenly started to make sense, as well as where I was heading in the future. I don't think most of us consider "how we got here." For the most part, we only agonize or rejoice about the here and now. But if you carefully think back to your most distant memory, hopefully from that point you can start to piece together the events and decisions, both small and grand, that changed the course of your life.

When I completed this exercise, I looked at the list of events. Of course, my DESERT STORM experience was one of the unique, if not pivotal, moments in my life. I came to regard it, however, as just a single data point, one that never would have occurred if some of the other seemingly routine life events had not taken place. Something even as simple as a chance meeting or arriving someplace five minutes early can change the course of this mighty river we call life.

So if you are reading this book because you want to live vicariously the life of a fighter pilot and experience the action of real combat, then you might want to skip straight to Chapter 8, and hopefully that recounting will be worth the price of admission. But I decided when I started to write this book, that if I was going to do this, I had to do it my way.

I want the reader to recognize the common bonds of our humanity, regardless of what we end up doing as our "life's work." The only way I could evoke this was take you back to the beginning ... well, not the actual beginning (like the day of my birth), but to some of those crucial moments in the life of a young boy who grew up in northern California and eventually flew with Eagles. Even so, my life did not "end" (literally or figuratively) over the sands of Iraq in early 1991. There was another path for me to realize and follow, and that is actually the most important discovery I have made in the last 20 years. If the engagement with the Iraqi Foxbat pilot had never happened, I don't really know where my life may have ended up, any more than how the preceding events led to the violent clash of two warriors southwest of Baghdad.

Not all of this history is positive ... it couldn't be, it shouldn't be. A life without struggles or challenges does not lead to personal growth. The hard ground we fall on is also the same firm foundation we use to push ourselves back up and continue on. The difference in outcomes lies in how we view life's hardships, whether with resentment and bitterness, or with a sense of gratitude for the place we have arrived, along with the determination and confidence to overcome anything life throws our way. This was my struggle also, and in that sense I felt it necessary to lay bare all the fundamental darkness that resides in my own heart (and in our collective humanity) and the challenges and frustrations I have faced along the way, in particular in the final years of my Air Force career, and even after.

My hope, though, is that readers can make a correlation between my life and their own, seeing the similar obstacles and disappointments along their individual journey with a more affirmative glow of appreciation. I am fairly confident that my episodes of greatest struggle and challenge ended up being the times of utmost personal growth.

Some 99.9% of what I have written here comes from memory and recollection. No recounting can ever survive the passage of time perfectly or allow for the different reminiscences of others involved in the events. If people, places, or events I mention in this book don't match with how others remember them, then I am sorry for that, but not apologetic. Once again, this is my story, not somebody else's. They are more than welcome to write their own book.

I also have no intent to "call out" anybody for the manner in which they chose to live their lives, even if it possibly affected my own life. We each have the singular burden of choice to carry with us. But as I have alluded, I believe that everything happens for a reason, and whether each event creates value in our lives or not depends on what we do after it occurs. For that reason, I appreciate everybody and everything that have come into my life, whether that connection was positive or painful.

I want to thank Steve Davies for encouraging me to write my personal historical account, which he felt other people would like to hear, and Douglas "Disco" Dildy for helping fill in some of the unknowns of the Iraqi Air Force (IrAF) pilots that came out to do battle that day in 1991. I also want to thank military history author Mike Guardia for his help connecting me with Casemate Publishers and for their willingness to take a chance on a first-time writer. As expert writers on aviation and air combat, Davies, Dildy, and Guardia have authored some of the most accurate accounts of my squadron's DESERT STORM exploits, along with other works, and I appreciate their support and encouragement on this project.

I also have to thank my fellow fighter pilots, friends, and my family ... all of them, but in particular: my father, who taught me how to fly; my older brother, whose "tough love" forged some steel will in me; my wife Sako, who always supported me in all my endeavors; and, to our kids, Sakura and Lucas, who did not always have the benefit of the most attentive father, but accepted my love anyway.

There are too many other people to thank. Doing so would bog down the intro to this book, so I will keep it simple. Thank you all (you know who you are).

CHAPTER I

The Wonder Years

"Clear prop!" ... the command barely squeaked out of my pre-pubescent voice.

It didn't sound very convincing, but as I pushed the starter button my father advanced the throttle ever so slightly and the Piper PA-18 Super Cub roared into life with a shake and the soon-to-be familiar smell of Avgas (aviation gasoline) exhaust. I didn't really know what to hold on to, or what to do, but Dad told me to keep my hands lightly on the control stick between my legs and the sliding throttle lever on the left side panel, so I could follow his movements. He also told me to do what I could to help him hold the heel brakes, restraining the powerful but light-framed Super Cub from rolling forward. I dug my heels so hard into the small square pegs on the floorboard just under the rudder pedals that I was concerned that my feet would at any moment break through and hang dangling underneath the plane.

I was excitedly nervous, which was my usual state of mind any time I was about to try something new, especially something new that might involve heights and the possibility of imminent death (or so I had imagined over and over in my fitful sleep the night before). I really didn't understand, however, why we had to get up before the sun, which as it crept slowly over the Sierra Nevada Mountains to the east was throwing a very long shadow of the Super Cub out in front of us.

I wasn't much for waking early on summer days, and I never had a morning appetite when I was young. This morning I did manage to get down a few bites of stale powdered donut and a half-glass of milk, although that did not do much to fuel my confidence in my constitution. I was well known as a child for my motion sickness, which interrupted many a family road trip, forcing my parents to pull over to avoid my puking in the car. This was probably my biggest fear—that my father would somehow have to "pull over" in mid-air to allow me to upchuck. But for some reason, today, I did not feel the cold fingers of apprehension crawling over my gut. I was so busy taking it all in that the thought of a vomit-covered lap had not even crossed my mind ... yet.

We were at the Stockton Metropolitan Airport in the Central Valley of northern California. My father knew that the cooler summer morning air would provide for a smooth first airplane ride ... and this was my first ever ride in my youthful memory, in a small civilian airplane. I have been told that my father had previously taken the whole family up in a small plane before, but I was a baby at the time and had no recollection.

Mark Tollini was my father. He had been a private pilot since a young age. Cutting his teeth on a similar but less-powerful Piper J-3 Cub, he had a love of flying that he was eager to pass along to me and his oldest son Mark. Today was my turn. For Dad this was a sort of renaissance too. He had long been involved in general aviation, as an accomplished Airframe & Powerplant (A&P) mechanic, but a wife and three kids had complicated any opportunities to continue flying. General aviation was expensive and normally the dominion of the country club elite.

Fortunately for my father, he had established himself as a government service (GS) civilian at the Sharpe Army Depot in Lathrop, just south of Stockton. The US Army used the depot to repair the multitude of helicopters and other small aircraft returning from the Vietnam War with battle scars. As such, Sharpe Depot (now called San Joaquin Depot) had access to surplus aircraft. So, with other interested members, a flying club was established. Depot workers or the active-duty military members could access the club and fly their aircraft at ridiculously cheap rates. This was, to my father's and my own great fortune, how he was able to afford to fly again.

This Piper PA-18, call number N6738C, affectionately known as "Three-Eight Charlie," was one of the club's first aircraft, lovingly refurbished and made airworthy by club members, including my father. And now, Three-Eight Charlie wrapped its steel tube and fabric airframe snugly around me in the front seat and my father in the back. The "solo" seat of the Super Cub was actually in the front, and even though I was obviously not qualified to be the "pilot-in-command" my father was used to flying from the back seat, which was the solo position for his old J-3 Cub. So, today he would tell me what to do with the controls and knobs to which he didn't have access. A high level of trust was required, I thought, but it was another good way to keep me busy and my mind off of my unpredictable stomach.

The Super Cub was a tail-dragger, meaning that it did not sit upright in a conventional airplane manner with a tripod nose wheel. Instead, the aircraft tipped back on two main fixed landing gear, with a small wheel at the tail attached to the rudder pedals in the cockpit to steer the plane on the ground left and right. Thus the nose of the Super Cub jutted up in the air, making it difficult to see straight ahead. For this reason, as we taxied out to the active runway we snaked our way along, making S-turns in order to visually clear the path immediately in front of us. I was reminded that this was the same technique that many old World War II fighters, such as the P-51 Mustang and P-47 Thunderbolt, often used to taxi their aircraft on the ground.

As we held short of the runway, I helped my father apply the brakes once again (I'm sure he didn't really need my help, but it made me feel at least somewhat useful) as we went through a series of flight control and engine power checks to insure nothing catastrophic would occur during those critical few moments when an airplane is just getting airborne and is at its most vulnerable.

And then suddenly we were on the runway and ready to go.

My father told me before about something called P-factor: the asymmetric torque from the thrust of the propeller, which would cause the airplane to want to pull to the left. The correct counter to P-factor was to apply smoothly a small amount of right rudder to keep the aircraft going straight down the runway. This correction would be held until the tail lifted off the ground, putting the plane in a level attitude, at which point the P-factor would decrease to negligible levels and the plane would behave true to form.

Let me tell you, it's easier to explain than it was to learn or perform. Today my father was flying, however, and his aim on the runway was straight as an arrow. The little Super Cub abruptly lurched forward, smoothly accelerated, and when the tail lifted as advertised I could see the world in front of me again. As I moved my head slightly over my right shoulder to say something to my father, I noticed the aircraft's shadow part ways with the earth. We were airborne, and I was liberated. I felt as I had somehow been here before. It was so natural.

I was a bird again ... learning to fly.

***

2405 Del Rio Drive, Stockton, California: my home for the better part of my early childhood and my only memory of such, since we had moved there while I was still a baby. I guess the best way I can explain my early life is in reference to the 90s TV show, *Wonder Years*.

I was THAT kid. I was Kevin Arnold.

Born in the mid-1950s, I grew up basically on the same timeline as the TV show. I wore the same crazy 60s and 70s wardrobe, tried to have long hair (which caused constant fights with my conservative father), and experienced the turbulent but exciting history of American culture during that period. I even had pretty much the same family dynamics: the perpetually grumpy father; the well-meaning try-to-keep-the-peace mother; the sweet but much older sister; and the classic older brother who felt his sole purpose in life was to beat me up at any opportunity that might arise, or for no reason whatsoever. The only thing I didn't have was a childhood sweetheart like Kevin's Winnie Cooper. I never actually had any kind of girlfriend for that matter, until after high school. I was painfully shy.

The neighborhood was classic 60s Americana. The 'burbs. Scraped from the rich peat dirt of the California Central Valley, Stockton was just like so many small towns and cities that populated postwar America. My school, John Tyler Elementary, was literally a stone's throw away—they built the school right behind the open cyclone fence that bordered our backyard. I could walk out of my front door, cross our front lawn, turn left, walk 50 feet, and pass through the gate of the schoolyard. BONUS! It probably saved me 15–20 minutes' sleep every day and, unlike most kids, I almost always walked home for lunch. I don't think I ever took a bag lunch to school until junior high. A cafeteria lunch was a special treat, for which I would sometimes ask my mom to give me money so I could eat with my best friends.

My brother Mark and I had plenty of neighborhood friends and a wealth of places to explore. Right behind the school, about two blocks' walking distance from our house, was the Calaveras Canal: a high-walled levee built to control the floodwaters of the almost sea-level San Joaquin Delta region and also to provide irrigation water for the rich Central Valley farmland. This was our Wonderland. Catching lizards, bugs, and the occasional gopher snake. Fishing for Delta catfish or crappie on the side of the levee. Finding "secret" hideaways that nobody else knew, where we could tell ghost stories.

One block down from our street, rows and rows of houses had been bulldozed to make way for the central California freeway, Interstate 5 (I-5). But for many years the fields and old foundations lay dormant as the enormous public works project sat idle. This area soon became overgrown with tall mustard plants and enormous thorny sticker bushes the size of a small house. These were our covert labyrinths and fortresses, where we would play from sunrise to sunset during the long and beautiful blue-sky northern California summers.

Before the age of computers, Internet, satellite TV, and cell phones, the neighborhood had its own lines of communication. With a network of family and friends, everybody always seemed to know what was going on and what were the important happenings. One uncharacteristically warm February day, there was a definite buzz and a different vibe going around on Del Rio Drive. You could feel it immediately as you walked out the door. Something BIG was coming.

Our friends, the Long family, who lived catty-corner from us, were almost always on top of the significant news and I am pretty sure it was youngest brother Clay Long who told me that day, "The Beatles are on the *Ed Sullivan Show* tonight! You gonna watch it?" Well, hell, nobody missed that 1960s Sunday night family event. The *Ed Sullivan Show* came on right after *The Wonderful World of Disney*. Normally, Sunday night dinner was over, dessert consumed, and the dishes done by time *Ed Sullivan* came on, and the whole family watched it every Sunday. Why would this one be any different? How could I possibly miss The Beatles, who had become my heroes of musical coolness in just a few short months in early 1964.

I will never forget that moment. I just sat mesmerized by the mop-top haircuts, the mod-style clothes, and that sound. It was different than anything I had ever heard or ever wanted to hear. All I remember was I wanted to be close to that ... somehow ... someway.

We learned all The Beatles's songs, waited for each new album, and tried our best to replicate their hair and style. They were just sooo cool. My dad hated them! He complained that they looked like girls and they couldn't sing. My father and I would have a long, drawn-out battle over culture and change. Eventually, I would win. I always knew that in some way music would be a big part of my life, and those classic pop and rock songs would be the measure of my years and memories.

*****

My family was dysfunctional. I just didn't know it until many, many years later. But, then again, I think every family is probably dysfunctional in some way or another, some families to the extreme, and some at barely perceptible levels, except to the trained professional. My family was probably around the middle of that scale. But we always had each other.

We were definitely a typical middle-class family, but probably just barely in the "middle." We were hanging on to our class status only because Mom and Dad both worked full-time. Our mother, Corinne Tollini, was a 6th grade school teacher at John Adams Elementary in a different part of town. I was *so* happy I did not have my mom as a teacher; I knew she would not have cut me any slack.

Family trips were normally whatever we could fit into a one-day drive and a tight budget. (I rarely ever left the borders of California until I was an adult and on my own.) These family adventures usually started with some kind of drama and often an argument between my mother and father, to the extent it would seem we wouldn't go at all. Then, all of a sudden, we would be in the car and on our way, with no air conditioning and constant adolescent bickering and whining about "how much longer" and "when are we going to eat." And then we would arrive.

*****

Disneyland, circa 1965, was truly a "magic kingdom." Nothing like it existed anywhere on Earth, or in the Universe as far as I knew. One summer in the mid-60s, after a long 10-hour drive through the central California heat, we ended up on our first family trip to Disneyland. I was in Mickey heaven.

I'm sure it was an expensive holiday for my parents. We stayed in a cheap roadside motel not too far from the park. Ticket prices and eating out for the next couple of days had to put a pretty big dent in their pocketbooks, but our parents wanted to be sure we had a full and memorable childhood. I will always appreciate their sacrifices.

I can remember every ride and event we experienced. It was like a repeated Christmas Day every time we got to the front of a long line and boarded a ride that took us to a different fantasy world. If I could have stayed in Disneyland forever, as a modern-day Peter Pan, I would have. But, all good things must end. On the final day of our vacation, as we left the park for the last time, it was already late and with enormously long drive home ahead of us. I begged Mom to stop at one of the exit souvenir booths to buy some trinket, to cherish this trip for the rest of my life. I ended up with a small Goofy penlight. It was a splendid memento.

On the way home, my father made what he hoped to be our only pit stop for gas and a bathroom break for the trip home. I was "ordered" to go use the Texaco station's restroom and make sure to take care of "business," so we didn't have to stop again. And I did. Back in the car and on the road, it didn't take long for me to crash fast asleep in the back seat. Sleep always helped to shorten the trip home. At some point, though, as I was probably reliving the whole Disney experience in my dreams, I reached into my pocket looking to fondle my prized Goofy penlight. I bolted straight out of my slumber. My Goofy penlight was GONE!

I frantically searched my other pockets and all around the backseat of the car. My suspicion turned to my brother Mark, even though he was sleeping too. I knew Mark must have taken my penlight, but after pounding him out of his sleep and raising the ire of our mother, he convinced me he had not taken it. That left only one conclusion. I had taken the penlight out while I was sitting on the toilet.

Oh my GOD! Goofy was still at the Texaco station, which was now at least an hour or more in our rearview mirror. I began to bawl uncontrollably, asking for the gods to intervene and take us back to the Texaco.

To this day, I don't understand why my father turned the car around. If it had happened to one of my kids, under the same circumstances, I honestly don't think I would have done the same thing. I would have promised some lesser substitute to replace the toy, but not swung around and added the extra hours of a detour on top of the already heinous drive home. I will never forget what my father did for me that night.

We arrived back at the Texaco and I hurried into the one-stall bathroom, and? ... no Goofy. My treasured souvenir penlight was gone. I was convinced some other kid, most likely my age, returning from his own special Disneyland trip, had gone into the bathroom and found my Goofy light. And now my penlight was in that other kid's pocket, in another car, on its way home somewhere on California Central Valley Highway 99.

Bummer.

I am not sure if I made an audible or even silent vow that night, but after the Goofy penlight incident I decided I would never lose something truly important to me again. EVER. As a young adult, I would always check and double check to make sure I had my important possessions with me, like my wallet, or car keys, or whatever else I considered irreplaceable. This tendency probably developed into an almost obsessive-compulsive condition in my personality, but one that I think would pay dividends later in my life and in this book. Having a fluid mental "checklist" is an important part of being a fighter pilot.

My streak of retaining my personal treasures continued for the most part unbroken until 1982, while I was at Undergraduate Pilot Training (UPT) at Williams Air Force Base (AFB) as a young 2nd lieutenant (2Lt). I made a trip to the local Base Exchange (BX) to buy something. As I got out of my car, in uniform, I realized I did not have my flight cap. I had no idea where I might have left it. I was horrified at the thought of having to run the gauntlet of other higher-ranking officers or enlisted personnel and then having to render a salute when it so was obvious I was without "cover" and not dressed to regulations.

Worse, the fix for the problem—a new flight cap—could only be found in the very BX store I was headed for in the first place. With no other options, I held my breath, got out of my car, and bolted for the closest entry. Somehow, I made it unobserved into the BX and purchased whatever I had come for plus one brand new flight cap with gold 2Lt bars.

I vowed that day I would never lose a flight cap again. And I didn't. That same replacement flight cap remained with me dutifully through pilot training, fighter lead-in course, F-15 initial training, my first and second F-15 assignments, over 1,500 hours of flight time, numerous foreign countries, countless combat training exercises, and one war. That hat was pretty "experienced" to say the least.

I removed the flight cap for the last time on the order of a three-star general who told me he had never seen a flight cap quite like that. I don't think he meant it as a compliment. I donated Flight Cap #2 to the 12th Fighter Squadron (12 FS) "Dirty Dozen" bar on Kadena Air Base in Okinawa, Japan, where it had previously spent many happy hours. When the 12 FS was closed down in 1999, I confiscated my treasured flight cap and its glass-framed enclosure. It now sits above my desk in my current workplace, still a reminder of many great memories, and ... the Goofy penlight incident.

***

Summer days in northern California, and specifically on Del Rio Drive, were glorious. The scorching hot Central Valley summers were naturally tamed during the night by the air flowing over the cool Pacific current that passed along California's northern coastline. Creeping through the Altamont Pass and over the Livermore hills, this crisp dry air mass would settle across the San Joaquin Valley. The mornings would normally hold on to their therapeutic breezes until late morning, and allow a long, deep slumber under the shaded windows of the small bedroom I shared with my brother.

We were normally nudged from our prolonged awakening by the smells coming from the family kitchen just outside our bedroom door. Bacon from my father's pre-work breakfast, our mother's toast and jam with coffee, and often the smell of a pot of our grandmother's apricot preserves as they slowly simmered on the stovetop.

Lazy days normally started with a stretch of TV reruns that were not quite old enough to be called "classics" yet, but we already knew they were: *I Love Lucy*, *The Beverly Hillbillies*, *The Andy Griffith Show*. Then we'd have something to eat that normally sufficed as both breakfast and lunch (before the concept of brunch was introduced), which would give us the energy to start our daily endeavors. We would venture out, or our friends would congregate near our front-door screen, and we would begin reaching a communal consensus on what we were going to do that day. More often than not, our summer days consisted of neighborhood pick-up games of whiffle ball, or sandlot football (in the winter), or some other street or schoolyard game, frequently made up. The other obvious choice was to go to the levee and transform ourselves into Cowboys 'n' Indians, or into our favorite World War II heroes from the TV show *Combat*.

The levee had many visitors from different "tribes" of neighborhood kids, but we tended to have our own territories and activities and we would not meet very often. Since the authorities had plowed the rows of houses for the new freeway, a natural divide existed between our east side John Tyler Elementary neighborhood and the west side neighborhood whose kids attended a different elementary school. It seems now like the stories of prehistoric times, when natural divides separated people and cultures. We knew there were other kids "over there," and that they were probably like us. We maybe even knew the names of a few or had met them on rare occasions up at the levee. But we had no real connection to them ... until one day.

I don't remember what time of year it was, nor do I remember exactly the year, but I do remember it was during my early grade school days. There was suddenly a very dark vibe that descended across Del Rio's happy abodes. It seemed to emanate from the air and ground around us. We seemed to detect it in the same way that animals feel an earthquake traveling across the planet, even before it's known by ignorant humans.

A young boy from the "other" Del Rio tribe, across the great divide of mustard plants and old house foundations, had drowned in the Calaveras Canal. We didn't really know his name or exactly what he looked like, but just the same, we knew him. He was Us.

It was just too close to home to ignore, but it could have easily been one of us, my neighborhood friend David Anderson, my brother Mark, or one of his friends, or even ... me. We did not know how it happened until whispered conversations at the family dinner tables were clandestinely pieced together by us kids. He was a younger brother who had tagged along on the tribe's Huck Finn adventure for the day, which was to build a makeshift raft to ford and fish along the cool and dark Calaveras Canal. Somehow the raft tipped or flipped, and as the remainder of the kids swam to the safety of the muddy banks, the younger brother went under and never surfaced.

We heard horror stories regarding the effort to locate the young boy's body, and a term I had never heard before called "dragging the river." After asking my father what that meant, he told me that they use a boat and drag a rope with a huge weighted hook on it until they snag something, or the body, and bring it to the surface. I could only picture the indignity of not only drowning but also being skewered by what I envisioned as an enormous fishing hook. How could a family endure such a tragedy?

Something changed, and it changed from that day on. I imagined what it would be like to give up all the "treasures" of life we enjoyed: our family and friends; our favorite TV shows; our favorite dinners and desserts; and our summer days. The fairy-tale suburbs of Del Rio Drive became tinged with the reality of life. I couldn't recognize what it was at the time, but now I know it was the realization of my own (and our collective) mortality. You never think about death as a kid until something like this creates a link between your own life and present death.

Many years later, I would see the movie *Stand By Me*, based on Steve King's short story *The Body*. The conclusion of that movie represents the "last day" of youth for the kids who, much as in my own childhood adventures, went on a summer escapade to find the rumored body of another kid killed by a train. The culmination of the adventure was the end of the magic days of summer. Thrust upon them was the realization that they would all grow up, leave the neighborhood, and someday they would die too ... some sooner than others. From then on, nothing would be the same.

The day we recognize our own mortality, and that this particular lifetime must end one day, is when our human delusion and suffering truly begins.

***

It's funny how a casual decision, made in a split second, can often make a profound and enduring impact on our lives. For me, one personal defining moment (of many) came around the same time as the Calaveras incident, although I can't remember now if it was before or after. Doesn't matter, really.

Our family had a generation of cousins on my mother's side who became a big part of our early years. The nine cousins, which included my brother and older sister Joy, were spread out fairly uniformly in age, so that not much more than a year separated any of us from the next older or younger cousin. This meant that when we had our regular family holidays, like Thanksgiving or maybe Christmas or Easter, they were very special events that still hold a permanent place in my heart and memories.

My uncle Kenny (my mom's brother) and Aunt Marilyn (Kenny's wife) had recently moved their family to a new community of homes in the East Bay foothills of California called Pleasant Hills. I would learn quickly during one of our first family visits to their new location that there wasn't much "pleasant" in them th'ar hills.

On this particular day I was in their garage with my younger cousin Craig, and I spied one of their bikes leaning against the wall. I asked Craig if I could ride it and of course he said "sure." As I remember, it was a typical "kids" bicycle, something beyond an early trainer but not as big as the 10-speeds that most teens would ride. Regardless, it was mobile and I was a bit bored so I took it out for a spin.

I'm pretty sure the Pleasant Hills community established its name based on the fact that the homes were built all along the rolling hills in the neighborhood. I did not have to travel very far from my cousin's house to find a rather large and somewhat intimidating downhill grade. From the top it looked to me like an Olympic ski jump, and my first run down the slope came with a good helping of back-pedal pressure on the brakes, but as I neared the bottom of the hill I let loose and felt a rush of adrenaline kick in as the small bike quickly accelerated.

I was not normally one to throw caution to the wind, but having cheated death once, I decided it seemed fairly safe and proceeded to make several more runs down the monster hill as cousin Craig looked on. Each time I allowed the speed to increase from a higher starting point on the hill, and I would excitedly push the bike back to the top to start another run.

I think I will always regret the finality of these words, but after another tiring trip walking the bike to the top of the hill, I remember turning to my patient cousin Craig and saying something like, "… just one more time." As I broke over the crest of the hill, instead of braking at all, I began to pedal as hard as I could to add extra acceleration to the bike. I was going so fast now that I could not even pedal fast enough to keep up with the pull of Newtonian Law. The rows of houses and the cracks in the sidewalk sped by in a blur and I felt an enormous rush of exhilaration, until …

Nearing the bottom of the hill, and probably nearing terminal velocity, I remember there was a slight wobble in the handlebars of the bike. This bipod machine I had picked up in the garage was apparently in need of some minor maintenance, and the bolt that tightens the handlebars to the head tube and the front wheel fork was loose. It happened so fast I don't think I ever saw it, but at some point the fast-rolling front tire rotated itself 90 degrees sideways and instantly became a brake.

I imagine it was quite a sight for my cousin and anybody else who was on the street that day. In today's world somebody with a video camera or smartphone would have instantly posted it on YouTube. As for me, all I remember is a moment of weightlessness as I flew over the handlebars, and suddenly … BANG! … and then momentary darkness. I knew I had abruptly stopped, but I didn't know how or why, and then I was picking myself off the asphalt.

The next thing I remember was the taste of salty warm blood in my mouth, from which I bent over and spit into my hand. In the pool of bright red blood were several pieces of white enamel chips, which were the remnants of my two permanent front teeth. Damn! I had just grown out those beautiful teeth less than a year before, and now there they were in little pieces in my hand. Apparently, however, I was much worse off than just an oral injury, as I could tell from the look on my cousin's face as he reached me at the bottom of the hill. I had also scraped off a good portion of my chin on the pavement, and now an ample supply of blood was flowing from the flap of skin hanging off of my lower jaw. The family holiday was over in a trip to the emergency room.

With stitches and nice scar on my chin, I would recover quickly, but the permanent damage to my front teeth would plague me for many years to come. I am not sure if the level of dentistry in the 60s was advanced enough, or if my dentist had a sadistic twinge and just wanted to teach me about the dangers of hill surfing, but I ended up with two tremendously large white enamel caps as my front teeth. I'm pretty sure Bugs Bunny would've been jealous, but as for me, I became severely self-conscious about my appearance, a malady that lasted all the way through junior high and well into my high-school years. I cannot say for sure that this was the primary factor that contributed to my social shyness, in particular with girls, but it did play a big part. In the end, maybe that was not a bad thing.

CHAPTER 2

Middlefield Avenue

Near the end of 7th grade, my parents had at long last reached sufficient financial stability that they decided we had "outgrown" our blessed little delta-track home on Del Rio Drive. Thus began the search to do what all good Americans did in the 60s and 70s. Upgrade. Whether it was buying a new car every three or four years, or getting the next larger and nicer home, conspicuous consumption was something that everybody took for granted ... I guess then, and still today.

Now, I cannot say my brother or I was too excited about this prospect. First, we would be leaving behind our beloved neighborhood and friends. The other fear was that of totally changing schools, or even school districts. As it turned out, though, our fears were unfounded. Mom and Dad found a home that remained in the same high-school and junior high-school zoning, and was even close enough that we could ride our bicycles back to the old neighborhood, assuming there might not be any "real" kids in our new environs.

The landmark moment of the move, though, was when our parents took Mark and me to check out the new house. It was ENORMOUS. Although it was not a "new" home, the previous owner was an architect and had added and modified the home extensively. My brother and I would still share a room, but it was probably four or five times larger than our tiny 8 × 8 we shared on Del Rio Drive. Our beds were so far apart we didn't even really need to talk to one another or acknowledge the other's existence. This was a perfect situation for two teen siblings. From that point on, we could not begin the moving process fast enough.

From my perspective, the timing of the move seemed a perfect fit with the natural flow of life, since I was no longer a grade-school kid. My shift toward adolescence and an expanding social environment fit right into the new neighborhood and a clique of new friends and experiences. I met and became friends with a lot of kids from school and the neighborhood, but the two who would have the greatest influence on my life were Steve Franklin (whom we normally just referred to as "Franklin") and my other friend Brad Koster (whom I always called Bradley, as his mother would often do).

Franklin and Bradley each held a different connection and importance in my life. Franklin lived directly across from our new home. As I remember, he came over just moments after we first arrived and, after introducing himself, invited me to ride our bikes to school together the next day. We became fast best friends from that day forward, and even in the ups and downs of teen relationships it would be quite a while before life events would intervene.

Franklin was my key to unlock the neighborhood dynamics and to help me quickly expand my social circles in a new tribe. This is how I met up with and became friends with Bradley, and Odis Smith and his brother Chester (who lived directly behind our fence line). Even with the expanding circle, however, for several years Franklin remained my closest friend and confidant.

Franklin was a different kind of kid. He was a towhead (blonde-haired) with bright blue eyes and an infectious smile. An only child to over-aged parents, Franklin reminded me of an adolescent version of the young (at that time) actor Jon Voight. Franklin was also a diabetic, and he had to watch his diet carefully and give himself daily insulin shots. I don't know if his medical condition created an awareness of a likely limited lifespan, but it seemed that Franklin was determined to take advantage of every day and live life to the fullest. He was a "boy on fire," sometimes literally.

I could probably write a novelette with all the "Franklin" stories I have, but I will boil it down to this—I can honestly say that Franklin was a kleptomaniac and a pyromaniac, but not in a publicly destructive way. He would steal things—*all* kinds of things—I think mostly just for the thrill of stealing them. Franklin once stole a full-size pellet rifle from a Montgomery Ward department store sporting goods section. He stuffed the rifle down his pants leg and sidestepped with a limp, ostensibly looking at the aisles of goods, until he made it to the door and was out of the store.

Franklin also loved anything that involved fire or explosives. He used to make his own smoke bombs and cherry bombs. Surprisingly, he never burned down his house. He did, however, destroy a bed full of linens when a homemade smoke cartridge prematurely ignited and turned itself into a mini-bomb, which exploded just as he threw it onto his bed and covered it with his bedding. His mother never did figure out what happened to his sheets and covers, since he covertly ditched them in the Smith Canal two blocks from our home.

Franklin also had a penchant for a new product line of refillable butane lighters and refill canisters, which he would steal from the corner drug store on a daily basis. This new obsession came much to the chagrin of his cat ... poor critter, who had the hair on one whole side of its body completely singed off when Franklin wanted to experiment (for a reason known only to him) to see if he could refill his lighter with butane while it was lit. The resulting ball of fire in Franklin's hands was tossed across the bedroom and happened to land right on top of his sleeping cat.

Mrs. Franklin had to wonder "why the cat's hair was singed off," to which Franklin convinced her "it had probably just got too close to the heater." Hah!

Finally, our trusting friend Odis was the victim of another Franklin experiment, in which he experimented to see if he could ignite butane sprayed onto Odis's t-shirt before it evaporated into the air. The first few attempts were unsuccessful, but by this time Odis's t-shirt was plainly dripping with the now-liquid vapors. Another attempt at ignition resulted in an inferno that burned Odis's eyelashes and eyebrows clean off of his face and singed the front part of his crew cut into tiny little balls of scorched hair.

As tight as we were, something happened with our friendship as we reached our junior and senior years of high school. Now, as I look back, I can only feel ashamed how it all went down. As cars became an ever-increasing influence in our lives, our circle of friends expanded with our new mobility. Another "friend" came into our group at this time and the dynamics created a negative influence in the older bonds of neighborhood friendship. Schisms soon surfaced. I don't want to name names or give any credible notoriety to this interloper, but it taught me an important lesson in life.

No-Name was the kind of kid who had to whip up resentment toward another member of the group in order to elevate himself to what he perceived as a higher ranking (or even to the "alpha" member of the group). His target was Franklin, and in just a few short months we all fell under No-Name's spell. Franklin was painfully ostracized from the very tribe that he had actually been responsible for cultivating.

I didn't recognize this until it was too late, and I am not even sure if Franklin recognized what was happening or why it happened, but it was an awkward neighborhood from this point forward. Franklin found a new set of friends and continued on with his life, but I am pretty sure the whole affair probably pushed him even farther toward the reckless life course that he chose to pursue. Once again, death would pass ominously close to my door.

Late in our senior year, a now-familiar dark vibe surrounded our once-peaceful quarters. Neighbors gathered whispering in doorways and on sidewalks, as the news broke first to Mr. and Mrs. Franklin and then to the rest of us. Steve had been driving back home from a trip into the nearby Sierra Nevada Mountains and, probably speeding as he was prone to do, lost control and slammed his small pickup truck into a large tree off the roadside. He was thrown from the vehicle and died instantly.

***

By the early 1970s, and even more so after high-school graduation, Bradley had become a much bigger influence in my life, and that "other kid" (No-Name troublemaker) just faded into local obscurity, as those types of trespassers are prone to do. The most important thing I can say about Bradley is that when I use the term "best friend" I reserve that solely for him.

Bradley was always the "big" kid on the block, and I mean that literally—he was, and still is, huge. Always a couple of fists taller than the rest of us, Bradley also carried a lot of extra weight. He could have easily taken on the role of neighborhood bully, but instead he was the protector, the confidant, and the one who was just a little more experienced and worldly than the rest of us. Bradley was one year older and one class ahead of us.

As my high-school years came to an end and I entered into junior (community) college, I once again moved through a whole new set of friends and experiences, with Bradley as my mentor. Compared to Bradley, and probably from his viewpoint, I had probably led a somewhat sheltered life. It seemed that Bradley was determined not to let me continue on that course and it was his job to bring me out of my shell and to "smell the roses."

I will always be grateful to Bradley for both taking me under his wing and, more important, for not allowing me to stray into the same path that he and our other friends would choose to hold on to. Bradley seemed to sense that there was something "bigger" waiting for me, a life that wasn't going to be found by hanging out in the "hood" or being a Stockton "homie." And even though we will always be close, I know Bradley understood at some point that he would have to let me go on my way.

I have fond memories of those years. Much later in life I would listen to a beautiful song by Neil Young, *Sugar Mountain*. In this song, Neil tells the poignant tale of moving from the innocence of youth to the wide-eyed world of semi-adulthood. It perfectly fits with my memories of this time in my own life.

***

While I progressed through the normal pangs of teenager angst, I somehow managed to stay connected with my father and our shared passion for planes and flying. Usually strapped into my companion Three-Eight Charlie, we continued to take frequent flights in the Super Cub together. I became more proficient at flying, as my father would informally instruct me in takeoffs and landings, stalls and flight characteristics, navigation, and communications. It was not long before my father could pretty much act solely as a passenger and safety observer and allow me to manage all the flight duties as a pilot.

There was something about flying that freed me from the normal trials and tribulations of teenhood, and over the years that emotion continued regardless of what type of plane I was flying or why I was doing it. To feel simultaneously you are the "master" of your destiny while also being intimately connected and enveloped by the aerial environment you navigate, to me flight has always been a very spiritual experience.

We would journey through most parts of northern California, sometimes just joy-flying, or taking the aero club airplanes to air shows and other events, with takeoffs and landings from controlled and uncontrolled airports, and some very small and challenging runways at times. It was all for the better for developing my flying skills. The times I loved the most would be when we would "contour fly" through the rolling foothills between the Central Valley and the Sierra Nevada Mountains, a casual course that was defined less by navigation and more by the natural topography that lay just below us. Each river valley, small knoll, or large oak tree acted as our guide, showing us to where to point the Super Cub next ... dipping, diving, hard turn, side-slip, and full-power climb.

On warm summer day flights, Dad would often open Three-Eight Charlie's clamshell-style side doors. These were not like the regular car-type door most small aircraft have, but two top/bottom half-doors hinged horizontally. They could actually be opened in-flight and the slipstream would allow them to float freely open. As we were strapped securely into our seats, there was no possibility of falling out of the plane, but the warm northern Californian air would flow through the cockpit, and it offered the feeling of riding in a convertible with the top down.

Once a year, in September, we would travel by car to Reno, Nevada, to experience the Reno Air Races. If you have never seen this unique American event, I would highly recommend you do it at least once in your lifetime. The highlight of the annual show and race are the World War II-era "unlimited" class of aircraft. These are P-51 Mustang, P-38 Lightning, F4U Corsair, and F-8F Bearcat fighters that have been super modified but still possess their original thoroughbred heritage. The sound and feel of these aircraft speeding by the grandstand at extremely low altitudes and full throttle is something that I cannot describe in words ... you just have to be there.

During my teen years I was not much of a "reader," but I had decided to sign up for a military book club. You know, one of those "get 10 books [or albums, or whatever] for free, but we will send you a new book every month and if you don't like it just send it back (or pay us)" deals. So I ended up with a rather large collection of military history books.

Most of the books I was interested in dealt with the air war of World War II—the planes, the pilots, and their adventures and stories. For some reason, I never saw myself as having what it would take to be a "fighter pilot," but I lived vicariously through their amazing stories: Gregory "Pappy" Boyington, Richard Bong, Adolf Galland, and Saburo Sakai, to name a few.

In 1995, while attending the "Gathering of Eagles" event where I was assigned at Air Command & Staff College in Montgomery, Alabama, I had the good fortune and honor to meet Saburo Sakai, one of the leading Japanese aces of the Pacific War. He was a diminutive gentleman, but in great shape and spirit for his age (although he would pass away only a few short years later). He did not look like the steely-eyed killer that his autobiographical book *Samurai* made him out to be. I learned later that after the war Sakai had become a Buddhist and had misgivings about war and all the men he had shot down in combat. It seemed a bit incongruous for a fighter pilot to be a Buddhist and pacifist ... at least it did for me at that time.

That night Sakai-*Sensei* signed my copy of his book *Samurai*, which I had read with great wonder and amazement as a teenager. I've since discarded most all of my old military history and flying books, but Saburo Sakai's *Samurai* is still one of my prized possessions.

***

When I turned 16, my parents had promised to buy me a car (used, of course) as they had done for my sister and my brother before me. The limit was one thousand dollars, but I could get whatever I wanted if I stayed within this amount.

Even though drag racing, muscle cars, and "cruising the Avenue" in downtown Stockton (as accurately depicted in John Lucas's defining film *American Graffiti*) was what kids my age aspired to, for some reason I always pictured myself driving a classic sports car like an Austin Healey or Triumph TR-4. Unfortunately, these cars were normally well out of the price range I was limited to. But, after patiently waiting several months after my 16th birthday, my father came home from work one day and told me he had seen a nice-looking Datsun (precursor to Nissan) sports car on a lot, and it looked like it might be affordable. Cool. We were off to take a look.

The Datsun Fairlady 2000 roadster was the predecessor to the famed Datsun/Nissan Z-cars (240-Z, etc.). Unlike the later hardtop Z-cars, these were true roadsters with a soft rag-top and lines similar to other classics like the MG or Triumph sports cars. When we went to the used car lot to check it out, it was love at first sight. The vehicle was actually priced above the "first car" limit my parents had imposed, but somehow my father had bargained the salesman down to get the exact price we needed, and the next thing I knew I was driving my roadster right off the lot.

I loved that car. It took me through high school, college, and after ... all the way to my first year in the Air Force. Being a sports car it did have "issues" and required frequent maintenance and a couple of engine rebuilds, but this provided me with technical and maintenance skills that I would use later in life.

***

When high-school graduation finally arrived, I had probably reached that same "burnout" point that most kids do. Some reach that point too soon and just drop out, but I felt that was never an option for me, nor even desirable. I knew I would go to college, somehow, somewhere. But for now I was just happy that high school was over. High school was not necessarily a "bad" experience, but for me it was not much more than a daily drone of classes, homework, and not all that much else. I did well academically, but I was undersized and pudgy, with those big-capped buckteeth, and no other uniquely identifiable talents like sports or music, or whatever.

The summer immediately after graduation I grew a full 6 inches and hit 6 feet tall, mutating out of my awkwardness, but it was too late to help me in my high-school years. So, I was not one of the "in" kids, but more like a "fringe" kid—not completely rejected or ignored, but just hanging on to the ropes like a geeky admirer at a movie premier watching the cool kids walk by. It just felt I was in some kind of "daze" through most of high school.

Graduation night did not hold much meaning for me, other than another event marker in my life. My parents and family attended the ceremony at the University of Pacific stadium (we had a huge graduating class); I received my diploma, and then I proceeded directly to Bradley's bungalow.

"Bradley's Home for Wayward Boys," as he called it, was the back room of their family home and formerly the dwelling of his estranged father until he had finally moved out. When Bradley graduated the year before me, he took over the room and converted it into the party/crash pad for himself and all of his friends. Bradley was the ever-present host and this is where we would go to hang out and, well, drink. We'd all chip in some money and one of our older friends would get us beer, cheap wine, or whatever we wanted to drink.

I had paid to attend the graduation-night events at our school, but I was not that interested in seeing or partying with people I felt I hardly knew, even after having spent most of the last three to six years of my life within the confines of the Amos Alonzo Stagg High and Daniel Webster Junior High classrooms. I really wanted to celebrate with those whom I now considered my friends, and at Bradley's. So, I proceeded to get pretty lit up.

At some point in the evening, I decided "what the hell" and drove to the high school, just to see what was up. I remember now just bits and pieces of that night. It was a fine party. They had some good bands playing and some good food to eat, but it felt like ... well, it was still high school and I wondered what I was even doing there.

I do remember that the last person I talked to before I left that campus for the final time was Kevin Britnall. Kevin was my earliest best friend in elementary school, all the way from Kindergarten to 6th grade. Kevin and I had drifted apart after leaving John Tyler Elementary, and even though we were in the same schools and occasionally same classes until graduation, it was not possible, for some reason, to stay as closely connected as we once had been. Things change. Kevin would later become a Christian minister, using his kind heart to help others. I do remember having a good visit with Kevin, as we reminisced a bit. I'm sure he could tell I was drunk, but he didn't seem to care. As our conversation slowly ran out of steam I knew instinctively "This is it ... it's time to go."

But I didn't really know where I was "going" ... figuratively of course. I knew I was done with high school. I had vague ideas of college and that somehow I wanted to be a commercial airline pilot someday, but I also remember a somewhat empty feeling—what was the purpose of all the effort and pain of growing up? I got into my roadster and drove myself to the levee.

Don McLean's classic song *America Pie* has an eternal significance for me. My "levee" was the fantasy island where I grew up and explored the "world." During our sophomore year, *American Pie* was *the* big hit and we probably heard it played at least 20 times a day on the AM radio as we rode around in Franklin's ancient Oldsmobile. The song spoke of a time of innocence that was suddenly gone in an instant ... "the day the music died." Google it if you don't know the back-story to *American Pie*, but that night I felt I was living that song, and I drove myself to the levee, but ... on this night the levee was definitely not dry.

I was back in the old Del Rio neighborhood, on the same road that had led me to so many summer adventures as a kid, running alongside the Calaveras Canal where we played seemingly without end, and where that other young boy had drowned. I remember driving my car that night with reckless abandon, faster and faster over the narrow levee road, taking more and more risk at each and every turn. The exhilaration and adrenaline flowed just as it had when I barreled down the Pleasant Hills pike on my cousin's faulty bicycle. I think I felt the need to prove to myself I had something to live for. At exactly that same instant I perceived the terrible mistake I was about to make ...

As I approached one of the final turns on the levee road before it ended, the car started to side slip off the pavement toward the steep dirt and rock embankment that led straight into the dark and silent waters of the Calaveras. I mentally saw myself in my car, flying over the embankment and into the waters ... and then somebody eventually fishing my body out the Calaveras with that giant fish hook I had heard described to my childhood horror ... and my grieving parents wondering how something like this could have happened.

And then, BANG! The tires gripped back into the pavement almost as if I had willed them to do so, or as if some giant invisible hand had stopped my sickening slide. The car and my heart caught themselves simultaneously and I down shifted and brought the roadster under control and came to a full stop.

The child was gone. It was time to go home and start my real life.

***

My "mission" that summer (as directed by my parents) was to go out and get a "real job." I had "worked" through much of my teen years, but only odd-job things like mowing lawns and helping Franklin and Bradley with their paper routes. I really had absolutely no idea of how to find a real job, and I spent the first week or two of the summer just as I had always done ... sleeping late, watching re-runs, eating late, and hanging out with friends (at Bradley's). I was therefore told in no uncertain terms that if I wanted to continue living at home, it was get-a-job or hit-the-road. I started looking in earnest.

Now if you are over the age of 18, I have to assume you have gone through the experience of finding your first "real" job. I don't know how many times I was asked if I had any experience. C'MON! I was only 18. What kind of experience could I possibly have that would qualify me for a job other than mowing a lawn? It came down to the point that I decided I would just lie about my "experience" when the next job opportunity that came up.

Bradley, the connoisseur of all of Stockton's fast-food joints (and there weren't too many), turned me onto the fact that they were just about finished building Stockton's second Jack-in-the-Box drive-thru restaurant, and there were job openings. Initially I thought I would have no chance versus the potentially hundreds of teenage applicants bound to show up, but this time I worked a little magic on my application.

I was actually already a reasonably accomplished cook at home. I frequently made my own lunches and meals and came up with "gourmet" experiments that more often than not came out pretty good. I knew how to cook, but I just had to convince my future employer that I could cover burgers and fries. The previous summer I had lived with my sister Joy and her husband John while they home-sat at his parents' house in Costa Mesa, California. I did help out with cooking and kitchen chores there, so I just stretched the truth a bit and on my application I reported I was a fry-cook at J.J.'s Bar & Grill in Costa Mesa (J.J. as in Joy and John's.) I got a call two days later from the Jack-in-the-Box manager, passed my interview and training, and was soon wearing the ugliest orange and yellow polyester uniform shirt and paper service cap. This was it! My first real job!

I don't think I ever worked so hard in my life. I ended that summer with the "graveyard" shift. That meant showing up at 10pm, and working until 7am. The unique thing about this particular Jack-in-the-Box at the time was that it stayed open 24 hours. Actually, back then, it was the only place to eat in Stockton that was open 24 hours. That meant, come around 2am when all the bars closed, we would get every hungry drunk and stoner in Stockton coming to our drive-thru (fortunately our front doors were locked after 11pm), ordering jumbo jacks, tacos, onion rings, or whatever. All this going on with only myself and one other worker, and we also had to clean the entire joint totally, including the grill and fryers.

As my friends partied at Bradley's all night, I would have to head off to "Jack's" and do battle with sloppy drunks and grease-covered tile floors. I can still remember getting my first minimum wage check and thinking, "I am not going to end up doing stuff like this the rest of my life."

At the end of summer, as I was about to start my first semester of junior college, I walked into my manager's office and told him I was going to quit. He was actually crestfallen. I was a good worker and he knew it, and he had actually recommended me to the headquarters as a candidate for their junior level managers school. He told me one day I could have my own Jack-in-the-Box. Oh, boy. Actually, the manager was a nice guy and I genuinely appreciated that he had given me my first opportunity at real work experience. But, the main thing it taught me is that I did not want to do THAT. I was focused now on my real goal, and college and flying was the path to take me there.

I do have to note one other quick story about my Jack-in-the-Box experience ... I invented the Jack-in-the-Box Super Taco. No brag, just fact. There was a rule at the restaurant that we had to pay for whatever we ate, except for condiments and anything that came out of the fryers. I have no idea why this rule applied, but I just assume they figured "how much fried food could any one person eat." You have to remember, however, the majority of the employees were 18–19 years old. We could eat a lot of fried food, and we had the complexions to show for it.

Well, the only things that they had on the menu that were deep fried were French fries (of coarse), onion rings, fish filet slabs, and ... tacos. I loved the Jack-in-the-Box tacos. They were the little frozen kind made of just a corn tortilla and some kind of spicy minced mystery meat filling. I grew up eating those things at home. To make one to order, we would add a triangular half-piece of American cheese and a squirt of hot sauce. But, being a true "gourmet," I thought this to be totally inadequate, so I would go to the condiment bar and add some shredded lettuce and sliced tomatoes and bingo! A real taco!

One day on break I was chomping down on a couple of my taco creations and the manager walked by and said, "That looks good, are those tacos?" I told him "Super Tacos." I am not kidding, but not less than six months after I quit the "Box," I see an advertisement on TV for Jack-in-the-Box's new product: The Super Taco. And it looks just like mine! I bet that manager got a big promotion for that one, and I never saw anything for it other than maybe a new zit on my nose.

***

As I started into classes at San Joaquin Delta College, I had decided that my goal was to attend San José State University (SJSU). I had heard that SJSU had a great Aeronautics program and it sounded like just what I was looking for. I also found a new job working as a tow-truck dispatcher for the Triple-A (AAA) auto club in California. My father had helped with this one, because he knew someone-who-knew-someone, and I wound up with the job. It was a great job because I could work around my class schedule, and often there was enough dead time in the office that I could also study while at work. Perfect. In fact, when I was ready to transfer to San José State, the Stockton AAA office was able to set me up with the same job in their Santa Clara office, which was close to where I would live while attending the university. It's funny how things can sometimes just line up for you.

Since I was still living at home while I worked and attended community college, I was able to save a lot of money that I would use later to help pay for my private pilot's license. Plus, I was still with my "homies" and hanging out at Bradley's, and experiencing many new facets of life, including new friends, new music, and, well, the 70s' drug culture.

This is something I am neither proud nor ashamed of, but it was a fact of life in California in the 60s and 70s that pretty much everybody my age either did drugs regularly or experimented with them to some extent. I was, in fact, one of the last holdouts among my buddies, but eventually I did try it and came to appreciate some of the finer characteristics of good pot. It was a beneficial experience from the standpoint that as I moved from home life to college life, I came to realize that pot, or drugs in general, were not going to create any real value in my life. I could see that the real danger of drugs was not that we would become crazed addicts, but our lives would somehow go on "hold" and we would stop making progress and probably never realize our full potential. This is what I saw among many of my friends who pretty much just "froze" in time ... never getting that education, or the better job, nor even leaving their old neighborhood. I had other plans, and when those plans and priorities rose to the top, I never smoked pot again. It was a good decision.

The other part of that period of my life I am still attached to was the expansion of my musical experience. Bradley and our new friends, the Johnson brothers (Roger and Steve), introduced me to the Bay Area rock scene and bands and artists I had never heard of before ... Lou Reed, Jeff Beck, Montrose, Savoy Brown, Blue Oyster Cult, the list goes on and on. Over were the days of AM radio pop trash. We would go on frequent journeys to Winterland in San Francisco, to see the great promoter Bill Graham's awesome lineups of frontline rock bands and artists. My musical horizons were forever expanded and to this day I remember some of my best times were spent with my friends at those Winterland shows in the city by the bay.

CHAPTER 3

SJSU

I left home for school in the Fall of 1976. Having a job in hand, I was actually able to find a small one-bedroom apartment in Santa Clara, California, close to the AAA office where I worked and easy driving distance to San José State University (SJSU).

I find it amazing nowadays that so many kids take out student loans or money from their parents to be able to make it through college. To me, it just seemed natural to work, go to school, and support myself at the same time ... and also take flying lessons! I started my flying lessons to get my private pilot's license fairly soon after I had settled in at SJSU. Even though I had flown extensively with my father, he was not a certified flight instructor (CFI) and none of that flying time accounted for anything except experience. But I was very grateful for that experience, because it shaved a great deal of time and money off of my flying course.

I still remember my first CFI. His name was Bob Dillon, not spelled like the artist Bob Dylan, he pointed out to me on our first meeting. He understood after our first flight that I was already good enough to qualify in the absolute minimum time. He did a great job getting me my private pilot's license in just 35 hours of flight time.

Bob and several other CFIs I flew with (such as my good friend Jim Garbett) were great mentors because we were all trying to do the same thing: earn enough flying time and experience to get the great golden ticket—a major airline job. This was the Holy Grail of civilian flying. It was not an easy path, but we all made steady progress in that direction. Some made it, others fell by the wayside, and some, like me, found another calling.

SJSU and the Aeronautics Department I attended were great places to learn and still enjoy life and living. Even though I worked and studied hard, I can honestly say I had a blast in college. It was really where I first started to learn about myself and what I could achieve.

As I was finishing up my degree, I moved from my dispatcher position at AAA to working as an actual tow-truck driver for one of the contract service providers: Murray's Towing, in Santa Clara. Another great job and more invaluable experience. Driving a tow truck was like being a one-man problem-solving white knight. Pretty much everyone who watched you drive up was really happy to see you (of course, since they were generally broken down). We did not do "Repo's" or tow-aways, only emergency road service. Although many service calls were for routine dead batteries, etc., some events required ingenuity and determination to resolve. It wasn't "rocket science," but really it was one of the most gratifying jobs I have ever done.

What I anticipated was that, because I was making such good money driving tow truck, after graduation I would continue to do that job while I progressed with my flying credentials and compiled much needed flight time. That was the plan anyway, until another series of events changed the course of my life.

***

After my "official" graduation, I needed to spend some time in the Aeronautics Department during the summer to finish an extracurricular part of my degree, and that was an FAA Airframe & Powerplant (A&P) mechanics license. I had completed all the coursework as part of my degree, but still needed to complete the Practical (hands-on) portion of the licensing process. That meant some extra hours and days working with some of the professors on a project and also with the department chair, Dr. Thomas E. Leonard.

Dr. Leonard, or "T.E.L." as some staff called him, had actually gone to college with my father, so they knew each other pretty well. And, strangely enough, I was attending the SJSU Aeronautics course with Dr. Leonard's son, Rob. So we had a somewhat connected relationship during my years there. Early that summer, Dr. Leonard asked me into his office, and I just assumed it was to shoot-the-breeze and ask how my Dad was doing, or what my goals were for the future, etc., etc. To my great surprise, he offered me a job to teach one of the lower-division Aeronautics courses. I was astounded! T.E.L. wanted me to be a lecturer-instructor (I didn't have the qualifications or experience to be a true "professor") for the Aircraft Production Processes (AERO 25/26) class, which was a combination lecture/lab course to teach young aviators and mechanics the processes and tools for building and repairing aircraft. Every student had to take that course, and I would actually be the "Lead" full-time instructor, teaching three courses a semester while I had some experienced part-time instructors assisting me.

I was the LEAD instructor! Holy crap!

After saying "YES," of course, I came to realize (as did Dr. Leonard) that this was only going to be a temporary opportunity while I continued my pursuit of an airline "ticket" (i.e., wings), but still, I was going to make the most of it. The other thing I quickly realized was that I was going to be making less money as a university instructor than what I was making driving a tow truck. Oh, well.

To this day, I view that position at SJSU as one of the most important landmarks of my life. It was an opportunity that opened the way for most of the successes I would have throughout the rest of my career. It was not just the prestige of being offered something like that at such a young age (and without the aforementioned "experience" requirement), but the fact that somebody trusted me enough to think I could do it, especially when I had serious doubts myself about whether I could perform as a "teacher" of students who were basically my peers a few months prior.

Over the summer I learned the coursework, made up lecture outlines, practiced on the machine tools and tasks the course required, and got a lot of help from the other course instructors and professors who had been doing this for a while. When the Fall semester rolled around, I felt like I was pretty well prepared. I quickly found out I wasn't.

My early lectures were long-winded and disjointed. I had no practical experience not only in teaching, but even speaking in front of large groups of people. And not just people, but students who were counting on me to explain what they needed to know to pass the course and to use the knowledge and skills for later coursework. It was the first time in my life in which somebody else was really depending on me.

I pitied the poor Monday–Wednesday morning group of students that year, who always had to get the first go-around of my lecture or machine-tool demonstrations. By time I got around to the Tue–Thu afternoon group, it was the third time covering the same material and I found myself starting to get the hang of it. Somehow though, both my students and I made it through the first semester, then the next, and a couple more after that. I got better, and my students got better too. I improved not just because of the repetition and experience over the two years I was at SJSU, but because the students actually taught me how to become a better teacher.

This is one of the greatest experiences that I carried with me. By trying to find a way to connect with each individual student, and to figure out the best learning strategies for them, it totally expanded my self-awareness of my own talents or, more important, my own limitations and how to overcome them. The path to success in life was suddenly illuminated. I will be forever grateful to T.E.L. (Dr. Leonard) for the precious gem of an opportunity he placed in my hands, and my only hope is that I did not let him down.

And then ... I got married.

***

I wasn't really sure if I should talk about this, because it involves a close relationship with another person who has not been in my life for almost 30 years (as of the writing of the book), but I figure if I am going to chronicle significant events in my life it would be disingenuous to leave this one out.

Her name was Geri. We dated through most of our years together as students at SJSU, and our marriage coincided with the same year as my graduation and shortly after I started my instructor position at the Aeronautics Department. Everything seemed fine during our courtship, but no more than 48 hours after our wedding it all came crashing down. At the time I could not really figure out why things changed so much just because of a piece of paper that said we were married.

Years later I could begin to understand that I was just never able fulfill whatever it was she envisioned a husband to be. Maybe call it "buyer's remorse" on her part? Whatever it was, Geri seemed to be dependent on me to make her happy and unfortunately, I just was not able to deliver on that. Still, Geri was there in my life for five more years and would be my shadow through the next portion of this dialogue. While the marriage weathered many rough roads, Geri was very supportive in my decision to join the Air Force and through my training and into my first assignment.

But the most important thing I will always be grateful for is that Geri actually "introduced" me to my second wife, Sako, whom I have been happily married to for more than 30 years. It's a long story and I will find the time and place later in this book to bring it up again.

***

December 31, 1981; San Jose, California. It was New Year's Eve, and I had been invited to a party at the apartment of one of my former students. I had some trepidation about attending because I felt a little out of place and figured I might not know a lot of people. Yet if I had not gone to that party, that night, I would not be telling this story right now.

I was actually just walking through the front door of the apartment, where the party was already rolling, and as I entered the open doorway I came face-to-face with a fellow SJSU graduate and classmate, Mike Heddon. I had not seen Mike in almost two years since our graduation. At that time Mike and I would be what I considered as typical California "hippies." Not like the "real" hippies of the 60s, but just kids who had grown up in the 60s and still carried the hippie tradition of long hair and scraggly facial hair, and to some extent the dress. But we were just suburban spin-offs of the original, kind of like a bad sitcom sequel.

Like myself and many of our classmates, Mike was also focused on that far-away dream of becoming a commercial airline pilot, but facing the reality of a long, hard road to get there. Nearing graduation time, Mike had told me he was planning to join the Air Force and get flying time and experience that way and then move on to the airlines. I think I was surprised by Mike's strategy because like myself, I thought Mike had absolutely no desire to enter such a bizarre and foreign path like joining "the military" to reach this goal. Besides, he would have to cut off his long hippie hair.

As it turned out, Mike did not join the Air Force right after graduation. He would relate to me later that he actually got all the way to the enlistment center in Oakland, California, and just before he was going to take the oath to enter service he had to sign the final paperwork for enlistment. He couldn't do it. He just said "sorry" and walked away. Afterwards, Mike had actually found a job working for a company that manufactured small piston engines for light aircraft, Lycoming, I think. The last I had heard from Mike was that he was still in that job and I assumed he still had long (or at least longish) hair and was still aspiring to the airline business.

On this New Year's Eve night, quite to my amazement, when I ran into Mike he had really short hair! A military style cut, it seemed to me. After the usual greetings of old friends surprised to bump into each other, I asked Mike "Why the short hair?" and if he was still working for the engine company. To my shock, he said, "No, after about a year I decided go back and join the Air Force after all. I just finished Officer Training School [OTS] and I'm on my way to pilot training." I was flabbergasted, but also intrigued. Why would a guy that I thought was so much like myself really be interested in the military, even if it included flying?

Over the course of the next 20 or 30 minutes, Mike told me everything he could about OTS, the Air Force, and his expectations for pilot training and what he would be doing after that. He was really excited, and as he talked to me I was getting excited for him, and then something just clicked in my brain and the idea of joining the Air Force no longer seemed far-fetched at all.

That small amount of time was about all we had together that night; Mike was actually on his way out of the party as I was walking in. I would not see nor talk to Mike Heddon again for a couple of years, and when we did meet again Mike was flying KC-10s for the Air Force. (The KC-10 is an air refueling tanker version of the commercial DC-10 airliner.) It was a perfect fit to set Mike up to achieve his airline goal, which he would pursue after about eight years flying for the Air Force. He made it to the "show."

When I think back to that night, if I hadn't gone to the party, or if I'd arrived even five minutes later, I would have missed Mike. Funny how such a chance meeting, which may never have occurred if some small life event had changed my arrival time, would actually shape the course of a life.

CHAPTER 4

OTS and Chandler

From that auspicious New Year in 1982, the idea of trying out for the military quickly took root and started to grow like corn on a sunny California day. In fact, in the early spring as I was driving down Stevens Creek Blvd in Santa Clara, I passed by a military recruiting office. Instead of just driving by as I usually did, this time I pulled over, parked my roadster, and walked into the Air Force office.

I still remember this episode very clearly. As I walked in, there were two enlisted airmen at their desks. They were both sergeants, probably staff or tech sergeants, but at this point they could have been four-star generals and I would not have known. As I walked in the door, one of the sergeants asked if he could help me and I told him, "Yes, I would like to find out what it would take to go to pilot training?" Now, I have to remind you I was still carrying my California hippie persona, my hair was rather long (almost shoulder length), and I had a full beard. The sergeants just looked at each other and did their best to hide their smirks, but I got a rather clear feeling they were saying with their eyes "Yeah, right! Pilot training? You gotta be kidding me."

Well, they started off by explaining that I would first have to be selected for Officer Training School (OTS) and that would take a bachelor's degree. "Got one of those," I said. Then they explained how hard it is to be selected for pilot training, but I may want to apply for other positions too. "Not interested. Only pilot training." Then one sergeant asked why I thought I might be able to be a pilot in the Air Force. At that point, I pulled out all of my FAA flying licenses and ratings and laid them on his desk. The sergeant opened a drawer, pulled out some papers and (with a big smile on his face) said, "Well then, let's get started."

I don't think I had even really discussed the idea of joining the military with Geri. It had always been an option, but it was one she knew pretty well that I did not really want to pursue. That same evening, when I got back to our apartment, I told Geri, "Guess what I did today?" Actually, she was good with it all. We were not exactly going anywhere fast on the road we were on, and I think she liked the idea of the "adventure" of a military lifestyle. Whatever that was.

From there things started to move pretty fast. I told Dr. Leonard that I would not be coming back to teach the Fall semester at the Aero Department. I owed him a lot, but he was also really excited for me and for my new opportunity. The rest of the spring involved lots of paperwork, tests, medical exams, and all the other things involved in joining the military. I did well on all of them, and most importantly I had no medical issues that would keep me out of pilot training.

The last thing I did was go to my long-time hair stylist and have her chop off all my hair and get it as close to a military cut that she could. She almost refused to do it and I had to keep telling her "shorter ... shorter," but she finally did it. Then it was off to Lackland Annex, San Antonio, Texas and OTS.

I had no idea what I was getting myself into.

***

I don't remember much about the trip to OTS and Lackland Annex, except it was late summer and we arrived on an Air Force bus from the San Antonio International Airport some time (it seemed) in the middle of the night. As we stepped off the bus I can remember there was something "different" about Texas. It was the humidity. Growing up in northern California I had never experienced, felt, smelled, nor tasted humidity before, but for me it had all the characteristics of something bad. I would never get used to it.

Arrival was not really like the classic scenes from boot camp, where you step off the bus and people are yelling at you, but it was very military-like. We were ordered what to do, which was basically get bed linens, get to our rooms, get some sleep, and report in front of our barracks at 0600 ("oh-six hundred," or 6am). Oh six ... whaaa?

For some reason, and much to my surprise, I acclimated quickly to OTS. I am still not really sure why, especially when I started seeing fellow classmates take SIE—Self-Induced Elimination (i.e., quit). They were dropping like flies. Even some guys that had coveted pilot training slots were calling it quits after a few days.

I could not understand why, but I came to realize that a lot of these people were fresh out of college. Maybe some of them had never really held a job or been on their own. Maybe they lived at home all this time and Mom was taking care of them. I don't know for sure, but they sure could not seem to handle the intense (but basic) routines we had to follow every day. I believe my experiences and about three or four years "extra" maturity helped a lot. Oh yeah, I forgot to mention that I had entered the Air Force just under the age limit for starting pilot training, which was 27. Most of these OTs ("Oh-Tees"; Officer Trainees) were 22–24 years old.

OTS was (I surmised) like a condensed version of a military service school, in this case, the Air Force Academy. AF Academy cadets attend for four years. We had 12 weeks (they called us "90-day Wonders"), and every three weeks we moved up to the next class status. The first three weeks were like our "freshman" year, with

"Plebes" status, and we were treated pretty much with no dignity. But just three weeks later we were "Underclassmen," and so on. So if you could make it through the first three weeks, things improved pretty quickly thereafter.

It was not easy by any means, but I much preferred the 12-week version than thinking of doing this stuff for four years. And, after three or four weeks I really started to feel like I was part of something special, something bigger than myself or my own personal ambitions. I truly bought into the idea of being an Air Force officer and part of this organization. I also liked a lot of the people I was getting to know and the officers who were leading and teaching us.

We were assigned to "flights"—an Air Force term that probably relates to a platoon in the Army. The flights were co-ed and made up of about 12–15 people with different backgrounds, goals, jobs, and abilities. We had to work together and help each other. That was evident from the start and was true all the way to the end. But our flight? We were a strange bunch. A bunch of "Misfits" it seemed. Not a single one of us stood out individually. Throughout the class there would be individual and flight awards handed out on a regular basis, but The Misfits never won any. It was not for lack of trying, but we eventually accepted our fate, that we were just below-average OTs. Then a strange thing happened one day when we went to the Confidence Course.

The best way I can describe the Confidence Course is like the event challenges you see on the reality show *Survivor*, where an obstacle or task has to be conquered in a team format. At the start I think everybody in our flight of Misfits expected that it was going to be a physically and mentally demanding struggle that would end mostly in failure, but as it turned out, we nailed it! Every single event required intuitive strategy, teamwork, and knowing each other's strengths and weaknesses. We already knew none of us had any strong attributes, but we were also well aware of our weaknesses and somehow that become our strength. As we found a way to complete one demanding event after another (and they became more difficult as we progressed), we ended up becoming increasingly confident in our collective ability. In the end, we were the only flight in the class to complete every single event successfully. We surprised even our flight commander (the "real" officer in charge of The Misfits), and ourselves. The stamp of "teamwork" had been imprinted in our minds. We now knew that for the rest of the class and on into our Air Force careers we would create greater success by working together with a common goal.

Early on in the class one of my flight mates, who was actually a prior enlisted sergeant who had been selected to attend OTS, turned to me in formation one day and asked, "Which one of these guys you think isn't going to make it?" I didn't have to think too long and I told him "Lesneski." He said "Yeah, me too." Lesneski was a character. A classic! A really nice guy, but somebody who just did not seem to fit the idea, or mold (if there was one), of an Air Force officer. He was always a bit unkempt and disheveled. I am sure he took a shower every day, but he always looked like a sweaty mess. And Lesneski would fidget. He would fidget *all* the time. Not a great attribute when you are supposed to be in formation standing at attention.

Lesneski was always being called out by our flight commander. One day, while standing at attention in formation after going through some marching drills, Lesneski started one of his fidgeting fits and our lieutenant could not take it any more. He ran straight up to his face and with spittle flying out of his mouth screamed: "LESNESKI! WHAT ARE YOU DOING?!" To which Lesneski calmly replied, "I got a bug in my ear ... Sir." That was it. The formation broke out in laughter and the LT ("Ell-Tee"; lieutenant) could barely hold back his own snickers while he admonished Lesneski to "just stand at attention the next time and let the bug do whatever it wants to do."

Another time we were marching as a flight down the sidewalk on a long hill from our classrooms to our barracks, when somebody stepped on the heel of somebody else's black corfam service dress shoe. The heel broke loose from the shoe and then was accidently kicked by another marcher; it went sliding out into the middle of the road. Upon seeing this Lesneski broke ranks, went running out into the road in front of an oncoming car, and booted that corfam heel as far as he could. The car that almost hit Lesneski came to a screeching halt, and out popped the meanest LT flight commander on the base (nobody liked this guy, not even the other flight commanders). While the rest of us stood there in shock, the rabid LT ran up to Lesneski and beet red, with veins popping out, screamed, "O.T.! WHAT ARE YOU DOING?!" To which Lesneski honestly replied, "I don't know, Sir. I saw that heel out in the road and it looked like a hockey puck. I couldn't help it. I had to go kick it." Expecting a possible execution on the spot, all of us were amazed when the LT just looked at Lesneski in wonder and said, "Well.... GO PICK IT UP!" And that was it. The LT got in his car and drove off, and we continued our march to the barracks. We all felt pretty good about that. Lesneski earned some "hero" points that day for surviving the wrath of the militant LT, and for giving us a great laugh in the process. Plus we were all going to the Officer Training School Open Mess (OTSOM) that night to party and to get blotto. The OTSOM was the annex "club" that the OTs could go to on Friday and Saturday nights once we reached upper class level (the last six weeks) ... and we did, and there was much drinking and rejoicing there. Good times.

Soon OTS was coming to an end. We lost a few more friends along the way who could not hack the program, but surprisingly Lesneski made it. He actually made it *all* the way through, and passed his final tests and requirements. And then ... he quit! Yep. Lesneski came to us the last week before graduation and told the flight he was leaving OTS and would give up his opportunity for commission. We all told him he was crazy after all he had gone through and was only a week away from graduation. Lesneski explained he was supposed to enter the service as an electrical engineer, but they wanted to make him a civil engineer. He said he told them he didn't enter the military to "fix peoples' toilets," so they let him quit.

OTS was a great experience, but I was glad it was over. I was ready to experience the "Real Air Force." That's what all the prior-enlisted and our officer leaders called it. I didn't know what that meant, but it sounded somehow better. And I knew it included pilot training and beyond. I was going to be back in the air and flying again soon. And not just flying, but flying jets!

***

I had about a month of free time when I returned home to Santa Clara. Geri and I went about packing up and cleaning out things for our Permanent Change of Station (PCS) move. It would be the first of many PCS, at least for me.

All in all, it went pretty smoothly, and for never having lived a full day of my life out of California (except for the OTS stint) we soon found ourselves comfortably settled into a single-family military tract home on Williams AFB, Chandler, Arizona. The home was surprisingly cozy for a young couple with no children, and we had several other couples who would be part of our Undergraduate Pilot Training (UPT) class living in our neighborhood. The adaptation to military lifestyle was nearly complete.

It was not much more than a week later that our UPT class started and from there things got pretty busy, and fun. The first few weeks were spent in prep courses focused on getting us ready to fly our initial sorties in the Cessna T-37 "Tweet." The subjects included: flight physiology, which taught us about the hazards and precautions necessary for high-altitude flying; parachute landing training, in the event we should ever have to bail out of our aircraft; academics on basic flight principles; and the aircraft systems and procedures we needed to know just to start the thing up, never mind fly it. It seemed like these classes took forever to complete, but at the end we were split up into two separate flights, assigned a primary flight instructor pilot (IP), and walked out for our "dollar ride."

The dollar ride was so-called because, as tradition went, if you successfully made it through (hopefully without puking all over your IP) you were supposed to give him or her a dollar for the privilege of receiving your first flight. My assigned IP was Capt Bob Nunley and we had a good time on the flight. I didn't puke, but I have to admit it was one of the only times in my life I felt the tinges of air sickness. It was probably because Bob had the "stick" (was flying the airplane) most of time, and being a not-so-good passenger I was pretty much holding on while he put the nimble little turbojet through its paces with lots of aerobatic maneuvers.

Bob knew I had lots of previous flight time and already knew how to fly, so he also gave me some "stick time" and allowed me to perform some touch-n-go landings. The T-37 was easy to fly, handling very much like the light aircraft I flew previously, but obviously much faster and able to handle high "G" load aerobatics.

Many of the UPT students in my class had virtually no flight experience. We were mostly a class of previous civilians who had gone through OTS or recent college grads who had been Reserve Officers' Training Corps (ROTC) cadets. The average student had maybe 20–40 hours of flight time that they either paid for on their own, or they had gone through an initial training program at a little airfield called Hondo Field, where they flew with crusty old civilian IPs in traditional propeller-driven Cessna 172s, to teach them the absolute minimum-level skills they would need to continue on to UPT.

For these students, the first weeks of initial training in the T-37 were a huge challenge, and very quickly some of our new friends started to "bust out" of the program. Sometimes it was for airsickness that they just could not overcome, or they could not keep up with the pace of training and achieve the required proficiency levels. The program is intended to train the best pilots in the world, so of course it had to be difficult.

For me, it felt great and quite natural to be back in the air again. Central Arizona had beautiful flying weather and gorgeous landscapes of tan desert and rough painted mountains. The mornings and sunsets were most striking, and even the dry blazing heat of summer was a welcome break from the San Antonio mugginess. Every day I looked forward to walking into the flight room, regardless of how early we had to get up, and find out what the day would bring in the way of flying or ground training.

In our class there were a handful of students, who like myself, had a fair amount of flying time from civilian training. A few were already Air Force officers who were navigators or weapon system officers (WSOs) in fighter aircraft. For us, the T-37 program posed few challenges. Mostly we just looked forward to the flying time, to twist and turn through aerobatics and spin-recovery training, and challenging our IPs to who could land closest to a designated spot on the runway. The prize was a Coke from the loser.

The IPs liked to pull pranks on the students and they were usually pretty good about singling out the most gullible candidates (actually that was most all of us). Most of the pranks were traditions handed down from other IPs and performed whenever possible on all of the classes that came through UPT.

Fortunately, sometimes scuttlebutt would get out to the students to be on the lookout for certain kinds of pranks, but occasionally the IPs would catch somebody unawares and a good story would be told in the early-morning flight briefs. One such event happened to one of my flight mates, 2Lt Whipple (real name ... not kidding).

One day Lt Whipple was assigned to accompany an IP out to the Runway Supervisory Unit (RSU). The RSU was a small, trailer-like hut that sat out by the approach end of the runway. At that time, they were used Air Force-wide as a safety backup, containing an observer who watched as aircraft landed to make sure their landing gear were all down, or that there were not any other observed malfunctions or wrong configurations with the aircraft that might result in a dangerous takeoff or landing. At UPT bases, the RSU was also used to observe and grade student landings, and to warn students if their approach was dangerous and if they should "go-around" and attempt it again. For this reason, there were usually one or two IPs in the RSU plus a student, who was mostly there as a "secretary" of sorts to write down notes for the IP. If you were really lucky, you might get to shoot off a "warning flare" from the flare guns mounted in the RSU.

And here is how the story of Lt Whipple's RSU tour was related to us. On this particular day, a call came into the RSU from the real control tower, which was a good distance away across the two parallel runways. The IP answered the phone, and after a short conversation and a final "Yes, Sir," handed the phone over to Lt Whipple. "Lt Whipple, this is Capt So-'n'-So up in the tower and we need to do a light gun check. Have you ever done one before?" to which Whipple answered, "No, Sir." "Well, OK, it's pretty easy so I will explain it to you," the tower voice replied.

The device called a "light gun" actually exists in all airport control towers worldwide. They are hand-held spotlights that a project different colored lights that can be seen by pilots on or around the airfield. They are intended for use when radio communication is not available between the tower and the pilot (for whatever reason). A red light means "Stop," green is "Proceed, or OK/approved," white is "Standby," and a few other combinations of those.

The tower caller continued, "Lt Whipple, I want you to go outside the RSU and look at the tower and when I flash a red light put up your right arm. Red for right, OK? Green light is left arm. Yellow light is left leg, and white light is right leg. You got all that?" Lt Whipple replied "Yes, Sir!" and ran out of the RSU into the middle of the field between two active runways for all the world to see.

If you think about this without the benefit of hindsight or scuttlebutt, you might just wonder why the guy in the tower wouldn't just ask the IP on the phone to tell him verbally what lights he could see while they were talking on the phone. But that just would not have been quite as much fun. In short order, Lt Whipple's right arm flew up into the air ... then back down. Then his left arm went up and back down. Then left and right legs ... and then ... you probably get the picture. Pretty soon Whipple was doing an awkward series of uncoordinated jumping jacks to the rapid-fire light gun test.

Upon re-entering the RSU, the barely composed IP told him, "Lt Whipple, the tower called and they wanted me to let you know that light gun test was best-seen-to-date." Lt Whipple left his RSU tour for the day with a sense of pride, until the next morning's roll-call and flight briefing and that IP's story-of-the-day offering.

For those who made it through the T-37 phase of training, the likelihood of "washing out" no longer lingered over the class. It did happen on occasion, but at this point the survival of the fittest had weeded out anybody that would likely have any big problems in the next phase, flying the T-38 Talon.

The T-38 was a whole other story. It was truly a *jet*. While the T-37 did have jet engines, they were embedded in an airframe that was more traditional, with straight fat wings and a short stubby body. For a jet it could not go that fast, normally around 200–300 KIAS (knots indicated airspeed, or about 230–350mph). The T-38, on the other hand, was a true supersonic jet, capable of a maximum speed of Mach 1.3 (or 1.3 times the speed of sound), but normally flown at typical fighter jet cruise speeds of 400–600 KIAS (741–1,111mph). And it looked fast—very sleek, tapered, with small swept-back wings and tail.

The T-38 was actually designed and produced back in the 1950s to train the first supersonic jet pilots in the famed Century-series fighters such as the F-100, F-102, F-104, F-105, etc. These were big, fast, and dangerous airplanes that killed a lot of both experienced and inexperienced pilots along the way. The T-38 was intended to build the skills (or weed out those that didn't have them) before pilots were assigned to the Century fighters.

So, the T-38 was a handful for anybody in pilot training. It really evened out the playing field at this point because, except for maybe the former fighter WSOs (back-seaters) in our class, nobody had ever flown anything like this. It flew and handled smoothly, but because of its speed it was easy to "get behind" the jet and not be prepared for, or thinking about, what was coming next. Also, because of its small wing and control surfaces, it could be very dangerous in the critical phases of takeoff, and most especially landing. The stall speeds were very high and the stall characteristics were not always predictable. This meant that the margin for error during the landing phase was limited, just like it was in those fast Century-series fighters it was designed to replicate.

The first month told the difference. I did in fact struggle in a couple of phases early on, but with good instruction from my IP, Capt Ken Dressell, I quickly caught on and surged back to the top of my class. A few of the others with previous flight experience fell back and never recovered, and a few who had struggled with the T-37 now gained confidence and passed them up. In the end, we were all just trying to complete the course and graduate, but for many of us we also wanted to graduate at the top of the class, or DG (Distinguished Graduate—Top 10%). The reason for this is that the DGs normally received the first or second choice of what type of aircraft they wanted to fly after graduation (and maybe even base location). It was going to have a big impact on our flying careers and the fulfillment of our desires. The IPs also stratified our abilities status in the class as "Fighter Qualified," "Instructor Qualified," or "Heavy Qualified." Fighter Qualified generally meant you were in the upper 30–40% of the class and could be trusted right away to fly alone as the single pilot-in-command of a high-performance fighter aircraft. Fighter Qualified students were also Instructor Qualified, which meant you were good enough to be selected to come back to UPT and be an instructor to new classes of students, just as some of our IPs had done. All students who graduated were Heavy Qualified, which generally meant they would fly first as co-pilots on large transport, tanker, and bomber aircraft, where they could build flight time and experience and eventually take over command pilot duties.

For me, originally I wanted to fly a "heavy" type aircraft to prepare myself for an eventual airline career, much as my friend Mike Heddon had accomplished. But, somewhere even before UPT, probably while at OTS, I had changed my mind. Going back to my childhood fascination with World War II fighter aircraft, I thought, "Why not fly fighters?"

While I was in T-37 training one day, my IP, Bob Nunley, asked me what I wanted to fly and I quickly fired back "F-111." Bob got kind of a sour look on his face and said, "Noooo ... you don't really want to fly that." I grew up in the 1960s and the General Dynamics F-111 "Aardvark" was one of the few "fighters" I knew about. It was better known as Secretary of Defense Robert McNamara's "failure," because he had tried to force all the services to design a single modern fighter to replace all others. "What transpired instead was a plane that was not really an air combat fighter at all, and wasn't much good at anything but going really fast, and really low, and dropping bombs. And that is what it became, and the only service to actually buy any was the Air Force.

There were, however, some brand-new Air Force fighters that were just coming into service. I had only recently begun to hear and read about them: the single-engine General Dynamics F-16 Fighting Falcon and the twin-engine/twin-tail McDonnell Douglas (now Boeing) F-15 Eagle. Bob Nunley loved the Eagle. It was his dream to fly the F-15 once he finished his IP tour at Williams. And he wanted me to fly the Eagle too; he thought I had the ability to get that opportunity. We would go back-and-forth on occasion about this, and I would hold fast to my guns and tell him I was determined to fly the "One-Eleven." He would often bring photos and other information about the Eagle and leave it around for me to see, but without much apparent impact, although I was starting to take a liking to the looks of the Eagle. It certainly looked like a fighter.

Then, one day, Bob finally found a way to convince me to capitulate.

We were flying together on a cross-country flight from Williams AFB to Peterson Field in Colorado. The cross-country was a navigation exercise, and it included a couple of separate "legs" (routes) to practice navigation procedures. One of the legs took us through New Mexico. With a map strapped to my leg to monitor our progress and verify our location visually, Capt Nunley asked me, "Where are we now?" I looked at the map, checked my instruments, and then rolled the wing over to look down at the ground. I said, "Looks like we are over Cannon Air Force Base." Bob said, "That's right, we are. And what do you see down there?"

"Mmm ... I see a runway ... and a few buildings ... and not much else." (It's barren high desert around Cannon). To which Bob replied, "That's right! That is Clovis, New Mexico. And Cannon is an F-111 base and that's probably where you will be assigned if you take a -111." That was enough for me. From that point on I had my sights set on an F-15 Eagle.

I did have competition to get that Eagle, and in my flight one of my primary competitors was somebody with whom I had also become pretty good friends—Larry Pitts. Larry had previous civilian flight time like me and an added bonus of having flown helicopters for the US Army for a while. So Larry and I were considered odds-on favorites to get the DG awards and our first choice. I assumed that Larry was going to seek an F-15 too, so I settled my expectations on the possibility of an F-16 if things just did not work out. In the end though, Larry decided he actually wanted to stay in the Phoenix area for family reasons and the best way to do that was to ask to remain as a UPT instructor. That was a no-brainer for the school because they wanted the best-quality instructors they could get to stay there ... for me, it opened the door for my Eagle.

***

Although there are a great many anecdotes from UPT, there is one story in particular I need to tell of our time at pilot training. This occurred during the final phases of T-38 training as we moved toward graduation.

There was a "war story" many of the IPs told of a young student pilot who had been killed when he crashed his T-38 at night into the Superstition Mountains, just east of Phoenix. The story was recounted as a precautionary tale of what "not to do," especially when flying at night or in adverse weather on flight instruments without sight of the ground or terrain. As the story goes, just a few years prior during a night-phase training sortie, the student pilot was flying his T-38 at a relatively low but safe altitude near the base, practicing his night landing approaches. While under radar approach control, he would listen to instructions from the ground controller on when to turn and what altitude to fly, and when to start his approach. On this night, the ground controller apparently either forgot to tell him to climb to a higher altitude or forgot to turn the T-38 from an easterly heading to a southerly track back toward Williams AFB.

Flying at night, without the ability to see the rising terrain clearly and without heeding minimum safe altitudes for that area, the young student pilot slammed his T-38 straight into the side of one of the higher peaks in the Superstition range. He was killed instantly. The story made an impact on us, and during weather and night missions I always made sure I knew what the minimum safe altitudes were wherever I was flying.

While an IP was telling us this story one day he turned to another IP and said, "Hey, didn't you go up to the accident site during the crash investigation?" The other IP said, "Yeah, and I could tell you how to find it." For me and a couple of my good friends, it was all we needed to hear to start a weekend adventure. We wanted to find the crash site.

We planned to make it a day trip. Go to the Lost Dutchman State Park and follow the trail (and the IP's "detailed" instructions) up into the Superstition Mountains, find the crash site, maybe pick up a souvenir of a small aircraft part to prove we were there, then head on home to our wives. That was the plan, anyway.

The Superstitions (as the mountain range is often called) and the Lost Dutchman Mine are part of western folklore and each has its own mystique and legend. The Superstitions are not extremely high peaks, but the terrain is rather rugged and some trails are not for inexperienced hikers ... such as us. On the trip were myself and four of my UPT class buddies: Darwin Frevert, Gordon (Kuch) Kucera, Kurt Skadeland, and Mark Catherman.

Kurt Skadeland drove that day. We entered into the Lost Dutchman State Park late morning and found the trailhead at the foot of the mountains, just as it had been described to us (that was a good sign). Kurt parked the car, we all got out, and we started up a very shallow grade that made this adventure seem deceptively easy. Nobody was truly dressed for occasion, it should be mentioned. I think I came the best prepared with a pair of strong brown leather high-top boots that had decent lug soles for climbing and hiking (I used to wear these when driving tow truck). Kurt had on a pair of tennis shoes, I believe, and everybody else was more or less wearing "street" shoes; I think Darwin may have even been wearing cowboy boots. Clothing was mostly shorts or jeans and short-sleeve shirts—we expected it to be warm that day. The only water we had was a bota bag somebody had brought, which probably held a quart-and-a-half of water. That's it. We really expected a "walk in the park," I think.

It did not take very long for the terrain to steepen and the walls of the mountains began to loom over the top of us. The IP who gave us instructions said there would be two very distinct "forks" in the trail and at the first one we had to stay right, and at the second one we had to stay left, and then just continue straight on the trail until we found the crash site.

It seemed simple, and sure enough after 10 or 15 minutes of walking we found the first fork, and off to the right we went. About the same amount of time later we found the second fork and we veered left. We were on our way ... until after about another 10 or 15 minutes we came to a third fork.

What the fu ...? Did we accidently take a fork that wasn't really a "fork," or did the IP leave out the third fork, and if so, which way do we go now? We had a 50/50 chance of choosing correctly, as long as we had not made a mistake on one of the earlier forks. There was no way of knowing for sure, but we decided going left was our best bet. So we did.

From here the terrain got very rough and the trail became less clear and viable. It was hot, everybody was hungry and thirsty, and some of the guys were having big problems climbing in their footwear. We decided to stop for a break and take a rest, but at the end of the break a few of the guys said they would like to turn back. It was a true "turning point" in our adventure, which was about to end in failure.

Kurt and I were still in pretty good shape and able to continue the trek, so we agreed we would go farther to find the crash site and then come right back down, figuring it would take us no more than another 30 minutes or so to get to the top of trail. So, we told the other guys that they could wait at the rest point and we would meet them on the way down, or they could just go back to Kurt's car and wait for us there.

Everybody agreed, and Kurt and I even let them keep the bota bag of water, figuring it was going to be a quick climb and return. That was a mistake.

As Kurt and I continued, it became apparent that this might not have been the correct direction to go at the previous fork. Pretty quickly, the trail evaporated and we found ourselves slipping and sliding on the side of a fairly steep gradient that was all shale rock. It was a physically draining struggle for both of us to get across that obstacle, not to mention fairly dangerous. Lost footing on the loose shale rock could have meant a 200–300-foot slide down the mountain.

Finally, we made it through the shale hazard and found ourselves near the summit of several small peaks, but we had no idea of where we were, or where the crash site might be. It seemed we might actually have bypassed it somehow by taking the wrong turn and that it was likely we would never find the wreck. So Kurt and I continued to the top of the nearest peak (which was more of a small plateau) so we could get our bearings and find the trail down to meet back up with the rest of the guys.

When we reached the top, we had quite a view. The entire Phoenix Valley lay at our feet out to the west, and the Sun was falling toward the horizon. It was late afternoon now and the shadows of the Superstitions were quickly engulfing the trails below, but we thought we could see a way down and the place where we figured we might have left the others.

By now, Kurt and I were thoroughly spent. It felt like we were dying of thirst. The idea of finding the crash site was no longer a priority or even attractive at this point. Just getting off the mountain before dark, and taking that first drink of water, was all we could think about, so we prepared ourselves for the trek down the mountain.

At this point, as I turned to follow Kurt toward the route down, I felt a pretty sharp stabbing pain on the side of my foot. Fearing a possible rattlesnake bite, I looked down and saw I had brushed my foot against a small cactus that had these huge 3-inch needles, and at least two or three of the thorns had penetrated the leather uppers of my boot. I froze in place and told Kurt, "Wait! I stepped on a cactus."

It actually looked worse than it really was, but I had to sit on the rocks and slowly take off my boot and remove the needles. They had just barely poked into the skin and did not really draw any blood. I was just glad it was a cactus and not an Arizona rattler. Kurt sat down and was waiting patiently for me to fix my issue, while casually looking around the peak's plateau, which had been somebody's recent camp site. While I was just finishing putting on my boot, Kurt said, "Hey, look. What's this?" as he reached down into the shadows of a dark rock crevice about a 6 inches wide, and pulled out ...

A SIX-PACK OF BEER!!!

Not only a six-pack of beer, but a *cold* six-pack of beer that had remained in the frosty shadows of the chilly Superstition Mountain nights. It must have been left and forgotten by some previous campers.

Kurt and I just looked at each other, and broke into what was probably the most ridiculous laughing, screaming, jumping, and dancing celebration ever witnessed by just two people. We started yelling down the side of the mountain toward where we thought the other guys were still waiting, "Hey, we got beer! We got beer!" Then we discussed our next decision. "We should drink it! Drink it all? No wait! Let's drink two each and take the last two beers back to the others to prove we found it and then they can share those." That was the plan and that is what we did.

Now, I have had beers on a hot summer day, maybe after mowing the lawn or some other physical activity, and in those situations the beers always taste better. But nothing, absolutely nothing, will ever taste better that the two beers Kurt Skadeland and I guzzled down on top of the Superstitions that day. Nothing.

With the remaining beers in our pockets, we found what looked like the best trail to head back down. But no sooner had we started along the path, when we noticed across from the trail the sheer face of the side of another small peak. And something didn't look right. On this flat vertical wall, there was a large white mark, almost like somebody had thrown a gigantic bucket of white paint against the cliff. Kurt and I looked at each other a little funny, as if we had the same thought, "What could have caused that and how did it get there?" Then I think the light bulb came on for both of us. Our T-38s were painted all white.

Kurt and I looked straight down from where we stood, staring into a deep gulley at the bottom the opposite cliff face. Down there we could see lots of little metal pieces and some bigger items we recognized easily as parts of a T-38. We found our crash site, but now it had more of the feeling of a gravesite.

As our eyes followed the white mark back toward the direction of Phoenix and Williams AFB, Kurt and I could imagine the flight path the young student pilot had likely taken. Remarkably, his T-38 had perfectly passed between two much higher peaks and would have made it clean through if it had not flown head-on into this last peak. And it missed clearing it by only 30 or 40 feet. Fifty feet higher, or 10 degrees right or left, and the young pilot would still be alive, probably serving his first assignment in a different jet, maybe in a different country, maybe with different-looking mountains. Who knows? But many unknowns and what-ifs surround flying; it's probably why so many pilots are a superstitious lot.

Kurt and I made our way fairly easily down to the remains. It was obvious that the investigation team had scavenged the most important parts of the jet to determine the details supporting the cause of the crash. Items like the flight instruments and controls were gone, but left behind were very large or heavy parts too difficult to get off the mountain, including the wings and engines, which now looked like large versions of crushed Coke cans. It was a somber place to be, and Kurt and I now felt the need to respect it as a place of rest for the young officer. We found a few small pieces of aluminum tubing and other parts and put them in our pockets and left everything else undisturbed. Much less gleeful than 10 minutes before, we started down the mountain.

The trek down was easy. We quickly found the trail we were supposed to be on originally and it was obvious now that we made a wrong turn somewhere. Even though it was getting dark quickly, we made good time at almost a trot downhill as the trail was very accessible. Soon Kurt and I were at the junction where we had left the others, but they were nowhere to be found. We assumed they had taken our suggestion and were happily waiting for us at Kurt's car. We couldn't wait to show them the jet parts and the beer.

Within 20 minutes we were back in the park at the trail entrance, but there was nobody at Kurt's car. Now, the dilemma began. Where were they? Did we actually mistake the place where we left them and they are still waiting for us up there? Did they get worried about our not returning sooner and go looking for us?

Kurt and I decided neither one of those options were likely based on how they were dressed and their desire to quit the mountain. They must be somewhere in the Lost Dutchman Park, so Kurt and I got in his car and started driving around. We could not find them anywhere. We checked a few different campsites, asking if they had seen three guys wandering around. We stopped at the ranger station at the entrance to the park, but he said he had not seen anybody.

Kurt and I really did not know what to do as we continued driving around the park. We were almost ready to head home, hoping that somebody had called one of their wives to pick them up, when Kurt peered over the hood of his car from the driver's seat and said, "What is that on the hood?"

Kurt stopped the car and we both got out and looked at the hand-scrawled writing in the dusty hood. It said "Go out the park, turn left on the highway, find the nearest place that sells beer. We will be there."

And we did and they were. There was much rejoicing.

***

All the training was over, and the big night was here ... Assignment Night.

This was probably the greatest event at UPT, since it was what all the hard work and training had been moving toward. The night was put together as a special occasion, highlighting the fact that up until that point, we didn't really know for sure where we were going next and what kind of airplane we were going to fly.

For the most part, some of us—especially those graduating as fighter qualified and at the top of the class—might have had an idea of what aircraft they might get. In my case, most of us had already shown our "cards" and declared our first choices to each other months before. I knew several of the guys competing with me at the top of the class were going to choose an F-16 over an F-15, and I was totally fine with that. So by the time we got to Assignment Night, I was pretty sure I was getting an F-15, it was just a matter of where to?

The way the night went down was that we were all in a small auditorium with our classmates, our IPs, and our families. All the aircraft and locations were written down on a big board at the front of the room. As each newly graduated pilot's name was called, he/she was given a piece of paper with their assignment on it, then they would go erase that assignment from the board.

It created a bit of suspense, as some people's first choices either remained or disappeared from the board.

There were two F-15 assignments on the board and when I saw that I was pretty relieved. I was pretty sure that only one of the other top grads and myself had put an F-15 down as a first choice. One of the Eagles was to Eglin AFB, in the beautiful panhandle town of Fort Walton Beach, Florida. The other Eagle was to Kadena Air Base in Okinawa, Japan. I had no idea where Okinawa, Japan, was, and it sounded way too far away and too much like a jungle outpost. Geri and I were both pulling hard to get the Eglin Eagle.

It didn't happen and I ended up with Kadena.

I think Geri was disappointed (not that she had any say in the matter) and for me it took a small amount of glow off of the big night, but I was still truly excited to get my Eagle assignment. I congratulated my other classmate on his Eglin Eagle as well as all of my classmates for whatever they ended up with. Just to make it through the entire adventure was quite an accomplishment.

It wasn't until the end of Assignment Night event that I talked to my IPs Bob Nunley and Ken Dressel. Later, as I talked to more pilots during the next phases of training, I realized that I had actually grabbed the "golden ring" or the precious nugget of assignment night. Little did I know that one of the best-kept secrets of the fighter pilot community was that the finest place to fly and train in the F-15 Eagle was in Pacific Air Forces (PACAF) theater, at Kadena AB, Japan. The future would prove this to be true.

CHAPTER 5

The Dirty Dozen

Before I could actually get to my first assignment, I had a lot of other training to complete. First it was off to Holloman AFB, in Alamogordo, New Mexico, where we entered Fighter Lead-In Training (FLIT). This was about two months flying the T-38 Talon again, but this time with emphasis on learning basic fighter maneuvers and tactics.

It was really stimulating to start going beyond fundamental tasks such as takeoffs, landings, formation flying, and aerobatics. Now we started learning how to "max perform" our aircraft, often flying in relationship to another aircraft, and how to start using basic element (two aircraft in the same formation) fighting tactics. The T-38s did not have a radar or anything resembling a weapons system, but at this point we did not really need those distractions. We were already learning things we had never done before.

After FLIT was over, I headed straight to the F-15 Replacement Training Unit (RTU) at Luke AFB, Arizona. This was where first-time F-15 pilots, or previous F-15 pilots returning to the jet after an extended layoff, would go to get their initial or refresher training.

Having my F-15 RTU as temporary duty (TDY) at Luke AFB seemed like quite a convenience, because it was just across the Phoenix metropolitan area from Williams AFB. So, I would stay in temporary quarters at Luke during the week and then on the weekend I would go back to "Willie," where Geri was still living in our home from UPT. The only bad part about this arrangement, which I did not really see or understand at the time, was that while I was going home each weekend, the other five future-Eagle pilots in my RTU class were hanging out together and "bonding," i.e., tearing up the town. I would come to understand later how important it was to build these deep bonds of trust among unit brethren. It was not too big of a deal, since we were all going off to different bases and squadrons after RTU, but I felt like I missed out on something special.

I would find myself challenged again as I stepped up to the next level at F-15 RTU. There was so much more to learn; not only the basics of flying the Eagle (and working all of its complex flight systems), but also how to operate the multifaceted radar and missile-based weapons system, at the same time as acquiring basic-to-advanced air combat tactics. I guess the best comparison is when you read about NFL "rookies" showing up to the first training camp and talking about the speed of the game, different terminology, and learning a complex playbook ... same thing.

We were given plenty of classroom academics and flight simulator training before we ever stepped close to an actual F-15 on the ramp. Still, nothing can ever totally prepare you for your first ride in an advanced fighter such as the Eagle. I was excited for the day to arrive, and apprehensive.

I am not sure I can really remember much detail of my first Eagle sortie. It was a very basic "fam-ride" (familiarity sortie) intended mostly to make sure I could safely start, taxi, take off, and land my Eagle, while learning the local area and airfield procedures. I flew an F-15B, the two-seat version of the early model F-15A, which was what the RTU at Luke used for training (the newer model F-15C Eagles were just starting to arrive in operational squadrons worldwide). This meant I would have a safety instructor sitting right behind me to assist and advise, much as my father did for me on my very first flight.

I do remember the feeling of climbing the very high ladder into the cockpit. As I eased into the seat and the crew chief helped me strap in, I was thinking "Holy crap! I can't believe I am going to fly this thing!" The other thing I remember was taxiing up to an F-4 Phantom near the runway. I was looking down at the F-4, which I had always considered to be a rather large jet, and saw that we just towered over it. The aircraft now appeared as if it was a miniature version of the classic Vietnam War fighter.

If there was one other thing I recollect about my first flight (and flights) was actually how easy it was to fly the F-15. As opposed to the tricky nature of the T-38 in UPT, the Eagle takeoffs, landings, basic maneuvering, and such were simple tasks that were easily mastered on the first flight or two. Other than the speed and complexity of some flight systems, I almost felt like I was flying in my old Super Cub, Three-Eight Charlie. I guess the Eagle was designed with flyability in mind, so the hands-on flying would be second nature in order to spend more time and effort on employing the weapons systems.

It was learning how and when to use the radar and all the switches on the control stick and throttle that took time and experience to master, and even then, it was a constant challenge to maintain a high level of proficiency. Combine the technologies with the fast-paced and rapid-fire decision-making of air combat tactics, and it was easy to become mentally overwhelmed during these early stages of training.

I did well at F-15 RTU, but I was not Top Grad. That honor went to Capt Thom "T-Mac" McCarthy. He was a previous T-38 UPT IP who got his dream assignment too. He had quite a bit of fast jet time already under his belt and caught on quickly to the accelerated world of air combat training. He was better than me at that time.

By the time we got to the final phases of RTU, though, I felt like it was all starting to click. The world and the air combat environment started to "slow down" a bit, to where I could start to apply what I was learning on a more intuitive basis and not have to think consciously about what I was going to do next. The world started to slow down a bit ... or so I thought.

***

One more training stop during the summer of 1984 was to Fairchild AFB, Spokane, Washington State, for Survival, Evasion, Resistance, and Escape (SERE) training. It was two weeks long and the acronym pretty much spells out what it is. All I can really say about it was that the weather was nice. Fortunately.

After completing all my required training, I returned to Williams AFB, where Geri and I packed up for the second time and made another move, this one much longer.

It was the last week of August 1984 that I first stepped off the "Freedom Bird" military charter aircraft onto the Air Mobility Command (AMC) tarmac at Kadena AB. It was a sunny day, late morning, and all I can remember is feeling I'd been punched in the face with a hot, heavy, wet towel. The heat and humidity was stifling and like nothing I had ever experienced, even in Texas. I had to wonder how people could possibly live in a place like this, but soon we were in an air-conditioned car driven by our sponsor, Capt Greg "Odie" Neubeck.

Odie was an F-15 pilot in the 12th Tactical Fighter Squadron (TFS), also known as the "Dirty Dozen." I had been assigned to the 12th TFS and Odie and I had already been corresponding by mail (not e-mail, it wasn't invented yet) over the last couple of months, since he learned he would be my sponsor. His job was to help us get settled, find a car, a place to live, and acclimate into the squadron so I could begin my training as soon as possible. Odie was a great sponsor and he would remain a lifelong friend.

Within a week or two, Geri and I had settled in enough that I could spend more time in the squadron and start my initial Mission Qualification Training (MQT) in earnest. This is where the rubber meets the road.

When I first walked into the squadron I knew right away something was different and special about this place and about "the Dozen" (as we often called the 12th TFS). There was an air of both confidence (but not arrogance) and sincere community in the unit. It was like everybody was looking after each other and trying to make them better at their jobs.

Everybody I met from the get-go was great, but there was also this invisible barrier of some kind. It was a slightly palable feel of "not belonging" or not being part of the "club" yet. I soon came to realize that I would have to earn that belonging through my performance in the air. The first part of this process would be to complete my MQT training, because we were not really Eagle pilots until that was accomplished and we received our "tactical call-sign," the moniker that will follow us through our entire Air Force career and beyond.

One of the first people I met in my MQT training and on my initial flight was Capt Craig "Sumo" Adler. Sumo was the 12th TFS' weapons and tactics officer. The weapons officer (for short) is a graduate of the elite US Air Force (USAF) Fighter Weapons Instructor Course (FWIC) at Nellis AFB, Nevada. It is the Air Force version of the Navy's Top Gun program. The graduates become their unit's lead tactical instructor, responsible for promoting the highest level of tactical skills within the unit. More than any other pilot in the squadron, they are charged with preparing the unit for combat.

I had no idea at this point what a "weapons officer" was, but I do remember Sumo and I going out on my first flight at Kadena and him just kicking my ass in 1 versus 1 (1 vs. 1) basic fighter maneuvers (BFM). Coming out of RTU, I thought I was pretty good at BFM fights, but I realized (too late) that at RTU they always gave some leeway to the student so he had at least some chance of success in order to learn.

Here in the operational world, that did not exist. Nobody would ever give you any "slack." There was a saying, "Slack is a pair of pants with one leg. It doesn't exist!" Your enemy in combat would never cut you any slack, so why should anybody else during training for combat? In individual air combat, there can only be one victor.

Over the coming months and couple of years I would be fortunate to have Sumo and many other great instructors and flight leads teaching me everything they could about air combat. Some were better than others, but I learned something from everybody. Eventually, though, I would come to look at Sumo and the role of weapons officer as something to aspire too. I did not see myself ever being that accomplished, but I was going to try. I had brought some natural ability with me from all my previous experience and the recent RTU training, but that was not good enough. And I soon found out, with some not-so-subtle kick-in-the-butt guidance from my leadership, that I needed to expect more from myself and work harder. My first year flying the Eagle in the Dozen I would say was "average." I did well but nothing to distinguish myself, although that would change soon.

Another thing that happened in that first year is that Geri and I separated and then divorced. Geri was not happy in Okinawa. The life of an officer's wife is not an easy one. Some people thrive in it, and others never really feel comfortable in that role. Geri and I had been having problems all along anyway, even well before I entered the Air Force, and now we were 6,000 miles away from home. There was a lot going on in our lives and most of it was not conducive to maintaining a happy married life.

That next summer, Geri wanted to move back to Arizona and continue her education, working on a Masters at Arizona State University. I told Geri, "If you move back we will probably end up divorced." She did, and we did.

That was a big moment in my life. The day after we went to the courtroom in Arizona (I had traveled back to the United States to take care of this event in person), it felt like this enormous weight had been lifted off of my shoulders. It wasn't just that I was "free and single" now, it was more like I had been playing some kind of game or "role" for so many years that was not really me. It wasn't just the marriage, but everything I had done in my life up to that point. I felt like maybe I wasn't always doing it for myself or the way I wanted to do it. I was doing it for somebody else, or doing it how I thought other people expected me to. That weight was gone. I felt emancipated, like there was something big waiting for me.

***

Right after I finished MQT two things happened. First, I received my tactical call-sign: "Kluso" (the fighter pilot phonetic spelling of Clouseau, of Pink Panther Inspector fame—I guess somebody thought I looked like the character). Second, I was selected to go on the next squadron training deployment to Exercise COPE NORTH at Chitose AB in Hokkaido (northern Japan) near Sapporo. Only about half of the squadron pilots would get to go to this smaller-scale flying exercise, so I felt fortunate.

At COPE NORTH I would learn for the first time what it is like to be on a squadron deployment or TDY. It was all flying and drinking, and not necessarily in that order. There were almost none of the distractions of normal home-based duty, so we could concentrate solely on air combat training, in this case against the Japan Air Self Defense Force (JASDF) fighter aircraft and their very capable pilots. When we weren't training, we were out at night with all our squadron mates and most of the Japanese fighter pilots at the Eagle Bar in downtown Chitose, drinking pretty much everything they had behind the bar. It was while I was at the Eagle Bar, learning to sing fighter pilot songs and other ribaldry, that I met a very quiet young Japanese woman who seemed a bit out of place amongst the craziness.

Her name was Mayumi, and she was a friend of the bar owner Yoshiko (a stunning middle-aged woman with a Cleopatra style haircut). Nothing ever happened between myself and Mayumi (I was still married to Geri at the time also), but we did develop a short friendship that included some time away from the Eagle Bar just to talk. Even though there was a significant language barrier, I felt I could be myself with this young woman, and I consequently discovered a fondness for Japanese women and Asian women in general. I have always wondered why this is ... maybe a past lifetime in this part of the world?

I soon got more chances to get great training and expand my "social" awareness in the Western Pacific. Not long after our return from COPE NORTH I was sent with a small cadre of pilots to sit "Alert" at Osan AB, Korea.

***

Alert posture in South Korea felt like war. Osan AB (near Songtan City, just south of Seoul) still carried the feel that the Korean War never ended, which it hadn't. It was all barbed wire, defensive gun emplacements, aircraft parked in hardened shelters, and AF Security Forces personnel carrying big guns and grim faces. It just felt like bombs and bullets could start flying at any moment, and I was taught early on to take this business seriously.

We always had two F-15C Eagles "hot-cocked" and ready to roll on a no-notice alert posture ... the traditional "scramble" order. Normally 4–6 pilots would rotate every two weeks into Osan, so over the course of a year everybody would spend about a month's total time on alert in Korea. Each alert event normally consisted of 24 hours on-duty, 24 hours off-duty, and an occasional 24-hour tour as the "standby pilot"—in this role he would have to come in if the first two jets scrambled and prepare the third spare Eagle to be ready to scramble if needed. He would also perform errands, such as ice cream runs to the Baskin-Robbins store on base, for the alert pilots. Alert duty was great, because once again you had nothing to do but be prepared to go to war at a moment's notice, or do the other things fighter pilots do: drink and party.

The "ville" right outside of the Osan main gates was like a little adult carnival. Lots of bars and clubs to drink at, pretty Korean "juicy girls" (bar girls) to talk to and flirt with, and soju tents where you could hang out at the end of the night and drink Korean OB beers and eat barbequed street food with hot chili paste. It was probably good we could only stay in Korea for two weeks at a time.

The actual alert tour was usually nothing more than hours and hours of watching the same VHS video-taped 80s B-movies over and over again, until you could memorize all your favorite lines from *Caddy Shack*, or *Used Cars*, or the introductory duo-logue between Rob Lowe and Jim Belushi in *About Last Night*. But there was nothing that would get your heart and adrenaline pumping faster than hearing the "BWAAAAA—BWAAAAA—BWAAAAA" of the claxon horn in the alert facility going off to announce a scramble. Even if it was a "practice" scramble (which about 98% of them were), and even if you had forewarning of it coming, the instant that claxon sounded it would be like all hell broke loose.

We normally stayed dressed in our flight suits and even G-suit during the day (and I often did at night too) because there was no time to don clothing or boots. If you were not out the door within about 10 seconds, the alert vehicle full of crew chiefs, weapons troops, and pilots would be speeding on its way to the jets about 150 yards away (and then you would have to hoof it yourself).

On one fateful day at Osan, I had the idea to set up a practice scramble with the senior operations duty officer (SODO) to give us a launch opportunity, because I had a new pilot with me and he had never scrambled before. I kept it a pretty good secret because everybody but me would be surprised when the claxon sounded. I found that was not necessarily a good idea.

I was near the Operations desk as the alarm went off, and I had to run back to a hallway to grab my flight (parachute) harness hanging on a peg. But as I entered the open doorway to the hall, I ran smack head-on into a very large weapons troop who just knocked me straight back on my ass, and said "Sorry, Sir" as he continued running out the door. So, I was the last one out of the alert building and there was the alert truck with everybody on board just starting to pull away. Somebody yelled for the driver to "STOP!" as I lunged toward the open tailgate, with some troops and my wingman trying to grab me to help me in.

This was the middle of winter in Osan, however, and there was about a 3-inch layer of ice frozen on the bottom of the truck bed. So, I did not stop when I passed the tailgate ... I just kept sliding and smacked straight into the front of the truck bed. And right then, somebody yelled at the driver, "GO!"

The driver of the alert truck punched the gas, and I reversed course this time, exiting halfway out the tailgate when somebody grabbed me before I hit the pavement, at which point somebody again yelled at the driver, "STOP!" and, well ... you probably get the picture. At that point, the poor airman driving had me yelling at him from the truck cab back window, "SLOW DOWN! It's only a practice!"

I learned my lesson.

It was not long after my *Cope North* tour, and finishing up and surviving my first Osan alert tour, that I was told the entire squadron was deploying to Clark AB in the Philippines. I was going to my first (of many) COPE THUNDER.

***

COPE THUNDER was the RED FLAG of the Pacific Theater. The name RED FLAG is probably better known to the general public, but all composite force exercises of this type (meaning very large exercises with many different types of tactical aircraft and units participating) were identified as FLAG exercises, whether the word "flag" was in the name or not. RED FLAG was at Nellis AFB in Nevada, MAPLE FLAG at Cold Lake AB in Canada, and so forth. The main difference in this instance (at least in the 1980s) was that COPE THUNDER was bigger and better than any of the others. It was why the Pacific Theater was known as "The Home of Large Force Employment."

The idea behind the Air Force FLAG exercises was to create as close as possible a true combat mission environment that had the size, structure, planning, complexity, and (simulated) adversary threats we would likely experience in any kind of modern air campaign or war. The exercise was normally two weeks long, with 10 total flying days. By participating in at least one of the two daily events (two events per day, AM and PM) at the end of the exercise a pilot would have completed 10 "missions." This number of missions was a critical number for young pilots. Historical statistics of air combat over many years and wars demonstrated that surviving the first 10 combat sorties exponentially increased overall survival rate and also increased combat effectiveness.

Flying for three years in multiple COPE THUNDER exercises and missions, I experienced both quantitative and qualitative improvement factors. Part of my development came with just becoming a more experienced fighter pilot, but the lessons learned there in the Philippines compounded to create a true depth of skills and knowledge, and a surplus of the fighter pilot's most essential quality—"SA," or situational awareness—something you cannot learn from a book or from simple training tasks and exercises. I would come to value this precious training when my opportunity for real combat rolled around in 1991.

My very first COPE THUNDER as a new wingman was close to a disaster, at least in the first week. I was barely holding on every mission, trying to do the most basic tasks, stay with my flight lead, use my radar and weapons system to simulate "kills" against aggressor aircraft, and hoping to avoid an airborne collision with so many jets buzzing around. On my first three THUNDER missions, before the end of each mission I would somehow lose sight of my flight lead. Knowing the contingency rules for this type event (a fighter, no matter how good the pilot or the jet, is always a more vulnerable target when flying alone without mutual support) I would latch on to the nearest F-15 flight I could find to continue to fight, or return to base (RTB) after the mission.

I felt that since I had performed reasonably well during the mission and came home with another Eagle, that I wasn't doing so bad. But one evening, as I was walking to my room in Chambers Hall, Maj Jeff "Jiffy Jeff" Brown called out to me as I walked by his open door, and said, "Hey, hey Kluso. Come in here. We want to talk to you." I walked into the room and there was Jiffy Jeff, along with a couple of the more experienced flight leads, drinking beers. Jiffy himself was what I would consider your "classic fighter jock." He had been raised in the post-Vietnam era by other jocks with lots of combat experience and he had been an F-5 Aggressor pilot (some of the best USAF pilots who fly aircraft and tactics to simulate enemy capabilities). He was also an "international ambassador," and by that I mean he had always been flying fighters overseas—he had never been assigned in the States. My hero.

Jiffy and the others mentioned to me that they had noticed I kept coming home without my flight lead. I confirmed that and just kind of shrugged it off. Jiffy said, "I want you to listen to this," and he started to play a cassette tape that had a recording of the in-flight radio calls from a long past mission over North Vietnam. I don't know how Jiffy got this, or how the recording was made to begin with, but from the sound of it, it may have been re-recorded and handed down over the years from one fighter pilot to another, to insure the lessons of real combat would not be lost.

I listened intently, not knowing what I was going to hear, but I could tell from the tension in the radio voices that this was what combat must sound like. It was a real combat mission, with flight call-signs I did not recognize. It was apparently some kind of fighter sweep or escort mission and I was waiting to hear the excited declarations of "tally ho" (enemy aircraft sighted), or Fox 2 (infrared missile shot taken), or "splash" (enemy aircraft shot down). I heard something quite different.

The flight was being managed expertly by the flight lead or mission commander. The flight may have even been on its way home to celebrate another mission accomplished and nobody shot down or lost. Instead, there is an excited call from "Blue 4" (I will use Blue as generic call-sign in this case, since I can't remember the actual call-sign)—number "4" normally reserved for the fourth (or last) jet in the formation, often flown by one of the younger or more inexperienced pilots. Blue 4 calls that he sees some "bandits" (enemy fighters) right below their flight, heading in a different direction. The Blue lead commands Blue 4 to maintain formation, but instead the young wingman breaks off on his own to attack a superior force of enemy fighters.

The radio quickly degenerates into frantic calls from Blue 4 as he is quickly swarmed by the enemy fighters and is soon overmatched with no help coming from his flight mates, who have now also been drawn into the frantic fight. Blue 4 is separated from the rest by the enemy pilots, just like a pack of wolves separate the youngest and weakest from the herd. The last thing heard from Blue 4 is not much more than a whimper over the radio, as he now knows his fate is sealed. At that point an unknown veteran voice comes over the radio and, without a hint of emotion, keys his mic and says to Blue 4, "Shut up, and die like a man." That radio transmissions end at that point.

Standing there stunned by what I had just heard, Jiffy turns to me and says, "So, Kluso. Are you going to lose sight of your flight lead tomorrow?" I said, "No Sir, I won't," and I didn't ... that day, or the next, or the rest of the exercise. In fact, since that time it was an extremely rare event for me ever to lose sight of my flight lead, and even when I became a flight lead I made sure to never lose sight of my wingman.

A cold hard fact that has been forgotten and relearned, usually through misfortune, is that a single fighter jet is not an effective combat unit and is more of a liability than anything else. The enemy will grow a brave heart when they know they have a solitary American fighter pilot alone in his aircraft. Even if they should lose a pilot or jet of their own, they will attack confident of downing such a precious prize as an American fighter. If there is another supporting fighter within visual range, then the enemy will begin to lose his courage and doubt his own ability to be victorious. It's called Mutual Support, and it is the bedrock of air combat tactics. I learned that lesson at my first COPE THUNDER, and I would never forget it.

We would normally attend two or three COPE THUNDER exercises each year. That was a lot, and much more and far bigger than similar FLAG exercises my compatriot Eagle pilots were training to perform back in CONUS (Continental United States). Typically our "Blue air" (or friendly forces) missions would be 50–60 aircraft of all types, with a full squadron of 16–20 F-15Cs providing the air combat sweeps and escort for the strike packages (fighter-bombers).

Sometimes we would send two full squadrons of Eagles from Kadena down to Clark for what they called a "Large Force" THUNDER (like they weren't already large?). For these missions we would launch 80–90 aircraft packages, with sometimes 32–36 Eagles. It was truly impressive. Just watching the launch and recovery operations was a testament to planning and determination, enabling so many aircraft to take off from and return to the single Clark AB runway. It would be rolling, formation takeoffs (two jets side-by-side), using afterburners and absolute minimum spacing (10 seconds) between formations. How we did not kill anybody doing this, I will never know.

Over the months, and years, and missions, I grew from that "sheepish" wingman, into an element (2-ship) flight lead, then a 4-ship flight lead (still as a 1st lieutenant), then eventually as air-to-air mission commander. The latter was the ultimate reward for me as very young captain on my first Eagle assignment, entrusted to plan, brief, lead, and debrief my fellow fighter pilots on this enormous stage.

I was thrilled ... until my first actual mission commander opportunity, that is.

I had seen it done many times before, I had worked my way to the top qualifications in the squadron, and now I thought I was ready to be a mission commander. I just had to impress one person to pass my qualification check-ride, and that was the 12th TFS weapons officer, Sumo Adler.

I planned the event on my own the entire day/night before, got up early, gave my brief to the pilots, we stepped to our jets on a beautiful Philippines morning mission, flew the mission and ... we kicked ass! I walked back to the squadron debrief room after finishing up the mass debrief for the day, covered a few odds and ends for the mission that I thought we could improve on, and then asked if anybody had anything else? And they didn't, so I thought that was just about it.

Now all I had to do was wait for the glowing accolades from my mentor, Sumo. I even told Sumo that it was OK if he debriefed me in front of all the other squadron pilots; after all, they could probably learn from this how to "do it right." Sumo said "OK," and then he ripped me a new asshole. Sumo told me that not only did I BUST (fail) this mission (and would have to do it again), but it was probably one of the worst mission commander events he had ever seen. Wow! Was I ever caught off guard? And now I had to take this caustic debrief in front of the rest of the pilots.

Sumo said that I might have had a good plan, but I had kept it all in my head and I did not clearly "build a picture" for the other flight leads and pilots of the critical events, timing, and flow of the mission. Sumo said the *only* reason we did well that day is that the other pilots were experienced enough to take up the slack for my lack of leadership. I might not be fortunate enough for that to happen on my first real combat mission. I had to do better and at the end, I agreed with Sumo's assessment.

About six months later, I would be back at what would turn out to be my final COPE THUNDER before I left Okinawa for my next assignment. I was even more experienced now and I had much more mission commander time under my belt from the previous THUNDER and other large force exercises like COPE JADE and TEAM SPIRIT in Korea. I had the opportunity to lead a large Offensive Counter Air (OCA) strike package in the final week of this THUNDER. We had been flying with the Royal Australian Air Force (RAAF), who had come up from "Down Under" to join us for this THUNDER. The Aussies were great pilots both on our team and as adversaries, but for the last week or so we had been having trouble getting our strike aircraft to their targets unscathed. It seemed that no matter what plan we came up with, the adversaries always knew what route and formation our strike aircraft were taking, and they would find a way to strip off the Eagle escorts and be waiting to pounce on the undefended strikers.

Trying to figure out why this was happening and how to counter it, I did a little intelligence hunting and discovered that the controllers in the E-3 AWACS radar control aircraft had access to both the Blue (Friendly) and Red (Adversary) Air Tasking Order (ATO), which contained the flight information and electronic Identification Friend-or-Foe (IFF) data for all the aircraft. So, they were sitting comfortably at 1-G in their airborne command and control platform with perfect situational awareness of where all the friendly and adversary aircraft were, and they could tell the adversary fighters which part of our formations were the strike aircraft.

Now, some people would say this is "cheating," but I would say that anything is fair in combat. ANYTHING! And two can play at that game. In fact, even though you would hope the real enemy would not have access to our critical identification plans, the reality was that during Vietnam this did often happen, and frequently with the same results—loss of aircraft—but in the case of war, that meant jets down and crews lost or captured. I had heard and read about a famous mission once, when Colonel Robin Olds (a famed fighter pilot already in his own right) decided to turn the tables on the North Vietnamese Air Force. Col Olds changed around the call-signs and electronic identification codes of his air-to-air fighter sweep and escort jets with those of the more vulnerable strike aircraft. He also chose ingress routes and formations to make his fighters look on the enemy radar like they were unprotected strikers. It worked, and the US fighters decimated the responding North Vietnamese MiGs.

So on this day, and this COPE THUNDER mission, I decided to do the same. My problem was how to get the controllers to use bogus call-sign and IFF information since they already had access to the ATO.

As mission commander, I was responsible for assembling a mission card (a single sheet of letter size paper) that had all the vital mission data on it, to include participants, type of aircraft, call-signs, IFF codes, routes, and targets. On this day, I made copies at the copy machine and handed them out to pilots for the mission brief. And then, I took out another mission card I had made, walked over to the copy machine (which was shared by all the participants at COPE THUNDER, the "enemy" included), made the copies (which I later threw away), and purposely left the original in the copy machine. The difference was that the card I intentionally left in the copier had all the *wrong* information on it. My intent was that the "adversary" mission commander would find this card, hand it over to his radar controller, and inadvertently place the bait on the hook. That is exactly what happened. When I stopped back by the copy machine before we stepped to our jets, the faux mission card was gone. The trap was set.

To further complicate the adversaries' problem, much as Robin Olds had done 20 years prior, I changed my flight routes and formations. The striker F-4 flights had often been flying in a "box" formation (two aircraft line-abreast in front, followed by two aircraft line-abreast behind them, looking like a square box) down the inland route of COPE THUNDER airspace to the Crow Valley bombing range. This time the front box of "F-4s" would actually be a 4-ship flight of my Eagles, ready to use their AIM-7 Sparrow radar missiles to blow away the Aggressor F-5 combat air patrol (CAP) from beyond visual range (BVR).

Meanwhile to the west, over the water, I had an eight-ship of Eagles, to which I added a 4-ship of my Aussie F-111 friends. The F-111s would line up side-by-side in a wall formation with my Eagles making it look like an air-to-air sweep from the west and unprotected strikers from the east. At the right time, the Aussies would drop out of our high-altitude formation and dive down to skim the wave tops at high speed all the way to the target.

It could not have worked any better. All of our strike aircraft reached their targets untouched, and our Eagles laid waste to the adversary formations. Coming back into the mass debrief, the adversary pilots were just shaking their heads, not sure what had just happened to them. The best part was when the adversary AWACs controller got up to debrief his performance and started to regurgitate the faux mission card plan I had left behind in the copy machine, convinced that he had known exactly where all the F-4s and F-111s were. His own adversary pilots started barking out counters to highlight his lack of SA, "NO, those weren't F-4s there! They were Eagles and we got mauled by them?" and "NO, that was not a fighter sweep to the west, there were 111s there, but by time we got there we couldn't find them and we were getting shot by Eagles."

It was a glorious way to end my COPE THUNDER days. I had several pilots on my side and even the Aggressor mission commander come up to me and say, "That was the best THUNDER mission they had ever seen." I felt like I would have made Sumo proud.

I cannot leave the topic of COPE THUNDER without talking about the Philippines.

***

There was something very special about the Philippines. It was not just that it was a tropical paradise. It had this cool vibe that I just cannot describe. Everything felt relaxed and easy there. It had a special tropical smell. Not a "bad" smell, but just a smell of comfort and respite, like you might feel on an easy summer afternoon lounging in the shade. And then, there were the Philippine women.

I am not sure I have ever been around women that were so pretty and feminine, but also seemed like they were your best buddy too. Almost like they would rather be hanging out with the guys than with other girls. Of course, the Philippines had bar girls, and dancers, and sex shows, and an active sex trade, and I have to admit in my single days I tried it all. But it was in the Philippines that I fell in love again for the first time after my divorce with Geri.

Her name was Marriette. She was a shy but precocious waitress at the Chili Pot, one of our favorite food and beer hangouts in Angeles City (the ville outside the Clark AB gates). We had a long-range romance that unfortunately did not withstand the test of time and distance. I know I broke Marriette's heart (even though she has since forgiven me), but I will be forever grateful to her for filling a void in my spirit after a rough divorce and for helping me build confidence that I could trust my heart to somebody else again.

In late 1987, I took off from Clark AB for the last time, and RTB'd to Kadena after my final COPE THUNDER before I left for my next assignment. I thought I might have a chance to come back, if I could get a return assignment to Kadena (which I did in 1991 right after DESERT STORM), but it would not turn out that way.

In the spring of 1991, I was back at Kadena with the Dirty Dozen (again) and we were just a couple of days away from deploying down to Clark for the final COPE THUNDER of the '91 training season. Then Mount Pinatubo erupted, or more like, exploded. The once-dormant volcano just west of Clark AB, right on the edge of the Crow Valley bombing range, showered ash and debris all over the base. Clark was quickly evacuated, and the US military forces would pull out of the Philippines permanently (Subic Bay and Cubi Point naval facilities, up for lease renegotiation, would also close). It was the end of an era, and an end of the best air combat training exercise in the US Air Force. Ever.

***

In 1986, I had just pinned on the rank of captain when I was told I would be joining a small group of Kadena pilots for a trip to Nellis AFB for a two-week Dissimilar Air Combat Training (DACT) exercise. After that, I had been hand-picked to attend Raytheon AIM-7 Sparrow (missile) school near Boston, Massachusetts. The AIM-7 school was quite an honor because we normally only sent one pilot per year from each squadron, and it usually meant we were being groomed for bigger and better things like, maybe, the Fighter Weapons School. So I was pretty psyched, but also a little curious about why the full group of us were flying all the way from Japan to Nevada just for some DACT?

DACT is always a fun mission. It means air-to-air training against "dissimilar" Air Force (or other service) fighters, like F-16s, or F-4s, or F-14s, instead of our normal everyday training of F-15 vs. F-15. But at Kadena we did a lot of DACT on a regular basis, including flying against the Philippine-based F-5 Aggressor squadrons quite often. So why go all the way to Nellis?

One thing I knew is that we were going to meet up with some of our home-based jets that had flown the entire way from Okinawa to Tyndall AFB, Florida, for the

William Tell Air-to-Air Competition. On their return trip, the Kadena William Tell team would stop over at Nellis, and while they took a break for a couple of weeks, myself and the other pilots would fly those jets for this DACT event.

We started to get inklings that this trip was not an ordinary event not long after we arrived at Nellis. After we had received an indoctrination mission at Nellis to learn about the local area and procedures, we were told to show up for a special briefing at the end of the day ... and "Don't be late!" When we all sat down in the large briefing room that day, we knew something was different.

First of all, the room was more of a vault, with combination locks on the door, not just an ordinary office-type room. Second, there were pieces of paper in front of each us, which we had to sign to commit ourselves to absolute secrecy. It was clear that we were going to get briefed on something very important, and highly classified. We just didn't know what.

In walked a couple of fighter pilots whom I had never met or seen before. They were wearing a special patch on their shoulder that resembled something like our Aggressor squadron pilots wore, usually a patch with a big red Soviet Union-style star. But these patches were different and said "Red Eagles" on them.

Red Eagles? Like F-15 Eagles, or something? It did not take long to find out.

The security briefing was a bit scary in itself. We would NEVER EVER be able to talk about this program to anybody else. NEVER. Even to the other pilots who were in the room with us that day. We would not be able to discuss what we were going to do and see, once we finished this exercise. HOLY CRAP! What was it? Were they going to tell us that Elvis was still alive and he was piloting his secret flying saucer in the Area 51 portion of the Nellis AFB ranges?

It was actually better than that.

We were being briefed into a highly classified program called CONSTANT PEG. The program was started a few years previously in order to train US fighter pilots against *real* Soviet MiG fighter aircraft. Real MiGs that were owned by the US government and flown by US pilots. I won't go into all the details about how the United States got hold of real MiGs and how this program started. Col Gail Peck, Jr. (USAF/Retired) wrote a great book about it: *America's Secret MiG Squadron: The Red Eagles of Project CONSTANT PEG.* I would highly recommend it to anybody interested in the details of this covert project. The reason I am able to tell you about it today is because several years ago CONSTANT PEG was declassified.

For us young F-15 drivers, it meant the chance of a lifetime (in lieu of real combat) to go face-to-face with a MiG. In this case it was the classic MiG-21 Fishbed (which our own Aggressor F-5s tried so much to emulate) and the somewhat newer frontline swing-wing MiG-23 Flogger. We were supposed to fly three total missions against a combination of one or the other fighters. On this trip, my MiG-23 mission got scrubbed (canceled) because my opponent's jet had some mechanical problems that day. That was a somewhat common problem with the MiGs (and their spare parts), which were obtained by backdoor methods and lots of cash. It is a testament to the maintainers and the pilots that they were able to fly these jets as much as they did. Even so, there were some accidents and a few brave pilots lost their lives.

I did, however, fly a 1 vs. 1 performance comparison and BFM (1 vs. 1 combat maneuvering) against the MiG-21 Fishbed. I was impressed. For a 1950s technology fighter, it was very nimble, accelerated well, and could "knife fight" very well. That means in a slow-speed, very close-in maneuvering fight the MiG-21 could easily defeat even a modern fighter like the F-15, if the US pilot was not careful. What it did not have was the thrust-to-weight ratio of the Eagle. So, instead of getting "slow" with the Fishbed, if the F-15 driver could maintain the "control zone" about 4,000 feet behind the MiG, and exploit vertical separation above the MiG, then the Eagle could easily win the BFM fight.

On my first attempt that is exactly what I did, and the Red Eagle MiG-21 pilot quickly "knocked off" the fight, knowing he was going to lose. My PACAF F-5 Aggressor friends had taught me well. The other thing I learned was how little gas and fighting time the Fishbed had. We were only together for about 15 minutes and used full-power afterburner for probably less than a minute of that time, and the MiG-21 already had to RTB to land. And we were almost directly over his base too—the top-secret desert strip in Tonopah, Nevada.

The next mission I flew was a 1 vs 2—myself versus two MiG-21 Fishbeds. This was much more challenging. The big fear was both being outnumbered and losing sight (or never seeing) one or both of the little fighters. Fortunately, as the MiG-21s split up to try to outmaneuver me, I was able to dispatch the first one quickly and then spotted the other about 3 miles away trying to sneak up on me. I max performed my jet to quickly turn my nose and shoot him with a simulated AIM-9L heat-seeking Sidewinder missile before he could even get his nose pointed in my direction. It was a BLAST!

I had many training experiences along the way that prepared me in different ways for combat. I have to say, however, that CONSTANT PEG was one of the most valuable single events to groom me for war. In war, fighter pilots (and even ground soldiers) were often reluctant to "pull the trigger" and shoot the enemy in the initial confrontation, much how a novice hunter will hesitate to kill an unaware buck deer the first time. To see and fight a real "enemy" aircraft went a very long way to ease the expected nerves, or "buck fever," often experienced the first time meeting the enemy in combat. Whatever the United States paid for those MiGs, it was worth it.

Shooting live air-to-air missiles (AAMs) during COMBAT SAGE and COMBAT ARCHER exercises was another great opportunity to diminish the likelihood of buck fever. At Kadena we were fortunate because almost every time we deployed to Clark AB, it included a chance to shoot live missiles at COMBAT SAGE. After I returned to the United States I had more opportunities to shoot both AIM-9 and AIM-7 missiles. By the time I had my first combat sortie, I already had about 11 live missile shots under my belt, and many, many more live 20mm air-to-air gun events. In combat, there cannot be any hesitation to pull the trigger (gun) or push the "pickle" button (missile). To wait even a second too long can mean the difference between a "good" shot or an invalid shot that has no chance to reach its target.

The other benefit of live fire of AAMs is to be able to observe the missile flight path and guidance to a target. With experience you can tell right away if a missile is guiding correctly or if it is having a problem and a likely miss. My live-fire experience would be a great benefit as my wingman and I blasted away in our first combat engagement.

***

Life in a fighter squadron is a unique experience. The camaraderie and esprit de corps are incredible, but it is a bond forged by life and death events, not just a desire to win.

Fighter squadrons have many traditions that are handed down, generation to generation, squadron to squadron, and airplane to airplane. But some things are traditional across the spectrum of units, specifically roll call and singing fighter pilot songs.

The modern-day USAF roll call may have actually started in the 12th TFS Dirty Dozen while I was there on my first tour. Maybe the Air Force had been doing roll calls all along, but I had not witnessed them before this day. Even later when I went to other units, they had never heard of "roll call," but they liked the idea.

Today, the fighter squadron roll call is a major tradition. It has taken on a life of its own, becoming more of a fraternity-like event than its original format, by intent or otherwise. In the Dozen we had our own squadron "bar" in the operations building. It was called the Tally-Ho, and it was nothing more than an old unused office that had a hand-made wooden bar, a few small refrigerators for cold beer, and a lot of squadron memorabilia. After the last mission of the day landed, the "beer light" would go on, which meant any of us pilots could wander down to the Tally-Ho and break open some cold beers or maybe of few shots of the famed rot-gut liquor, "Jeremiah Weed."

That is how our days normally ended. A couple of drinks, shoot the breeze and tell "war stories" or funny happenings from our day's training missions, then head home to do it again the next day. Fridays were a little bit different though. With a non-flying weekend ahead of us, most of us would stay late and really push-it-up on Friday nights. This is when the wild stories and fighter pilot songs would break out.

The first time I witnessed a "roll call" it was just a normal Friday night, and most of the squadron pilots were in the Tally-Ho drinking. Somebody asked somebody else, "Hey, where is So-and-so?" When we looked around to see there were a couple of the regulars missing, somebody yelled out, "Hey! Let's do a roll call and see who's NOT here."

So, somebody pulled out a squadron roster on a sheet of paper and started reading off names/call-signs. And we answered up, or otherwise it was noted that somebody "missed" roll call and next time they would owe a round of drinks to the rest of us (this part was to encourage everybody to show up on Friday night). That was the first roll call (that I know of anyway).

One particular Friday night, we had a visiting US Marine Corps F-4 Phantom squadron at Kadena and the Marine aviators were all invited to the Tally-Ho to join us for roll call. Those Marines could drink pretty good and we basically ran out of beer, and whiskey, and had to break open a huge sealed earthen jar of Japanese sake that a former commander had given as a going-away gift. It sufficed.

Along the way, we were sharing fighter pilot songs with the Marines, when a young Marine lieutenant broke into a song I had never heard before. It started out something like this:

"I am the Music Man. And I come from down your way. And I can playyyy!!"

(And then the other squadron pilots would respond with) "What can you playyyyy?!"

(And the leader would reply, sung loosely to the melody of "London Bridge is Falling Down.")

"I can play an Officer's Club shit-house dooooor ... Ohhhhh, Banga–banga–banga–bang, banga–bang, banga–bang. Banga–banga–banga–bang, banga–banga–bang, HEY!"

Then it would continue from there, adding different verses that usually had something to do with a musical instrument, like "pica–pica piccolo," or something insulting about other aviators or airplanes that did not belong to the unit or person singing the song.

It became quickly apparent that this was a great fighter pilot song, and it was one we unashamedly stole to make it into a Dirty Dozen tradition. We even added our own special verses. And, somehow, pretty soon (as other pilots left the squadron and handed over responsibility to lead the song) it became *my* song, and I would lead the "choir" through the many verses.

One of my favorite verses, and one to which I would add my own touch, would be saved to the very end of the song. Remember this was in the 80s and it was around the time (1984 to be exact) that Michael Jackson momentarily became a human torch when his hair caught fire during a pyrotechnic accident while filming a Pepsi commercial. So, as I delivered the final verse, I would challenge the choir "... and I can playyyyy."

"What can you playyyyyyy?"

"I can playyyyy, Michaeeeeeeeeeeeelllllllllllllllllllllllllllllllllllllllllllllllllllllllllllllllllll"

... and I would extend the end of the word "Michael" as long as I possibly could, with ultimate diaphragm control and people cheering me on, until my neck bulged red with veins popping out, and just enough breath remaining to squeeze out the final ... "JACKSON!!!"

Then, patting my head and rotating around in a circle, I'd sing "Fuckin-A my hair's on fire, hair's on fire, hair's on fire ... Fuckin-A my hair's on fire, hair's on fire! Hey!"

That final line was the killer. The place would always erupt in laughter and everyone joined in the crude imitation of Jackson trying to put out the flames. (Sorry Michael. I love you anyway.)

I would sing that song in many bars, in many squadrons, in many places and countries around the world. When somebody would want to hear it they would just turn to me and say, "Hey Music Man. Sing us a song." And then it would start, "I am the Music Maaaaaaaaaan!"

***

To the reader: This next section deals with subject matter pertaining to what young fighter pilots might do to entertain themselves when they are on the road with time on their hands. So, if you are too young for a PG-13 movie, or just a bit sensitive about subject matter of a sexual nature, then you might want to skip the next couple of pages. Fair warning.

As I already alluded to, the Western Pacific was a fighter pilot's paradise, not only for the great flying and training, but also for the wonders of "the Orient." I entered my life in the Air Force as a less than "worldly" person. I did not have many significant "romantic" relationships with women before I met and married Geri. So by the time we had finally divorced (and the six months of separation leading up to that), I was pretty much ready to light my own hair on fire.

I think I subsequently ended up getting a reputation as being a "wild man," always on the lookout for any "port in the storm," but actually over the next couple of years my dating and relationships were mostly monogamous. I did spend time with many different girlfriends and partners over short periods of time, but also stayed dedicated to Marriette in the Philippines and then later to another young and pretty Korean girl (in Osan). I'll just refer to her as Miss Choe. In between those relationships though, and during frequent TDY training deployments, I did get to experience some of the "jewels" of the Western Pacific.

On one such trip, we deployed to Hat Yai, Thailand, for a new exercise called COBRA GOLD. This was 1985, and it was the first time US Air Force fighter units had returned to Thailand since the end of the Vietnam War. It was a pretty big deal, and even for the "veterans" in the squadron the idea of going to Thailand (after hearing stories from the Vietnam jocks) to fly and party was something nobody wanted to miss.

The flying was great! Almost no restrictions, training against types of aircraft and pilots we had never met in the air before. And the nights ... well, they were even better. Now I am not going to go into lurid details of everything a young man can experience in Thailand. In fact, there was little that Thailand offered that we had not already seen or done before in Korea or the Philippines. But in Thailand it was (at least it seemed) much more open and available.

Right next to our hotel we had a "fish bowl." Not a bowl full of little orange colored fish, but a hotel-like massage parlor that really fronted as a house of prostitution. They called them "fish bowls" because when you walked into the lobby of the business there would be a huge picture window with a room full of beautiful women behind it looking out at the prospective customers. The women all had badges with large numbers on them and one only had to ask for the number of the woman that tickled one's fancy. Then it was off to a private room for a massage, or any of the "extras" if one chose to pay for those.

The nice part was that our squadron flight surgeon (doctor) actually went into this one particular fish bowl next to our hotel, talked to the owner and their on-site medical staff (which they actually had), checked out the girls to make sure they were "clean" and gave it his personal thumbs-up. The flight doc seal of approval! What a guy.

It was mostly the single guys partaking in the delights of nightly "massages," but some of us wanted to explore more of Hat Yai, so we decided to try what we had learned was the preferred way to find the best kept secrets of any city ... ask a cab driver. And we did.

In the local market area near the hotel, myself and a small group of some of the younger fighter pilots stopped a cabbie and asked where we could find some nice nightclubs with young women. We were actually looking for a real nightclub to hang out in and have some drinks for the evening, because we already knew where the fishbowls were and frankly those places became pretty boring after your 30–40-minute event was over.

The cabbie told us to meet him back at the same place around 8pm and he would take us. So, we all showed back up at the rendezvous spot on time, dressed for a night of disco dancing, packed into his cab, and off we went through the streets of Hat Yai, Thailand.

The cabbie seemed a bit nervous and he asked us several times not to tell anybody where we were going. We had no idea why, but we were all pretty much lost anyway, so it didn't really matter. And we started to figure out that there must have been something lost in translation when we made our request for a "nightclub" with "women." He must have just assumed young American men only had one thing on their mind.

Well, after a 10- or 15-minute ride through small streets and alleys, the cabbie stopped at an inconspicuous building with a plain single door. He told us, "Go in the door, walk down the stairs to a room, and wait there." Oh-Kaaay(?)

When we found the room, it was pretty barren. There was a small square wooden stage about 2 feet high, surrounded by four sets of bleacher-type seating on each side of the stage. There were also four or five TV monitors up above the stage, showing a continuous flow of soft-core porn. We all now realized we had just been dropped off at a Thailand version of a Far East sex show. It was not something we had never seen before because in the Philippines, at a place called the Nipa Hut, you could see one of the most famous sex shows in all of East Asia. So we were really not that impressed (and it definitely was not the disco or nightclub scene we had in mind), but we decided "what the hell"—we might as well stay to see the show.

We were shown to the bleachers by some very nice staff. They asked us all to pay the equivalent of $5 US in Thai Baht, and we were able to purchase beer and snacks too. It was almost like going to the movies. Then a funny thing happened. There were very few customers, mostly just the handful of us Americans, but about 10 minutes before the show started a literal bus-load of about 25 or 30 old Thai women came shuffling into the room and sat down in the bleachers around us. When I say "old" I mean like 50-, 60-, 70+–year-old grandmas. It was like a tour bus or something had let them off at the door, and I wasn't even sure they knew where they were or what they were going to see. They must have had some idea because some of them became very interested in the porn they were seeing on the TV monitors.

Then the show began.

We were a little disappointed at first. It was very much like the acts we had seen at the Nipa Hut. The "hot wax" girl who dripped liquid wax from burning candles over her naked body (Ouch!); the "beer girl" who would take a "bath" in beer and empty entire bottles into her vagina and "spit" it back out again; the "cash girl" who would squat on stacks of coins and have them disappear up inside her, only to distribute the change back out in small denominations; the "razor blade" girl ... well, I don't really want to describe this one.

One of the final acts did leave a big impression on us though; it was the "blow dart girl." This very pretty and healthy-looking Thai performer came out on stage with a thin, meter-long hollow tube. She was accompanied by a young man holding a large plywood board with lots of balloons on it, like you would see at a carnival game booth. We figured out pretty quickly she has a blow gun and that she was going to pop those balloons with some darts. We just don't know "how" ... so she quickly demonstrates.

The young woman takes a dart and inserts it in the tube, then lays down on her back, puts the tube into her vagina, rapidly compresses some apparently very strong pelvic muscles, and from about four feet away blows the dart and pops a balloon. Impressive, and the young woman receives an appreciative "golf clap" from the crowd.

The helper with the balloon board now moves a couple feet back on the stage, she lets loose again, and POP! goes another balloon. Wow, she's accurate too. Now the young man with the board of balloons is entirely off of the stage, a good 10–12 feet away from Annie Oakley. She winds up again, swoooshh ... POP!

So, how far can this girl really shoot for accuracy? Well, we are about to find out, because she is down to her last dart. Finally, the balloon guy moves all the way back and a couple of steps up into the bleachers next to us. He has to be at least 20 or more feet away from the girl, and there are only a couple of balloons left to aim at.

We all start making bets on whether she'll be successful this time, when blow dart girl takes a mighty windup, releases a loud grunt, and ...

The dart exits the tube like a bullet. It misses the board entirely, sailing over the top ... the customers in the bleacher behind the board duck (fortunately). The dart sails another 25 feet farther, and then impales itself in a large wood rafter beam in the back of the room. The whole crowd just pauses ... then in unison lets out a great, "Whooooooaaaaaaaaa!"

"Blow Dart Girl" gets a standing ovation.

After that, the live sex performance was extremely boring. We went back to our hotel.

***

While I had two serious relationships with women outside of Japan (Marriette in the PI and Miss Choe in Korea), I really didn't have much success in meeting or dating Japanese women in Okinawa. Maybe I just didn't know how or where to go to meet them, or maybe most were leery of dating American GIs? I don't know why, but it just didn't seem to happen for me. I did actually start to date casually a very pretty young Korean woman nicknamed Yumi, who worked on base on Kadena. It took me a while to catch on, but I would finally start to wonder how somebody who was Korean could be working on base in Japan? Plus, Yumi would never invite me to her place; she always wanted to come to my apartment.

I was slow, but not an idiot ... eventually I realized she was actually married, probably to another GI or airman on Kadena. So that relationship would come to an end, but I have to thank Yumi, and also Geri for that matter, because they would both introduce me to Sako, my future wife.

The Geri connection to meeting Sako was something I did not even realize until later, when it was Sako who told me about it. While Geri was still with me in Okinawa, she got a job on base working for a travel agent that booked foreign travel and tours for military members and their families. One day I stopped by Geri's work to ask her if she wanted to go to lunch. Geri introduced me at that time to her two Japanese co-workers, Chinami and Sako. They were both cute young Okinawan girls, and that was about it.

Fast-forward about a year later, Geri and I are divorced now, and I had just started to date Yumi (before I found out the details of her secret life). Yumi told me she had a friend who wanted to meet American guys, so we decided to set up a double date. I asked one of my single squadron friends, Rich "Spad" McSpadden, if he was interested. Spad said, "Sure!"

So that is where I met Sako again—she was Spad's double date.

The evening went pretty well, but for some reason from the moment I had met Sako I found myself very attracted to her. This might have been bad form, since Yumi seemed to sense this and she was obviously jealous. (Hah! Jealous? She was married herself!) But I pretty much left it as momentary infatuation, because after all I had set Sako up with my friend Spad, so I was not going to make any advances.

The one thing I didn't know, or remember, was that Sako had worked with Geri and that we had met before. For whatever reason though, Sako remembered and she knew exactly who I was. She just didn't know until now that Geri and I had divorced.

When the evening ended, Yumi and I dropped Sako off at her car off-base and said goodnight, and I assumed that was the last I would ever see of her, although her face and her smile would stick with me, through many more girlfriends and other dates. I could not get Sako out of my mind, and for some reason unknown to me, Sako felt the same.

When Spad was leaving Kadena for his next assignment I decided to ask him if he still had Sako's phone number and if he would mind giving it to me. I knew Spad was not interested in Sako, because he had never called her for a second date, so it was no problem and luckily he still had her number. But even with her number in hand, I could not get the courage to call her ... what could I say? I felt like I was in high school again ... afraid to call a girl to ask her to the school dance.

What I didn't know was that Sako's friend Chinami had my phone number from having worked with Geri. And they had even called me at home once at Sako's request, but got scared and hung up as soon as I answered the phone. Hmmmm.

Fast-forward again, and it is about six months before the end of my first tour at Kadena. It's coming up fast and I don't really want to leave Okinawa and the squadron. Although it's been the best couple of years of my life, I have this weird empty feeling like I am missing something. Like there is destiny beckoning—something or somebody I am supposed to find here on this assignment. This was probably why I had entered into serious relationships with Marriette and then Miss Choe, but I came to recognize that they were not who I was looking for (or who were looking for me). It was somebody else, but I had not found her yet. Or was it Sako? How would I ever see her again?

It was a Saturday night and I decided to meet up with some of the guys at the Kadena Officer's Club bar. It was a pretty regular thing to do when we were at home station, and the Kadena Club was always really hopping on weekend nights, kind of like the scene from *Top Gun*, in the bar. Guys in flight suits, women flowing in and out of the club, loud 80s music videos playing on the monitors.

Actually, I was kind of bored this night, just standing at the bar looking around. I was just about to call it an early night, when a small entourage of local girls walked right in front of me and I glanced down and recognized one of them. It was Sako, and she looked over and recognized me too.

I froze. I didn't say anything and she walked on by. Damn! I thought I might have just blown my chance, because Sako sat down with her friends and now there were a couple of guys at their table asking them to dance. I waited and watched, and then thought, "What's the use? Maybe I should just leave." Here was another of those moments where just the smallest decision would have an impact on the rest of my life, and hers also. Should I go say hi to her? Or just leave it alone?

I made my decision. I gathered up my courage, walked across the room, and said, "Hi. I'm not sure if you remember me, but …?" and I was met with a BIG smile. Four months later we were married.

***

My last year at Kadena was great! I felt like I had grown so much both as a fighter pilot and as a person. I had made it through the struggle of a painful divorce, but come out on the other end better for it. And, as I mentioned before, I really did not want it to end. It was like that first family trip to Disneyland. If there was only some way I could stay at Kadena in the Dirty Dozen forever.

But that is not the way the Air Force works. Every three years (on average) we are expected to make a PCS move. New base, new assignment (job), and often for fighter pilots the worst prospect … a new airplane (and not a fighter). I had already learned that it was almost impossible to receive a follow-on F-15 assignment. Most of my friends that had already left Kadena on new assignments were doing things like flying T-37s and T-38s back at UPT as instructors, or doing "Alpha" tours as air liaison officers (ALOs) with our Army brethren, or even worse, the kiss of death—a staff (desk) job.

I had actually planned ahead and campaigned for an assignment (if I couldn't get another F-15) that would be almost as much fun and challenging. The squadron commander for the F-5 Aggressor squadron in the Philippines had taken a liking to me through all our training interactions over the years, and he had offered me an Aggressor job when my F-15 tour was over. I was set. Flying F-5 Aggressors in the Philippines. Continuing to travel all over Asia to train other pilots like I had been doing for the last three years? That was my plan, until Opec Hess walked up to me in the squadron one day.

Lieutenant Colonel Dan "Opec" Hess was the squadron commander of the Dirty Dozen. When I had first arrived at Kadena, Opec had started out as my DO (Director of Operations, also known as the OpsO who is the second-in-command). Not long after, he would become our Dirty Dozen commander, and we would grow together through much of the assignment.

When I think of Opec he, probably more than any other officer or commander I've had, was the one I always used as my primary example of how to be an officer, and a leader, and a commander. I had lots of great leadership and commanders along the way, and I learned something from all of them. Even from the "bad" ones, I learned some good things or ways NOT to do things.

But Opec was special

That trip to Thailand I mentioned earlier. It was Opec's very first TDY as the new 12th TFS commander, and as I mentioned it was a very high-profile exercise. One would expect a brand-new commander to be a little nervous and maybe even rightfully conservative about how to conduct operations on the road. And, shortly after our arrival when the exercise opening ceremony was finished, Opec asked to meet with all of the pilots for a quick "commander's call."

We all assumed Opec was going to "lay down the law" for this TDY and we prepared to live with whatever rules Opec devised, although not exactly looking forward to it. What happened instead I remember very distinctly, and it made a huge impression on me for the rest of my career. Opec stood in front of all the Dozen pilots and said basically this, "Guys, we are here to fly and train with our Thai and US counterparts. I want you to fly hard and have fun. I have only one thing to ask of you. Please bring the jets home safe every day."

That was it! Bring the jets home safe every day! No rules! No restrictions! No admonitions or threats! Opec trusted us. Even though he knew a single accident or even minor incident could cost him his job, he trusted his pilots. WOW!

And everyday we flew hard ... we flew fast ... we pulled lots of Gs, and we brought the jets back to base in one piece. Because Opec had so much trust and faith in us, nobody in the Dozen wanted to betray that faith. We were our own best "police" and if we saw anybody stepping out of line and getting ready to do something stupid, then we would look after our own and make sure it didn't happen on Opec's watch.

It's not like that in the Air Force anymore. It hasn't been for a long time, and there are many reasons for it. I will get into that later in the book.

For now, Opec had cornered me in the squadron and wanted to talk to me. I had no idea what it was about. Usually he was the bearer of good news ... maybe a new, good-deal TDY I get to go on or something?

Opec said "Kluso, have you ever heard of Constant Carrot?" "Constant WHAT?" I said, "No, Sir. What is that?" Opec chuckled and said, "It's where they take a carrot and stick it up your ass!" Then he continued while we both laughed, "No, actually it's an Air Force program in which each year they give the wing one F-15 assignment that they can give to anybody they want, and the wing commander chose you as the Constant Carrot winner for this year. Congratulations!"

I was floored. I had just been handed a follow-on F-15 assignment. It was beyond my imagination that this could happen. The first thing I did was call the Aggressor commander in the Philippines and tell him I was sorry, but I would have to turn down the assignment he was holding for me. When he heard the reason why, he understood what the opportunity meant and he was very happy for me.

The next thing I did was tell Sako. We would probably be going back to the United States. It was not too long before I found out that we would be headed to Eglin AFB in Florida. The same base the "other guy" got three years prior on Assignment Night. Funny how things work out.

Before moving on to the next assignment, there is one thing I have to make clear about my first Eagle assignment in the Dirty Dozen. I know that for most pilots their first fighter squadron assignment is usually the most memorable. It's true for many reasons, but mostly I think it is because it's their first exposure to the fighter-pilot culture and the extremely close bonds of friendship and camaraderie that are nurtured in it. I can say the same about my own experience.

But my first three years in the Dozen at Kadena go well beyond that. I think I can make this statement without hesitation: I credit everything I was able to accomplish in my career—and I mean everything—to my first assignment in the 12th Tactical Fighter Squadron. I may have still gone to the same places, done the same things, fought the same war, etc., etc., but I would not have done any of it as well as I did without the opportunities and the mentoring I received in the Dozen.

Period. Dot.

CHAPTER 6

The Gorillas

Sako and I showed up at Eglin AFB as newlyweds. Literally we had "just married" the previous month before in Okinawa; we had not even had time to get her a permanent visa. She ended up being able to enter the United States on a valid tourist visa she still had in her Japanese passport. Not to worry, she went back to Okinawa a couple of months later to pick up her permanent visa when it arrived at the US Consulate there.

I was assigned to the 58th TFS ... the "Gorillas."

I don't know if I just got lucky, or if I had been "drafted" (hand-picked) for the Gorillas, but I was coming into the squadron as a highly experienced Eagle driver with instructor and mission commander qualifications. Most squadrons would kill for an experienced guy to show up basically "ready-to-go."

The 58th was unique in the F-15 air superiority fighter community because they were the very first F-15C squadron in the Air Force to get "MSIP" jets (pronounced "Miss-ipp"). This stood for Multi-Stage Improvement Program (MSIP).

To break it down into simple language, these were the newest F-15Cs coming off the McDonnell Douglas assembly line with significant radar, hardware, and software modifications to allow them eventually to integrate and employ the next generation AAM—the AIM-120 AMRAAM (Advanced Medium Range Air-to-Air Missile). We didn't have any AMRAAMs in the Air Force inventory yet, but once we did the Gorillas would be the first to get them.

What was significant about the AMRAAM is that it would be the first AAM to have its own on-board active radar (a mini version of a pulse-doppler radar like that found on the F-15). The AIM-120 would allow the pilot to fire the missile without having to continue to guide and support the shot all the way to the final intercept of the target. This was called "launch-and-leave."

When I arrived in the Gorillas, it was obvious that they had also "drafted" other experienced pilots and were building a dynasty of sorts. The squadron commander was Lt Col Frank "Paco" Geisler, and he can pretty much be credited with being the one who built the Gorillas into the squadron that would perform so well in

DESERT STORM. Paco was a legend in his own right. Having just recently come from the same 4477th Test and Evaluation Squadron (TES) "Red Eagles" that I flew against in CONSTANT PEG at Nellis, Paco was a fighter pilot's fighter pilot. He was known to do whatever it takes to get the job done ... and he did.

Another huge opportunity I had was to come under the tutelage of one more great FWIC (Weapons School) graduate—Capt Steve "Mongo" Robbins. Even though I had come to Eglin as a fully qualified instructor pilot, I was stripped of all of those qualifications and I had to start upgrade training from the bottom up. For most of the guys in the squadron (including myself) it did not really make a lot of sense, but actually I did not mind. Being in an upgrade program gave me priority on the flying schedule, and I would be able to fly with other instructors to learn and share techniques, and that included being able to fly a lot of my sorties with Mongo. I felt like I was being groomed to go to Weapons School, but I also knew I was still "young" and would have to wait my turn. In the meantime, I was going to soak up all the instruction and experience I could.

Things worked out well, and I quickly advanced through all the upgrade events (most of which had been shortened based on my experience). Finally, I was back in the Instructor Upgrade program and I was flying my final "check-ride" with Mongo. It was a 4 vs. 4 (4 × F-15s versus 4 × Adversary) Tactical Intercept mission against some F-16 Vipers who were visiting Eglin to fly DACT against the Gorillas. The 4 vs. 4 is kind of the "bread-and-butter" mission of the F-15 community. The baseline air-to-air employment entity for F-15s has always been the "4-ship" formation. If you could not do well leading a 4-ship, you generally could not progress to higher-level positions.

My coordination and 4-ship employment brief went very well (I'd had a lot of experience briefing those by this point), but the proof was going to be in the actual execution of the mission or how well we did against the F-16s. It was a bit of a grudge match when fighting Vipers, because the F-15 was considered *the* air superiority fighter in the Air Force, while the F-16 was a dual-role fighter that performed mostly air-to-ground strike missions. The F-16 pilots often carried a bit of a chip on their shoulders (not all, but many) about this, and maybe rightfully so, because the F-16 was a very capable air-to-air fighter in the hands of an experienced pilot. But they did not train to this mission as much as the Eagle community did, and they did not have the longer-range weapons (AIM-7 semi-active radar missile) that we had. But they could be good at drawing us in close and trying to get an Eagle into a "knife-fight" (within visual weapons range), where it was a much more even match.

I was not too concerned about doing well until, as I was checking my flight in on the radio prior to taxi and takeoff, and I found out two of my flight members were having maintenance problems and had "ground aborted" their jets. That meant they had cancelled their sortie due to a broken jet. There were no spare Eagles available for the now "grounded" pilots to fly, so it looked like it was going to be just me and Mongo against the full 4-ship of Vipers—2 vs. 4.

Those poor guys never had a chance.

With the best "wingman" in the squadron flying with me, I employed every trick I knew to keep the Vipers at bay, lure them into weapons parameters, avoid getting outmaneuvered by their superior numbers, and achieve simulated "kills" against all of the F-16s (a couple of times over) without them ever completing a single valid "shot" against either Mongo or myself. By time the four Viper drivers walked into the room for our debrief session, they already knew that they had taken a pretty good lickin'. What made it worse for them, though, was that they did not know until about halfway through the debrief that it was only Mongo and I out there giving them the business. They thought they got beat up by a full 4-ship of Eagles (which probably would have been forgivable), but when they found out we were just a 2-ship ... the Viper drivers all just slumped in their chairs. I did my best to be gracious for their efforts during the remainder of the debrief.

Afterwards, Mongo, as the IP of record, had his chance to critique me on my performance and regardless of how well I did that day, he still had some constructive criticism for me. That's just the way it is in the fighter world. There is always room for improvement, but I obviously passed the ride. A couple of days later I found the written grade sheet for that mission in my flight upgrade folder. I had never saved a grade sheet before on any of my upgrades, but this one I removed after the upgrade was over and kept it for posterity.

Fighter upgrade missions are generally graded on an alpha-numeric scale. The grade of "U" means Unsatisfactory (also known as a "hook") or a failed upgrade mission that would have to be performed again. From there the numeric grades went from 1 to 4, with 1 being "Below Average" (and generally, not good); 2 was "Average" and normally would be considered a solid passing grade; 3 was "Outstanding" and normally very difficult to achieve; and, 4? Well it was just there as the ultimate but unachievable goal. The last line Mongo wrote on my grade sheet read, "I have NEVER given an overall grade of '4' before, but I cannot think of any reason why this ride did not deserve it. Maybe I'm getting soft."

I think after that ride, Mongo and I both knew I was ready to go to Weapons School.

***

I still had more waiting and flying to do, though, before I would finally be selected to Fighter Weapons School, and once again to my benefit. Being the only F-15C MSIP squadron in the Air Force meant we were on-call to assist the 422nd TES (Test & Evaluation Squadron) out at Nellis AFB.

The 422nd was a special squadron tasked with evaluating and integrating new capabilities, technologies, and tactics before they would be accepted and employed in the rest of the Tactical Air Force (TAF). This was a great concept because it allowed a group of experienced and capable fighter pilots to make recommendations based on sound theories and actual in-flight testing to give the operational fighter community a "leg-up" on developing new tactics and procedures.

Without the 422nd, it could take years for different operational squadrons to accomplish the same evaluations, bickering between themselves about the best way to do business. The 422nd provided a good foundation for this process and helped streamline the baseline tactics development. The reality, however, is that full-scale combat tactics need to be established and trained to by the weapons officers at the actual operational squadron/wing level against regional threats and tactics. It is one of the primary reasons for the original establishment of the USAF FWIC. Unfortunately, that philosophy has changed over the years, and not necessarily for the better. I will discuss this later in this book.

So, from 1988 to 1989, the Gorillas were often out at Nellis with a group of pilots and jets to assist the 422nd with MSIP Advanced Launch & Leave Tactics in anticipation of eventual AIM-120 AMRAAM operational capability. Since the 422nd could only generally put up about four F-15Cs and pilots in the air at any given time, they needed the Gorillas's extra MSIP jets and experienced pilots so they could fly large-force tactics development of eight Eagles or more.

I was selected to go along on a lot of these trips, and they gave me opportunity again to fly with experienced IPs and weapons officers, and also to be the mission commander for some of these advanced tactics missions. Bonus!

Time and patience finally paid off, and in the summer of 1989, while I was out at Nellis on a 422nd test trip, Paco gave me a call and congratulated me on my selection to Class 89CIN for the Fall FWIC. I was going to Weapons School! But there were two problems. First, I had been selected to attend Squadron Officers School (SOS) that summer. This was an intermediate-level "professional officer development course" that most fighter pilots thought of as a total waste of time. It would not prevent me from going to Weapons School, but it would impact the important preparation time and flying training that the squadron would want me to go through before heading to Nellis. Paco said, "Don't worry about that … I will get that shut off." Cool.

The second problem was that Sako was pregnant with our first child, and her due date was smack in the middle of Weapons School. This was my problem, and it was a big one. The Weapons School is an intense four months (at that time, now it's six months) conducting the highest level of fighter pilot training in the Air Force. It's really "doctorate" level training for fighter pilots and requires 100% time and focus. It's a TDY also, meaning they don't provide housing and extra support for spouses or family members. Most pilots would not bring their wives or families with them.

I did not want to leave Sako alone back at Eglin either. Being a Japanese spouse, she really did not have in Florida any close friends (and definitely no family) that she could count on to support her, or get her to doctor appointments, or to the hospital when the baby was on its way. We decided that the best thing for her to do was to go back to Okinawa to be with her family and use the US military hospital facilities on base there. It was hard to have that kind of separation with our first-born due, but I had some comfort knowing she was with family. I would later go pick her up right after I graduated from Weapons School and bring her and our new baby daughter Sakura back home with us to Florida.

***

I drove four days cross-country from Fort Walton Beach, Florida, to Nellis AFB, Nevada, in late August 1989. I had been to Nellis many, many times, but I had never driven there. It was a nice (but long and lonely) road trip across the southern half of the United States.

I checked into billeting (our apartment-like rooms on base) and no sooner had I dropped my bags that one of my new classmates was knocking on my door. Actually, he wasn't "new" at all ... it was Russ "Job" Handy. Job and I had shown up at Kadena basically at the same time in 1984 as first assignment Eagle pilots, and Job had also done good work impressing the leadership there. He actually received the previous year's CONSTANT CARROT award, and his follow-on Eagle assignment was to Langley AFB, Virginia. Just like me, Job waited his turn and finally got the call to attend Weapons School. Our career paths would be almost strangely identical all the way up to the point where I left the Air Force and Job stayed in to eventually become a general officer.

Job told me another one of our classmates was already at Nellis and he took me upstairs to meet Scott "Scooter" Brown (it seemed like almost every fighter pilot with the first name of Scott ended up with a "Scooter" call-sign). Scooter and I seemed to click right away. Not sure why, because we had not known each other at all before this, but I just took a liking to his personality and dry sense of humor. Plus, Scooter was always "up" for a good time and didn't mind coming up with great ideas of things to do to keep us amused.

The first thing Scooter suggested was that we go to the Class Six (the base liquor store) and buy a bunch of beer, whiskey, and Jeremiah Weed (that nasty sweet liquor we all pretended to like), in anticipation of the remaining classmates arriving. So, we put notes on their room doors to meet us up in Scooter's room, hit the Class Six, brought back the booze, and soon there were six of us getting this whole Weapons School tour off to a great start! How hard could it be anyway?

The other classmates were Charles "Bones" Shugg, T.G. "Krazy" Kyrazis, and Mark "Link" Stevens.

We proceeded to get plastered that night and decided early on that if this Weapons School thing was going to be as much of a "ball-buster" as everybody said, at least we were going to have fun (while getting our balls busted), and we set about doing just that.

As a class of six, we bonded quickly and pretty much became inseparable—"attached at the hip," as they might say. Whether supporting each other through the coursework and flying events or finding different ways to "light our hair on fire" in the city that never sleeps, we spent virtually every day and night out together for the entire four months. Other than actual combat, I cannot think of any other setting or affair like Weapons School, which provided a shared experience that all of us remember to this day.

At Weapons School we were the students, and we were known as (or called) "FWUGs" ... Fighter Weapons Up-Gradees. We accepted the term as a badge of honor, and like other FWUGs before us, the Barnyard IPs (Barnyard was the nickname for the F-15 Division of the Weapons School) expected us to make a name for ourselves, somehow. We started that process early when Class 89CIN met the Barnyard instructors for the first time. We already knew some of these guys, and for the most part they were all our heroes. These were the guys who had been our squadron weapons officers. We had looked up to them for all these years, trying to get to the same place they were and earn the right to wear the coveted USAF Fighter Weapons School patch on our left shoulder. We were star struck.

Still, that did not prevent us from being cheeky. Somebody gave us a sheet of paper that we were supposed to fill out with our personal data, emergency contact information, and also to tell the IPs a little about ourselves. When asked, at the end of the document, to include what we think we do best, we all decided to put the exact same quote; "Walks on water ... except when partying." Actually, Link Stevens came up with the idea for that quotation, but it was in fact supposed to be, "Walks on water ... except when parting it." We had all just misunderstood him. We liked what we came up with better anyway.

Apparently, the IPs thought this was amusing too, because the very next day when we showed up at the Barnyard dressed in our full flight suits and boots, the IPs decided to take us on a base tour. So, they piled us into an Air Force step van, and drove us around the base showing us all the sites and places we should know about. What a great bunch of guys ...

That is until we pulled up in front of the base swimming pool and they ordered us all to get out. This was not looking good. Upon reaching the edge of the pool, the IPs reminded us of what we had written on our in-processing forms the day before. "Walks on water ..." So, they said, "Prove it!" In flight suits and boots, we each stepped off one-by-one into the pool and immediately sank to the bottom. The only one of us who had a chance was Krazy Kyrazis. As the rest of us formed a line in the water, and as Krazy stepped off the side of the pool, we each in turn placed our hands under Krazy's flight boots in an attempt to allow him to "walk on water." We did pretty good and Krazy actually made it about halfway across the pool, until he lost his balance a touch, wobbled, and fell in, much to the delight and laughter of the Barnyard IPs. I think we earned a little bit of their respect that day, at least on the ground. In the air would be another thing.

***

I *loved* Weapons School. It was hard and demanding, but our entire focus (and the focus of the Barnyard IPs) was on becoming the absolute best Eagle instructor pilots and weapons officers. We had nothing else to do or think about for four months other than that.

I think I had an edge on some of the other guys. Because of my experience at Kadena, and because of my other advanced-level opportunities at Eglin, I was really prepared for Weapons School. The first phase of the training was BFM or 1 vs. 1 maneuvering against another F-15 flown by one of the Weapons School IPs. I was fortunate because I was already a pretty good BFM'er, and I flew many preparation sorties at Eglin against some really good IPs, including Rob "Cheese" Graeter, one of the best BFM'ers in the Air Force. Cheese was another Dirty Dozen alumnus. He left Kadena just a few weeks after I arrived and went on to fly F-5 Aggressors and then with the 422nd at Nellis, before attending FWIC and then heading to Eglin. We would fly together a lot more in the next year after Weapons School.

I did well in the BFM phase, and regularly outperformed the Barnyard IPs. While some of my classmates struggled, I did not "bust" (fail) a single BFM mission, until the last one (or what would turn out to be my next to last). This BFM sortie was to be a "dissimilar" BFM fight against an IP in the F-16 Division. Ahhhh … our nemesis, Mr. Viper Driver.

On these sorties, our Barnyard F-15 IPs were actually on our side, really pulling for us to "spank" the F-16 IPs in order to maintain harmony in the universe. After pretty much having my way with the Barnyard IPs, I felt confident (as they did also) that I would take care of business. Unfortunately, we were both to be disappointed.

I was up against (whether by bad luck or design) the IP who was known as the best BFM'er in the F-16 Division. I realized it right away on the first setup where I started with the offensive advantage and he was quickly able to neutralize that advantage and prevent me from obtaining valid "shot/kill" parameters.

On the next setup, when I started out in a defensive position I was hoping to do the same to him, but instead I found myself fighting for my life. I was able to survive and hold off the more experienced Viper driver for quite a while, but at the very end I ran out of altitude, airspeed, and ideas, and he was able to get a valid simulated "gun kill" on me. The final engagement, from a neutral starting position, ended up staying neutral until we both ran low on gas and had to "knock-it-off" and RTB.

I did not perform terribly, but I knew my F-15 IP overseeing the mission was as disappointed as I was. I still had a chance, however, to "save it in the debrief," that is, if I could show I understood all the mistakes I had made and how to correct them I could still "pass" the ride. It was not to be though.

Sometimes our failures provide the best opportunity to learn. On that day I learned an important lesson about flying against a dissimilar airplane versus an experienced (and maybe better) pilot. I had started to become too relaxed flying against other F-15 pilots whose maneuvering and performance I had seen so many times over and over. I could almost guess what they were going to do next (or at least recognize it quickly) and know the exact timing and type of counter move to make each time. It had become too easy ... too "canned." On this day, when I met up with another pilot in a different airplane, I had forgotten the most important part of BFM—maneuver in relation to the bandit (the adversary airplane).

The importance of BFM in our training is not only for the 1 vs. 1 combat maneuvering aspect. It is also a critical building block to all higher-level training that follows. Some who don't really understand this, in particular senior leaders who imagine we will never again need close-in visual combat maneuvering due to advanced longer-range weapons, believe there is no purpose to continue this type of training. Contrary to this viewpoint is the fact that the essential link between BFM and the rest of our combat training is the high-speed, high-intensity, mental aspect of the process (even though it is very physically demanding also). In actual combat, "tempo" is everything. If you can get the advantage in tempo versus your adversary, whether in individual maneuvering or larger force tactics, then you are always one step ahead and can gain and hold the advantage. This all starts in BFM.

A fighter pilot not only has to know how his own jet can perform, but also the performance capabilities of the adversary. Then, he has to be able to assess quickly what the bandit is doing with his airplane (in relation to your own), all the while maneuvering at 5-Gs to 9-Gs, and sometimes twisted around looking almost directly back behind your own jet (like Linda Blair in *The Exorcist*). Next, but within milliseconds, he has to make a determination of what is the best counter maneuver (among several options), and even then, perfectly max perform his own jet to fly that maneuver, and while doing so simultaneously start the assessment process again, continuing until the outcome is decided.

It is this process of dynamic observation, decision, and implementation, and staying one step ahead of your adversary, that can be used in every other phase of training and combat. It is basically a microcosm of a bigger concept called "the OODA loop," for *Observe, Orient, Decide, and Act*, originally applied to the grander scale of combat operations. In this case, even in individual or small-scale combat events, the one who can control the fight by driving a more-aggressive and timely OODA loop will generally be the victor. Canned maneuvers and static tactics are doomed to failure over time.

I had failed correctly to analyze my adversary's moves, his energy state, and airspeed, where his jet had an advantage or disadvantage over mine, and my counter moves were a bit late or poorly performed. By the time I had come to the end of my debrief, my F-15 IP (Major "Doc" O'Neil) allowed me to come to my own conclusions and ultimately a more enlightened understanding of what I had done wrong and how to fix it.

Doc's example of instructional oversight also became an important lesson for my future as an F-15 IP and weapons officer. Don't just "tell" somebody what they are doing wrong and how to fix it. Instead, lead them to the point where they come to realize it somehow on their own. This is how to truly "teach" somebody anything.

The other lesson was to never underestimate your adversary. You have to assume that the pilot you meet in a 1 vs. 1 situation in combat is the enemy's best pilot. No slack and no mercy. I did well on my "repeat" ride against a less-fortunate F-16 IP.

***

The next phase of training was Advanced Combat Maneuvering (ACM), and in the Eagle community I had already come to recognize it was one of the weakest areas of employment expertise. Even in Weapons School, for some reason, it received very little emphasis.

The basic idea of ACM training is for an element (2-ship) of friendly fighters to work together either to defend/survive against, or quickly dispatch, a single adversary aircraft—it is 2 vs. 1. It requires practiced coordination for the two fighters to decide who is in the position of advantage (or who can gain it earlier) and who will be in the "engaged" fighter role, or who will be the "supporting" fighter. The engaged fighter is supposed to fly his "best" BFM against the adversary, either to get the quick kill or effectively defend himself as long as possible until the supporting fighter can provide help. A defensive fighter is *de facto* always the "engaged" fighter, since he must fly his best BFM to survive, neutralize, or separate from the bandit. The supporting fighter is supposed to stay out of the way of the engaged fighter, but constantly on the lookout for opportunities to get a kill on the adversary if the engaged fighter is defensive, or if the engaged fighter is not in position to gain an advantage and deliver his own kill. ACM requires a high level of tactical techniques and practice, as well as good communication between the two friendly fighters. It's not easy, by any means.

Even though this area of training has been a foundation of air-to-air combat training for many years, the advent of more modern and capable all-aspect air-to-air heat-seeking missiles and more reliable radar-guided missiles like the AIM-7 (or similar adversary counterparts) means it is much more difficult to survive in this combat environment even when entering the fight with a 2 vs. 1 numerical advantage.

A very dangerous zone exists within a 1–5 nautical mile (nm) circle of an adversary's nose, where he may be able to take a shot on either the engaged or supporting fighter. Even if the adversary ends up defeated, once a launch-and-leave weapon comes off his jet (if the adversary has such weapons), then one or both of the friendly fighters may also suffer in the engagement. This would be called a "mutual kill," and for our purposes, it's an unacceptable result.

The only way to deny a mutual kill opportunity for the adversary is for the engaged fighter to obtain an offensive advantage (behind the bandit, where he cannot employ offensive weapons) while the supporting fighter "stiff-arms" the adversary's mutual kill zone until the supporting fighter can find the exact opportunity to re-enter the fight, get the kill, and still be in a position to defend himself from the adversary.

Another important concept in ACM is only to enter the merge (a visual-range maneuvering fight) with an offensive advantage and, whether you are offensive or defensive, to end the fight quickly either with a fast kill or by separating from the fight as soon as possible. While everyday combat training emphasized a sterile 2 vs. 1 environment, the reality of combat is that we should always expect more bandits to be out there.

Once an Eagle starts turning-and-burning, its large size and wing planform makes it stick out in the sky like "dog balls." For this reason, my personal technique was to normally establish a "180-degree rule" for deciding if, how, and when to "throw out the anchor" for an ACM engagement. What that means is that if we could not enter the merge and dispatch the adversary within about 180 degrees of turn (about 15 seconds of time), then the best decision should instead be to disengage from the adversary. If the adversary chose to disregard your decision, then hopefully he would suffer the consequences of a poor choice and another friendly fighter would dispatch the bandit.

I credit my Aggressor friends, and the oversight of some great Dirty Dozen IPs at Kadena, for continuing to pound this theory into my head—never remain anchored in a turning fight any longer than necessary.

At COPE THUNDERs I learned to stay well outside of the fighter "fur balls," where many jets would engage in a swirling dogfight that looked like gnats gathering in a summer twilight. I would pick off the unknowing bandits as they spat out of the mature engagement, unaware that another Eagle was waiting for them. Maybe this was something like you might see on a National Geographic documentary on ocean baitfish; a fish is relieved to avoid an obvious marauder, only to swim straight into the mouth of another waiting predator.

I wanted somehow to work to improve the overall concepts of ACM in the modern air combat environment. With that in mind, I decided that my written thesis for my Weapons School graduation requirements would focus on All-Aspect Advanced Combat Maneuvering (AAACM). The basic concepts of what I wrote in 1989 are still valid today, but unfortunately mostly overlooked or forgotten. But, for my wingman and me, I would get a chance to test them out in combat over southern Iraq.

***

The "Art of the Intercept" is another area that has fallen into disrepair. The "intercept" is the complete execution of a tactic from the very beginning (or commit) to the (hopefully) successful end result. Sometimes "successful" does not always mean killing the adversary; it could just mean preventing him or her from completing the mission.

The commit phase would normally start anywhere from 40 to 80nm away (depending on many factors) and would involve multiples of 2- to 4-ship F-15 formations working together. The basic technical portions of the intercept involved delegating and locking individual F-15 radars into the bandit formations (called "targeting") to maximize firepower and take out as many bandits in one fell swoop with BVR weapons like the AIM-7 (or nowadays, the AIM-120).

The "art" portion of the intercept was to try to complete the intercept to a position of advantage (POA). To define POA loosely, it would mean to put the Eagle formation in a place and time where we would have an offensive advantage, but still be able to leave or defend ourselves if for some reason we would lose that advantage. This is the portion of tactical employment that has largely been replaced today by dependence on technological advantage of weapons and weapons systems.

The intercept only has a practical application when applied to the two most basic mission areas the F-15 Eagle would perform in combat (because "intercept" is not really a tactical mission area). Those areas are Defensive Counter Air (DCA) and Offensive Counter Air (OCA). DCA means flying in defensive CAPs to find and destroy or negate any enemy strike aircraft (i.e. those that carry bombs or other ground-attack ordnance) and any escort aircraft that might be there to defend them. The objective of such a mission area is to put the entire priority on killing the "bomb-droppers" or getting them to abandon their mission before reaching their target. The enemy escort aircraft should either be avoided, forced to split up their forces, or accept a position of disadvantage in order to protect the strikers. This is where the "art" part comes in—how to effect that end result?

OCA, for the Eagle community, was just kind of the reverse role of DCA. Then the job was to keep the enemy away from our friendly strike package, by either forcing the enemy to go through us to get to the strikers or force the bandits to make a choice between going after the strikers or the F-15 OCA escort/sweep. The "art" part of this mission area was to set up our POA by developing smart tactics and fluid and flexible tactical execution.

The age-old problem with becoming dependent on technology is that there are always counter-tactics and countermeasures that can negate technological advantage. This lesson has been relearned (the hard way) in every major area of combat throughout history. What generally cannot be negated or denied are the laws of physics and the imagination and courage inherent in the human heart and mind.

***

From my experience at Kadena, my "top off" training at Eglin, and my experience at Fighter Weapons School, I felt like I had reached a level of expertise unimaginable just five years prior. Having a class of very talented and highly capable fighter pilots around me, I was honored to be named the Outstanding Graduate F-15 Division for FWIC Class 89CIN. In fact, I would go on to be named overall Top Graduate of the Year (1989) and I was the Robbie Risner Award nominee for the F-15 Division the following year for the overall Top Weapons School Graduate for the entire USAF. (Note: I would not win that award.)

The one thing I had learned up to that point, though, is that "you're only as good as your last mission," meaning you cannot rest on your laurels in the fighter business. The search for continuous improvement in tactics, techniques, and experience is essential to combat success. And I had another challenge … it was now my job to prepare the Gorillas to go to war.

While I was in the 12th TFS at Kadena, there was a lithograph in the Dirty Dozen weapons and tactics vault (where we studied, planned, and briefed all our training missions). On the litho was a painting of a North Korean MiG fighter going down in flames as it was being engaged by an F-15. The slogan written on the litho bluntly stated, "The War starts TOMORROW."

That was always our attitude at Kadena. With only an armistice in place, the Korean peninsula was in a constant state of preparedness and under the expectation that war could break out at any moment (hence our constant scramble alert posture at Osan AB). We always carried that awareness around with us at Kadena, whether we were training at home or in Korea, or anywhere in the Pacific.

At Eglin, it was a little bit different. We were a "state-side" unit and not on "the tip of the spear" as we would say at Kadena. There were all the normal distractions in both the social and training environment of the squadron. Being "at home" in the United States meant family, hobbies, and individual desires that did not always promote a strong focus on combat training or cohesiveness. We were a little bit fortunate in the 58th because (as I mentioned before) we did have several experienced squadron leaders who had lived and trained overseas (even at Kadena), and we also had many unit deployments (TDYs) away from home base, all of which promoted a vigilant attitude.

Still, we were not close to "the war" or the possibility of such. Eglin's primary area of responsibility for contingency combat operations was in the European Theater. Our mission was to support NATO and the defense of Europe against the Soviet "hordes" from air bases in Germany. There was only one problem with that—peace was breaking out all over Europe.

***

The downfall of Soviet communism was actually occurring while I was at Weapons School (not that I had much time to notice). By the time I returned to the Gorillas in late December 1989, the Berlin Wall had already fallen and most of Eastern Europe was on the path to independence from what would soon be called the "former Soviet Union."

The "FORMER" Soviet Union … unbelievable.

Not that any of us were against a de-escalation of the not-so-Cold War. After all, only a crazy person or a sociopath would desire full-scale warfare just to get their kicks. But we did come to the realization that we in President Ronald Reagan's Air Force had been built up, equipped, and trained specifically to take on the huge and what we thought was indomitable Soviet military machine. We had no doubt that if the day came when we faced off with the Soviets we would win a conventional matchup, but there would be enormous devastation and we would lose a lot of our friends along the way. Worse, the greater specter was the likely escalation to full-blown thermonuclear war.

So all in all, we were happy with the turn of events. The only problem now was *who* would we focus on as a possible future adversary and how would we train against this fictional entity? We didn't know, and it made my job that much harder. How could I keep my young and inexperienced Eagle pilots motivated and working on the critical combat training events they needed to master?

Upon my return to Eglin, I made a concerted effort to develop a comprehensive flying and academic training plan to keep everyone focused on preparing for the possibility of combat, even though that possibility now seemed so distant. It wasn't easy to keep their attention and I remember often seeing a few pilots snoozing during my academic lecture sessions. Funny, a few short months later those same pilots would be regretting not paying more attention during my lectures.

Compounding these preparation issues, the Gorillas had also recently undergone a large turnover in experienced pilots and received an influx of "newbies," or first-time fighter pilots who needed to go through initial MQT and other upgrades. Whereas a few years previously the 58th was benefitting from the "Paco" years of drafting experienced flyers to help with the MSIP upgrade, now we were turning over pilots just like any other squadron would do.

Not that I did not appreciate the crop of young Eagle Drivers we were receiving. We had some really talented "youngsters" join the Gorillas: Joe "Corn" Hruska, Tony "E.T." Murphy, Bruce "Roto" Till, Mark "Nips" Arriola, and Scott "Papa" Maw, to name a few. Another welcome addition to the Gorillas was my old friend from UPT—Larry "Cherry" Pitts. Cherry (he got that call-sign after completing his MQT qualification in the Gorillas) had finished up his tour as a UPT T-38 IP and finally got to do what he had always wanted to do—fly the F-15. Much like me, Cherry also had a new wife and a fresh start. It was good to have Cherry there and he quickly picked up the essential skills to be a great combat wingman. In fact, Cherry would end up becoming my wingman of choice.

Fortunately, the 58th continued to pick up some great training opportunities at RED FLAG at Nellis AFB and MAPLE FLAG at Canadian Forces Base, Coldlake, and other DACT events. The youngsters were progressing quickly … and they would need to. Storm clouds were brewing.

CHAPTER 7

Tabuk

We had no idea how quickly our world could spin on a dime.

It was an early August morning and I had just walked into the squadron to start what I expected would be a routine day for the Gorillas. First things first, I needed to get a cup of coffee and at least one smoke. I had never smoked cigarettes for most of my life, until I went through the divorce with Geri. I am not sure why I ever started. Maybe I was bored or just felt a little rebellious and wanted to do something "different," but once I started it sure was hard to stop. Sako did not like me smoking and was constantly encouraging me to quit, and I did my best. I had actually cut back to just a couple of cigarettes a day and expected I could quit completely any time I wanted to. But, for now, a morning smoke and a cup o'Joe was what I needed.

What I saw that morning on TV as I walked into the Gorilla bar/break room made me quickly realize I had "picked a bad day to quit smoking" (to quote *Airplane*). Cherry was in the bar too, where we often met for the same morning routine, and he said something like, "Hey, check this out!" I looked at a CNN breaking news-cast and watched video as some Langley 1st Fighter Wing F-15s (with three full external fuel tanks for a long trip) were taking off and heading toward Saudi Arabia. The headlines stated that Iraq had invaded neighboring Kuwait and President George Bush (the first one) had ordered an immediate and aggressive response.

Holy crap! It only made sense that if this potential contingency operation expanded, the Eglin F-15s would be next "on call." And it did, and we were.

We were told by our leadership to prepare to depart for Southwest Asia, most likely Saudi Arabia, within days. We had no idea of what base we might go to, what our mission might be when we got there, or what to prepare for. Hell, the Middle East had never been in our sights as a possible deployment location. It was a mad scramble to garner any kind of intelligence about the Iraqi Air Force (IrAF) and whatever likely deployment location we could get.

What now occurred over the next two weeks would be a constant yo-yo of up and down deployment warnings then cancellations. It was nerve racking, because one minute we would be "leaving tomorrow," then the next it would get cancelled with an expectation of leaving in another week's time. Or it would be, "We might never deploy, so don't get too excited." I think I must have said "Goodbye" to Sako and our baby girl Sakura at least three or four times, only to return home with all my packed bags. It was not easy to do.

Finally, my new squadron commander, Lt Col Bill "Tonic" Thiel, told us one day that the fun and games were over and we were definitely deploying the next morning. This was it.

I was not chosen to fly an F-15 all the way across the Atlantic to our destination, which was now declared as Tabuk, a Royal Saudi Air Force (RSAF) base. Instead, I was supposed to be on the Advon Team (Advanced Party), with the intent that we would arrive early and help with the setup of our operations and make preparations to commence combat sorties.

It didn't quite work out that way. The deployment plans for so many different squadrons, personnel, and equipment trying to get to the Southwest Asia Theater had taxed both airlift and tanker assets and planning staffs. My airlift flight ended up being diverted to another base and then a layover at Dover AFB, DE. We ended up getting into Saudi Arabia a good day-and-a-half after our jets and other pilots arrived at Tabuk. So much for planning ahead.

The only good part about the Advon flight was that our flight doc, Capt Kory Cornum, accompanied us. Doc Cornum had brought plenty of "supplies" with him and that included some little blue pills called Restoril. He handed them out to myself and the other pilots to insure we arrived "fresh" in-theater.

I don't recall much of the long multi-layover flight, because I had a great sleep along the way. I would come to appreciate how much Doc Cornum was able to use his medical expertise to keep myself and all the other pilots fully combat ready regardless of our operations tempo. "Better life through chemicals" was the motto I believe.

Kory was actually married to an Army flight surgeon, Maj Rhonda Cornum. Rhonda would later be shot down over Iraq on a combat rescue mission and captured by the Iraqis. Afterward she co-wrote a book about her experiences, *She Went to War: the Rhonda Cornum Story.*

The initial panic to get forces into Saudi Arabia eventually cooled off a bit, as Saddam Hussein had apparently decided to be content with occupying only Kuwait for the time being and did not seem to be threatening to cross the Saudi border. Still, we knew that could change at any moment. But when I finally arrived on the ramp at Tabuk and was met by Tonic, he told me to relax as we were in a "Hurry Up and Wait" mode for now.

***

We were a bit lucky with the draw of Tabuk as our deployed location. Actually known to the RSAF as King Faisal Air Base, to us it was just Tabuk. Home primarily to a couple of RSAF F-5 fighter squadrons, Tabuk is located on the west side of Saudi Arabia on a high plateau just east of the Red Sea and the coastal mountains that border the ocean. This location provided a much more moderate and dry climate than the rest of the Saudi bases, which were sweltering in either high heat or high

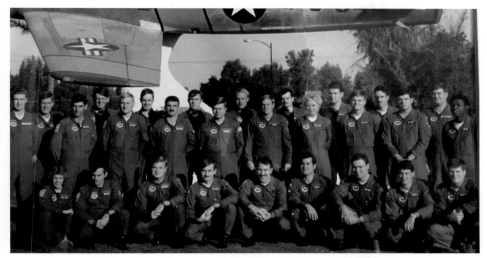

Class photo, Undergraduate Pilot Training (UPT) at Williams AFB, AZ, circa 1983. Kluso standing back row, 4th from right, directly behind his friend and eventual DESERT STORM wingman, Larry "Cherry" Pitts (right side of Kluso). Other friends from the famed Superstition Mountains/Lost Dutchman State Park expedition include Gordon "Kuch" Kucera (left side in front of Kluso), Mark Catherman (back row, first on the right), Kurt Skadeland (back row, first on the left), and Darwin Frevert (standing, fifth from the left). (Photograph courtesy of Larry Pitts, Williams Air Force Base, AZ, circa 1983)

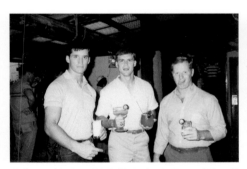

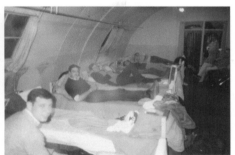

(*left to right*) Greg "Odie" Neubeck, Bruce "Phoid" Netardus, and Rick "Lips" VanDeusen, most likely in a Clark Air Base, Philippines bar. Odie was my sponsor on my first tour in "the Dozen" (the 12th TFS) at Kadena Air Base, Okinawa. Phoid and I would share a second F-15 assignment together at Eglin AFB, where we were teammates on the 1988 William Tell aerial competition team. Phoid would tragically die in a flying accident at Nellis, AFB, NV, several years later. (Photographer unknown, Clark Air Base, Philippines, mid-1980s)

Kluso's first taste of life on the road (TDY—temporary duty) with a fighter squadron. At Japan Air Self Defense Force (JASDF) air base Chitose (near Sapporo) for Exercise COPE NORTH. Barracks-style living and sleeping arrangements allowed for the ultimate bonding experience. Fly—fight—drink … rinse and repeat. (Photographer unknown, Chitose Air Base, Japan, circa 1985)

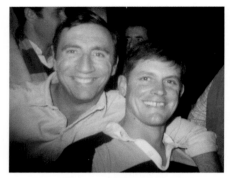

Two of Kluso's earliest fighter pilot mentors, Major Gary "Uncle Budge" Wilson, and Major Jeff "Jiffy-Jeff" Brown. Taking Kluso under their wing they (and others) would lead Kluso on the path of developing a professional approach to becoming the best fighter pilot possible ... and the culture of fighter pilot traditions. (Photographer unknown, Kadena Air Base, Japan, circa 1985)

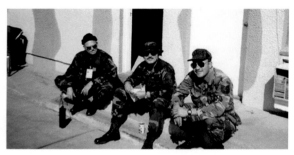

Chief Master Sergeant Matos (center) with his senior non-commissioned officer (SNCO) production supervisors at Royal Saudi Air Base (RSAB) Tabuk: (left) Master Sergeant Bernie Sweeka, and (right) Master Sergeant "Alex" Alexander. Working closely with Kluso during DESERT STORM planning stages they were able to assist in providing the highest air superiority asset sortie/mission rate in the combat theater, and revolutionize how to efficiently task combat air patrol missions in the future. (Photograph courtesy of CMSgt (Ret) Jose Matos, Royal Saudi Air Base, Tabuk, Saudi Arabia, circa 1990)

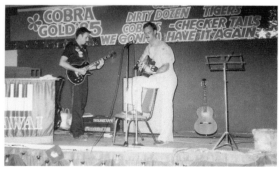

Displaying his love of music and live performance that would follow him into his post-Air Force life, Kluso (left) with his good friend Robert "Zombie" Scott. An impromptu performance at the End of Exercise party, Exercise COBRA GOLD, Hat Yai, Thailand. (Photographer unknown, Hat Yai Air Base, Republic of Thailand, circa 1986)

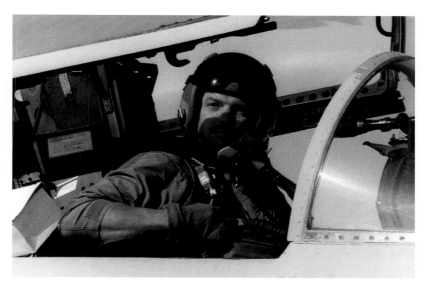

Kluso's wingman, Capt Larry "Cherry" Pitts, in the cockpit of his F-15C. Note the rifle scope attached to a bracket on the right side of the photo. This was known as an "Eagle Eye" and allowed a pilot to identify a potential hostile aircraft from a safer standoff distance. (Photograph courtesy of Larry Pitts, Tabuk Royal Saudi Air Base, circa 1990)

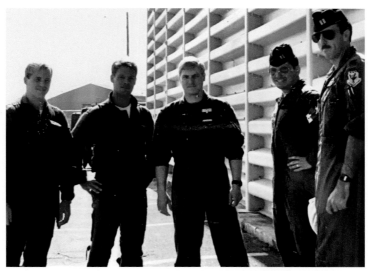

Kluso and members of an Osan Air Base (Republic of Korea) PARPRO Alert team. Ready to scramble two F-15Cs, at no notice, into the skies bordering South Korea and North Korea to protect US airborne reconnaissance aircraft from North Korean threats. (Left to right) Craig "Sumo" Adler (Kluso's first squadrons weapons officer, instrumental in Kluso's tactical progress as a fighter pilot), Tom "Mouth" Gemmell (young wingman, first Alert tour), Maury "Skins" Forsythe (similar first-tour Eagle driver, but seasoned from experience as an F-4 Weapons System Officer), unknown pilot, and Kluso (in his classic RayBan shades). (Photograph courtesy of Thomas L. Gemmell, Osan Air Base, Republic of Korea, circa 1987)

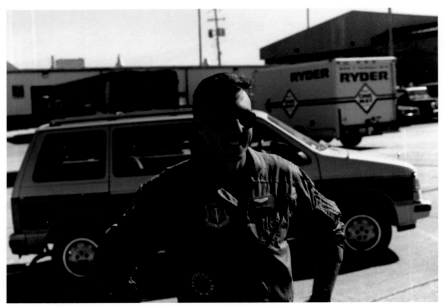

Kluso, shortly after his arrival at Tyndall AFB, FL, for the world-wide aerial competition William Tell '88 (note the special William Tell commemorative patch on Kluso's flight suit, below his right zipper pocket). (Photo by Theresa Hicks, 58TFS, Tyndall Air Force Base, FL, circa 1988)

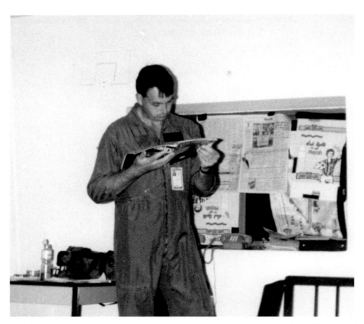

58th TFS assigned Flight Surgeon, Captain Kory "Doc" Cornum, in his deployed "clinic" (note *Stars and Stripes* newspaper clipped to the poster board in background). Doc Cornum was a hero to the deployed Gorilla pilots, following the creed "better life through chemicals," he was able to keep the pilots alert when needed during weeks of grueling 18-hour day combat duty cycles. Kory Cornum's wife, Major Rhonda Cornum, an Army Flight Surgeon, was shot down and captured by Iraqi forces during the course of DESERT STORM, later penning her story in her book *She Went to War: the Rhonda Cornum Story*, with Peter Copeland. (Photograph courtesy of Larry Pitts, Tabuk Royal Saudi Air Base, circa 1990)

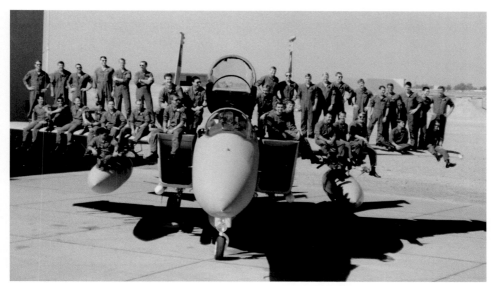

Pilots of the 58th Tactical Fighter Squadron (58TFS) Gorillas, deployed at Royal Saudi Air Base, Tabuk, Saudi Arabia, DESERT SHIELD/DESERT STORM 1990–91. Kluso, kneeling immediate left side of canopy. Notable other characters, Commander "Tonic" Thiel (foreground, sitting on intake, right side of canopy), Kluso's wingman Larry "Cherry" Pitts (standing on wing, second from left), Gorilla Flight Surgeon Kory "Doc" Cornum (tallest, standing on wing, fourth from left), 4-ship flight member John "JB" Kelk (standing right side next to Doc Cornum), Kluso's mentor "Uncle Budge" Wilson (standing, right side next to JB), 4-ship flight member Mark "Willie" Williams (sitting on wing, second from right). (Photograph courtesy of Colonel (Ret) William "Tonic" Thiel, Royal Saudi Air Base, Tabuk, Saudi Arabia, circa 1990)

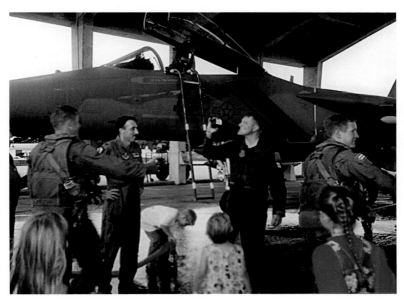

Kluso (standing, hands on hips) as 12th FS Dirty Dozen Operations Officer, joining in the traditional celebration of a pilot's final flight (fini-flight) in the unit. The wash-down and shared swig of a bottle of champagne exemplified the unique bond of fighter pilot's during their time together. Also pictured, Robert "Rodney" Seaberg (drinking from his fini-flight bottle). (Photographer unknown, Kadena Air Base, Japan, circa 1999)

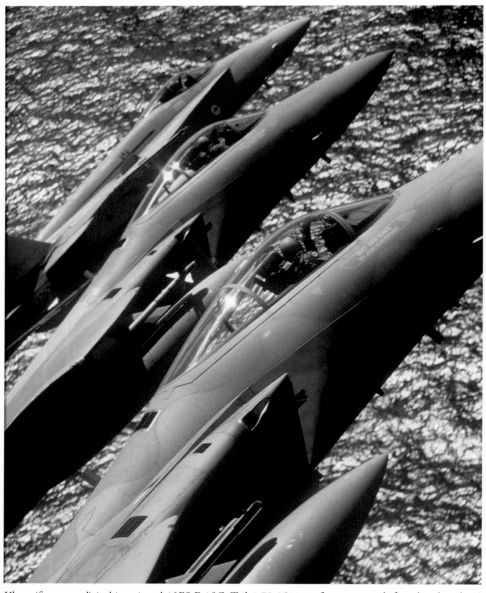

Kluso (foreground) in his assigned 12FS F-15C, Tail # 78-0511, in formation with friend and 12th FS Commander, Tim "Tex" Merrell (middle) and Royal Australian Air Force F-18 Hornet, low over the water off the east coast of Sydney, Australia. This was a special flight for aerial photographer Ned Dawson, in another 2-seat RAAF F-18, during the Dirty Dozen's final mission before standing down in October 1999. Note on the right side below the canopy are the names of Kluso/511's assigned crew chiefs, Staff Sergeant John "Burnsy" Burns, and Senior Airman Jason Aschenbrenner. (Photo by Ned Dawson, Williamtown Royal Australian Air Base, circa 1999)

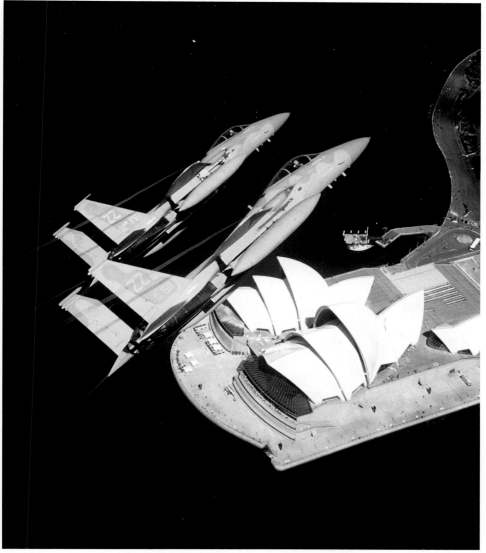

Kluso (foreground) in his assigned 12FS F-15C, Tail # 78-0511, in formation with friend and 12FS Commander, Tim "Tex" Merrell buzzing the famed Sydney Opera House. This was the same special flight for aerial photographer Ned Dawson, in another 2-seat RAAF F-18, during the Dirty Dozen's final mission before standing down in October 1999. It took five or six circular passes for the photographer to snap enough pictures for his satisfaction. The RAAF commander would report a multitude of complaints from the civilian population of Sydney, which the commander would just shrug it off in classic Aussie fashion. (Photo by Ned Dawson, Williamtown Royal Australian Air Base, circa 1999)

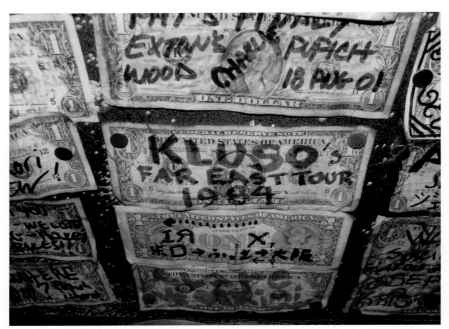

KLUSO DOLLAR, in the tradition of leaving evidence of existence by either a posted dollar bill or a squadron stick-on patch (also known as a Zap). This dollar is actually post-Air Force career, at Kluso's favorite bar and live performance venue, The Chicken Shack, Fussa, Japan (on Bar Row, just outside Yokota Air Base). (Original photo by Rick "Kluso" Tollini, Fussa, Japan, circa 2005)

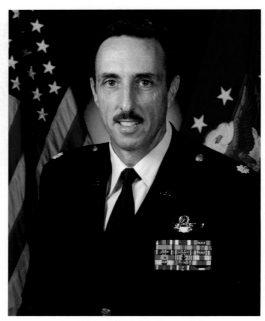

Kluso in his final official photo of his Air Force career, here as the 18th Operations Support Squadron (18 OSS) Commander, Kadena Air Base, Okinawa, Japan. (US Air Force Official Photo, Kadena Air Base, Japan, circa April 2000)

humidity conditions (normally both). The other nice thing about Tabuk was that it had an excess of old dormitory-type quarters that used to house expat British contractors. The rooms were far from Hilton Hotel quality, but compared to the hot, dirty, and dusty tents many other USAF units had to survive in, we had no complaints about the clapboard dual-occupancy rooms with communal bathrooms and showers.

The operational advantage of Tabuk was its unique location just southeast of the Israeli–Jordanian border. We were out of the "limelight" of some other units such as Langley's 1st Fighter Wing at King Abdul-Aziz Air Base (Dhahran), who were getting all the CNN coverage. Though it was not obviously apparent even when looking at a map, Tabuk had a closer straight-line distance to Baghdad than any other US units in Saudi Arabia. This would put us at an economical advantage over other units to get to and from the fight quicker with less refueling requirements. I made sure the combat plans people understood this, to our benefit.

Having arrived a bit late to Tabuk after a very long and roundabout flight routing, I was still getting acclimated. I had a couple of Restoril pills left over that Doc Cornum had given me, and I was following his instructions to use those to help overcome a large dose of jet lag.

I was the 58th TFS weapons officer, so it was my job to insure I could make recommendations to our squadron commander (Tonic) about how best to cover our Air Tasking Oder (ATO) responsibilities. It had been a busy day. I had to come up with plans and options how best to cover the Quick Reaction Alert (QRA—or scramble alert) we had been tasked to perform, and I also had to plan for the airborne defensive CAPs (Combat Air Patrol) we were soon going to be flying near the Saudi–Iraqi border. I was looking forward finally to getting a good night's sleep. The Restoril soon worked its magic and I was out like a light.

Somewhere in the middle of the night, I faintly noticed an ardent pounding on my room door, and I was barely able to come out of my stupor as I saw the outline of somebody standing over my bed. It was Col Rick Parsons, our 33rd Tactical Fighter Wing (TFW) commander. Even though we had deployed as a single squadron, with Tonic as our deployed squadron commander, Col Parsons had also deployed with us; he was the overall deployed commander. Was this by design and deployment orders, or had Col Parsons decided on his own that this tasking was too important to miss? I didn't really know, and it probably didn't really matter. He was in charge.

Col Parsons started to speak to me, "Kluso, Kluso … are you awake?" And I respond probably with something like, "Yes, Sir. I think so?" He said, "Okay, you need to get dressed and out on the ramp by 0300." That's 3am folks, and I looked at my watch and it showed 2.30am. Col Parsons continued, "There's a C-21 [a USAF Lear Jet used for liaison and senior officer flight support] coming to pick you up and take you to Riyadh. They are having a big planning conference there and they need somebody from the 58th to represent us. I'll drive you out to the flight-line … Are you ready to go?" What could I say … "Yes, Sir. I'll be ready in 5 minutes."

I grabbed a small flight bag and quickly stuffed in some underwear, socks, an extra flight suit, and my toilet kit. I was ready, I guess.

As Col Parsons was taking me out to meet the Lear Jet on the Tabuk ramp, he told me he did not have much information on what the meeting was about. He just asked me to use my best judgment and to brief him when I got back or call if I needed any help with anything. "Yes, Sir," I said, and I quickly jumped on the USAF C-21. In less than two hours I was in Riyadh.

I was met by a staff officer, a major, who took me to a four-star hotel in Riyadh, where I was issued a blanket and pillow and ushered off into a huge ballroom that had probably 400–500 other cots with sleeping troops. The major told me he would pick me up at 8am, so I was able to get about an hour of sleep and a great buffet breakfast on-the-house. That breakfast was a welcome event, because we had no chow hall established at Tabuk yet, and we had been surviving on Meals, Ready to Eat (MREs), the modern version of C-Rations, which are not bad but get old pretty quick. Fresh eggs, bacon (yes, bacon in Saudi Arabia), and great coffee. Ahhhh, if only I could stay in that hotel forever, but it was the only time I would be lodged to that level of comfort for the next five months.

Sure enough, at 8am I met the same major (who I think had been picking up and shuttling other officers for the same meeting all night long), and soon afterwards he was dropping me off at a very secure area of buildings that made up the RSAF Headquarters (HQ) which was also now the US Air Forces, Central Command (CENTAF) HQ in the middle of downtown Riyadh, Saudi Arabia.

After going through a series of security checks to receive an area access badge, I was tagged with an escort officer to help me get where I was going and to bring me up to speed on why I was there and what I would be doing. My escort was Maj John "Turkey" Turk. I preferred just to call him "Turk" because he was a big dude and I was not really sure he actually liked the "Turkey" call-sign that had been bestowed on him.

Turk was actually much more than merely an "escort" officer. He was part of the CENTAF combat planning staff, although he made it clear to me early on that he felt he was not really being utilized as such and that he had become more of a "gopher" than anything else ... hence the indignity of a major having to "escort" a captain like me (a lesser-ranking officer). But I really appreciated Turk's efforts and his desire to make me feel comfortable, as he could probably sense my awkwardness, with the enormous number of high-ranking officers floating around the place. It was probably for this reason that Turk and I ended up with a really good working relationship. He probably felt a bit sorry for me that I was only a captain, and that I was about to walk into the "lion's den." Little did I know what was ahead, but the professional bond that Turk and I quickly made would pay off huge for the Gorillas in a few short months.

***

After a full morning of guiding me around the facility and meeting some of the other lower-level planning staff members, Turk ushered me into an expansive conference room that had an enormously long table in the center, seating probably around 30–40 officers. Turk told me he would meet me after the meeting, and then "Good luck! And watch out for Buster." I was not really sure what he meant or why he felt the need to tell me that, and I had no idea who "Buster" was, but I would soon find out.

I located a spot on the side of the long table and sat down next to another F-15 pilot from the 1st Wing (Langley), Lt Col Dennis "Denny" Kremble. I did not know Denny previously, but I recognized his wing patch on his shoulder, which told me right away he was an Eagle pilot. I quickly latched on to him so at least I had some common ground with somebody in the room, because I was the only captain in this obviously very important meeting. The room was full of mostly full-Bird colonels (0-6) and generals. There were some lieutenant colonels like Denny, and only a handful of majors, who seemed to be no more than aids to the senior officers. There probably was not another captain anywhere closer than back at Tabuk, to the best of my knowledge. I thought surely Col Parsons had made a mistake or misunderstood his orders, and it was really supposed to be him at this meeting and not me. Regardless, I was here now and I was representing the 58th TFS (Deployed).

With a rustling of officers and staff, and a quick scramble to seats, the meeting was about to start as the "star" of the show arrived. It was Brigadier General Buster Cleveland Glosson, better known as just "Buster." I had absolutely no idea who he was, but I could tell right away all the lower-ranking officers gave him his due space.

I leaned over to Denny and asked, "Who is that?" And when he said, "That's Buster Glosson," at that point Turk's previous warning came into perspective, although, my initial impression was that he did not seem to be that bad of a guy. Buster was smiling and seemed in a good mood, and he appeared happy to be presiding over this obviously important meeting (though I still had no idea of what it was about).

Gen Glosson started off the meeting by telling us we were all here to see the initial operational plan for what would eventually become the air campaign for Operation DESERT STORM. If you can picture an old World War II movie, somewhere in an Allied bomber command operations center with a huge map that is unveiled to present "Objective: Berlin" … it felt pretty much like that. A large covered board had been placed at the far end of the conference table, and as a staff officer removed the butcher paper layer it revealed an extensive map of Iraq, with lots of targets, OCA packages, and DCA CAPs identified on it.

The briefer started into a synopsis of all the targets, taskings, and Allied air assets. The initial start to operations was intended to be a surprise attack in the middle of the night by a combination of land-attack cruise missiles and our new F-117 stealth fighters, taking out the Iraqis' main command-and-control (C2) radars and command centers to degrade their initial defensive air response. From there, our F-15C Eagles would spread out across the width of central and western Iraq would perform a pure air superiority fighter sweep (nobody to protect, just shoot down the bad guys) that would hopefully pick off any of the IrAF alert fighters that managed to scramble after the initial bombs and missiles exploded. From that point on, there would be an endless stream of large OCA fighter strike packages flown by all coalition assets, with escort and fighter sweep protection by the F-15s and F-14s (Navy). It was impressive and I was pretty excited by what I was hearing and seeing.

Most of the officers in the room were seemingly amazed and possibly a bit intimidated at the size and scope of the air campaign, and this was just Day 1 of the operation that was being briefed. But to me it made perfect sense and appeared to be doable even at first take. I could pretty much equate the opening day of DESERT STORM to combining two full weeks of a Large Force COPE THUNDER into a single night/day. There was nothing on the board that was much different than what I had been doing for so long now at THUNDERs and our Nellis/RED FLAG deployments (other than the novelty of the F-117 missions and capabilities, and much of their contribution was at night).

Once the brief was over, our job was to look over our tasking, figure out if there were any glaring issues or limitations to prevent our units from being able to perform our missions, and then to coordinate with any other unit representatives present to start the ball rolling on the long-range planning for this air campaign. This was just the "first draft" plan. We knew that as more units came in-country and the target priorities changed, so would the opening salvos of DESERT STORM. I would say, however, that what we had just witnessed was 80% aligned with what we would end up doing about 4½ months from then.

Denny and I set about divvying up the F-15 OCA and DCA taskings. The 1st TFW (Langley) had sent two full squadrons to Saudi Arabia and we just had our one full squadron representing the Gorillas (Eglin). So numerically, it appeared Langley could handle more mission taskings than the 58th.

The easiest thing to do was divide up most missions geographically, since we were at Tabuk in the far west and Langley was at Dhahran out to the far east side of Saudi Arabia, on the coast near Bahrain.

We pretty much ran a line straight from Baghdad (Iraq) due south to the Saudi border, with the intent that the 58th would own any DCA CAPs and OCA strike missions west of that line, and Langley would take anything to the east of it. Later on, before the war started, USAF F-15Cs from Bitburg, Germany, would also deploy in-country. We would split the difference and delegate a central corridor along that same line to the boys from Bitburg.

That was the easy part. The next part was to figure out if we could actually perform the missions. I knew from first glance that the sortie generation requirement (how many F-15s we could get into the air at any given time) was going to be a challenge and I would probably need more time and planning to make sure it could be done. But for now, it did not seem impossible.

It did not take too long, though, for me to find a huge Limfac (Limiting Factor) that could make the whole plan fall apart. There appeared to be a gap in how many air-refueling tankers were tasked and how many external fuel tanks (bags) we would have available for flight operations. The KC-135 Stratotankers were the USAF's (and in this case the entire Coalition's) workhorse refueling assets. The tens of thousands of pounds of jet fuel they could carry would be essential to support the long distances all the Coalition aircraft would have to fly to reach their targets, or for the defensive fighter CAP and C2 aircraft, like the E-3 AWACS (Airborne Warning and Control System), to stay airborne and on patrol long enough. Right now, we already knew there were not enough tankers in-theater, but more were on their way, so our hope was they arrived in time.

Another issue that nobody had seemed to notice was the lack of external fuel tanks (drop tanks) for our fighters, especially my squadron's Eagles. Just as in World War II, the advent of external drop tanks had extended the range and endurance of fighters such as the P-51 and P-47 over Europe and the Pacific, modern fighters would rely on them for the same reason. In peacetime training we rarely ever carried more than one or two "bags," as the external tanks were also known. If we did carry the maximum three-bag configuration, it was usually just for a long-range deployment trip from one base to another.

For most of the tasked missions in DESERT STORM, we would need to fly with three bags to meet our requirements for distance on the OCA missions, or loiter time in the DCA CAPs. This was fine, but we did not want to enter into any maneuvering fights or engagements with all that extra fuel and drag from the drop tanks. That is why they call them "drop tanks." The plan was that once we were committed to an engagement, we would immediately "punch off" (drop) some or all of our external tanks. The main issue was that the only tanks we had were the bags that were on the jets when they flew from Eglin, Florida, all the way to Tabuk.

So as the conference was starting to wrap up, Gen Glosson re-entered the room and sat back down at the head of the table and said, "OK, fellas. You've seen the plan, and you've had time to look it over. I need to know today if anybody cannot accomplish their tasking." From there they went one-by-one clockwise around the table and each unit representative would give affirmative confirmations that they were good-to-go, with, "Yes, Sir," and "No problems here, Sir," and "Can-do, Sir."

I was at the far end of the "clock," so I was one of the last to be called on. I had remembered Turk's warning about "Buster" and I was now aware of Gen Glosson's famed temper, so I took a really hard swallow and said, "Sir, we have a problem … and it looks like we can't do our tasking." Buster turned to me with a somewhat surprised look on his face (after so many positive remarks), as I imagined him thinking "who is the young CAPTAIN, telling the KING he has no clothes on?"

Buster barked "WHAT? What do you mean you can't do your missions? Why NOT?"

So I explained to him, "Well, Sir, we should actually be able to do all of our initial missions with no problem, but we don't have any extra drop tanks." Buster looked interested now, as I continued, "We have enough tanks for our initial tasking, but the first time we engage any Iraqi fighters we are going to drop our bags." (Buster nodded, understanding this part.) "So, when we get back to base, we won't have those tanks anymore. We need extra drop tanks to be able to do the follow-on missions. That's the problem."

Buster's demeanor suddenly changed. As he continued to face my way, the look of "interest" turned into a hard stare ... and then his face started turning red. I had heard of the term "beet red," but had only seen it one time before (the famed OTS Lesneski shoe-heel incident). It may have only been four or five seconds seconds of silence, but it seemed like an eternity. As Buster's face changed eight shades of crimson and his hair appeared to shine like titanium white, I began to sink slowly back into my chair hoping maybe I could just disappear. Even the other officers, feeling the discomfort in the room ("Who is the idiot who just said 'No'?") also started to shrink back to avoid possible collateral damage. Just as it looked as if Buster's stare was going to burn a hole right through my heart, and before his head exploded, he made a full turn to a colonel sitting on his immediate left and screamed, "YOU GET THIS YOUNG MAN HIS DROP TANKS, YOU GOT THAT?"

Wow! ... a last-second reprieve from the gallows. I don't know who that poor colonel was, but I sure was glad he was there to "cover the grenade." There was an audible exhalation from the whole room, and just like that the conference was over. I was on my way back to Tabuk with "The Plan." I was told before I left the conference that the DESERT STORM air campaign was "close hold," meaning only myself and my commanders (Col Parsons and Tonic) would have access to the details.

I had a lot of work to do, and for now I would be doing it entirely on my own.

***

Life at Tabuk was not too bad. All the pilots eventually moved from the original condemned dorms we were in to an old expat compound that was in a separate part of the base. The rooms were not really any better than the old place, but each had its own bathroom and shower; still two-to-a-room, but much more privacy and convenience.

My roommate for the duration of the deployment was Capt Rory "Hoser" Draeger. Hoser was actually a young flight lead in the Dirty Dozen when I first arrived at Kadena. We did not have a whole lot of overlap, because he also received a follow-on Eagle assignment to Langley, then on to Weapons School. Hoser eventually got to Eglin after I did and was assigned to the 59th TFS "Lions" as their weapons officer.

Hoser made the trip to Tabuk with the Gorillas because our expectation was that if a war did not start right away, the wing would probably swap out squadron pilots somewhere around the three-month point. Nobody wanted to stay in the desert any longer than necessary if there wasn't a war going on, and it was not good to keep a fighter squadron "on hold" for too long without normal daily training. Hoser was supposed to be the "continuity" for the 59th when they showed up at Tabuk. He would already know what was going on and could help his squadron transition more quickly. It actually never turned out that way, because the planned "swap out" was turned off by higher headquarters. They wanted everybody to remain in place in Saudi Arabia until this thing was over, whenever that was going to be.

I was actually happy to have Hoser with us though. I knew he was an outstanding aviator and, being from Kadena originally, he was somebody I could count on to lead some of our more difficult large-force missions. Also, we would need everybody we could get. Hoser and I were not "best friends" by any means, but we got along well together and gave each other "space" as roommates. Not too long after the war, I received news that Hoser was killed in a car accident. Apparently, he was a passenger riding with some friends when the driver lost control and went off the road. Very sad … and ironic to survive a war and be killed in a random accident.

There was not a whole lot to do at Tabuk. We did have some tasked flying missions, mostly at night, to fly out to an area south of the Iraqi–Saudi border and patrol in DCA CAPs to protect our E-3 AWACS and RC-135 reconnaissance aircraft, which were flying orbits as they kept an eye on what was going on across the border. We also tried to fly as many normal training sorties as we could, but these were difficult to do because we had to keep most of the jets armed and loaded in a combat configuration (live missiles). It's difficult to "train" when you're locked and loaded for bear.

So the highlights of our day were usually chow time and visits to the US Military Training Mission (USMTM). I use the word "chow hall" very loosely, because what was available at Tabuk was far from the standards we would find on any ordinary US military base. As I mentioned before, when we first arrived at Tabuk we only had MREs. Those portable meals had come a long way since the earlier wars, but the variety was severely lacking. Thus there was great excitement one day when we were told they would open a chow line for dinner that night. We all gathered early (more than 400 personnel) at a base auditorium and trudged excruciatingly slowly through the line to get our meal. It took about two hours for some of us to get to the front of the line, and when we got there we were truly disappointed to look at our plates. We each had the most pitiful-looking, scrawny piece of chicken (the thigh/leg portion only), a handful of plain rice, and a Coke. That was it. We actually all went scrounging for MREs after our first real "meal" in weeks.

Not long after that, I think some Air Force contracting officer must have showed up at Tabuk with a suitcase full of cash (they do actually do that at times), and soon we had a full-up chow hall that got better and better every day. The food at least resembled Western chow-hall cuisine and the portions were large enough to satisfy. Then one day an "auto-dog" arrived. An "auto-dog" (I have no idea how that name came into military jargon) was a soft-serve ice cream machine. Once we had the "dog" machine, we knew we could survive at Tabuk for the long term.

The USMTM (pronounced "Yu-suh-mitt-um") I mentioned was a high-walled secure compound off of the base in the actual town of Tabuk. There were many USMTMs across the Middle East and in other countries, and they were where US military foreign liaison personnel lived in-country to assist our allies with training and operations.

The USMTM in Tabuk had very nice apartments (for the residents only, not us), a great swimming pool, and its best asset ... a fully stocked bar! There was supposed to be no alcohol allowed on base while we were in-country, but the USMTMs were different. They were a little piece of "America" and had immunity from local laws and customs. So when the Gorillas first arrived in Tabuk all the pilots would head to the USMTM on any given night they could, that is until General Order No. 1 (GO#1) was issued.

GO#1 would (in my opinion) become one of the worst decisions ever in the annals of military history. It was issued by General Norman Schwarzkopf (the commander of US Central Command/CENTOM) and the order stated there would be absolutely NO drinking in the Kingdom. This was hopefully to show "solidarity" with our Saudi hosts and not insult their cultural sensibilities. Even most Saudis I met who heard about this no-drinking order thought it was crazy. They really didn't care if we drank as long as we behaved.

I now believe the long-term effect of this original GO#1 was that it tried to mandate good order and discipline via a "general order," rather than to establish this with good leadership and respect up and down the chain of command. From then on, any chance a commanding officer had to create an appearance of "good order and discipline" quickly and easily, he would just start signing out these types of "General Orders" and absolve himself of any responsibility to actually "lead" beyond that point. It was such a crock, and the troops could see right through it. I saw it as kind of the opposite of how Opec Hess treated us that first day in Thailand. Our leadership no longer trusted us. If you think there might be a problem with behavior and leadership in today's military, I believe the root cause goes all the way back to Stormin' Norman's original GO#1.

Well, they shut down the bars in all the USMTMs in Saudi Arabia. There were some really unhappy people. But being resourceful fighter pilots, we still found ways occasionally to get booze. One of the most ingenious was when one of our pilots received a huge stuffed animal in the mail from his old college roommate. We all looked at him like he must've had a really strange relationship with his roommate. What fighter pilot would want to receive a cute stuffed doggie? But when he accidently dropped the gift it made a tinkling sound. That poor stuffed animal did not last another 10 seconds as it was ripped open and out spilled about 30 airline booze miniatures. We tried to make those last as long as possible.

Somebody would always have a bottle of whiskey or something. One or our best assets was Doc Cornum. His wife Rhonda was stationed in Bahrain, where it was possible to purchase alcohol. So when Kory would come back from a visit with Rhonda, we would ask him if he had any "IVs" with him. Usually he would say "Yes" with a little gleam in his eyes. Normally, if we were sitting around the USMTM pool Doc Cornum would come around with an IV bag that he had filled with vodka while he was in Bahrain. Typically returning with two or three of these, we would have a nice little pool party as Kory dispensed the nectar into cups of juice we were drinking. If we couldn't drink, then we would find some other kind of chemical to put in our system; for most of us that would be caffeine and nicotine.

Cherry Pitts was my wingman (and good friend) and he had a room directly across from mine in the compound. Hoser didn't smoke and I never wanted to bother him with my bad habit, so I was constantly over at Cherry's room, and we would while away the hours of boredom by drinking coffee and smoking cigarettes all day long and late into the evenings. They started calling Cherry and I "The Chimney Brothers."

It went so far that Cherry and I (and some others) would smoke in the jets while flying our DCA CAP missions. I had found that I could use these little plastic powdered-lemonade drink cups (which had a foil lid) that fit perfectly between the light control panel knobs on the right side of the F-15 cockpit. So, I had a little ashtray I could use in flight, and when I was done I would just wrap the foil cover back over the top of the cup to prevent spillage. It was perfect. We didn't smoke when anything important was going on, but for a four- or six-plus hour mission boring holes in the sky, it was a nice "break" to look forward to every hour or so. If I ever took off without a pack of smokes and lighter in my G-suit pocket, I knew it was going to be a long and grueling flight.

***

Saudi Arabia was a strange country. I don't mean that necessarily in a bad way, but just that it felt "strange" being there. I had been in a lot of foreign countries, but this was the first time I had felt like such a "foreigner," like I did not belong there. The people were nice enough, and most of us even made friends with many of the Saudi pilots. But it just always felt like there was some kind of barrier, as if we were the houseguests that had impolitely overstayed our visit. Our hosts would never say anything to us, but I felt they probably really preferred it if we would leave, as soon as possible. And, frankly, I felt the same way.

***

I had work to do. Over the next several months I would often walk from our operations building all the way down the flight-line to our intelligence center, where I could have a secure room to myself and go over the mission taskings for DESERT STORM in solitude.

I had to figure out first of all if we could do all our taskings, and if so, if we could do even more. I had a yellow legal pad and I came up with a way to start managing pilots and airplanes. We had deployed to Tabuk with 24 Primary Assigned Aircraft (PAA) of F-15s and about 30 pilots. This created a ratio of 1.25 pilots per jet. This was a normal peacetime ratio of pilots-per-aircraft for training purposes. I would soon figure out that it was woefully inadequate for prolonged combat operations.

My first step in task planning was to create dedicated 4-ship pairings for the pilots. What this meant is that I created a selection of the flight leads and wingmen I would match up to fly together. My intention was that they would probably fly in these pairings both in training, the pre-war DESERT SHIELD missions, and finally for the duration of combat operations, if that came. The advantage of the pairings was that we would be so familiar with each other within each flight that it would eliminate the need constantly to brief and debrief missions. We would understand each other's strengths and weaknesses and know what to expect of each other in certain situations. The other advantage was that keeping each 4-ship pairing together made it as easy as possible to schedule the group and know what their availability was at a glance. I gave each pilot an alphanumeric number that signified what 4-ship he was in and the position he could fly in that 4-ship.

From there I gave each F-15 aircraft an alphabetic designation from the letter "A" on until I ran out of planes or alphabet. Since there were only 24 jets at Tabuk, I had enough letters. I would use these alphanumeric designations for the pilots and the jets and go through the air tasking order to try to get the most efficient use out of each. What I found was that I kept running out of pilots, and while I had enough jets to fulfill the basic mission requirements it seemed like a very inefficient way to task the sorties.

The planners were relying on their peacetime training and exercise experience where the emphasis was always to generate as many sorties as possible, i.e., "turn" the jets (that means refuel, rearm, and ready for next mission) as fast possible and have the pilots fly their butts off. The only problem is that peacetime training and exercises normally only ran on an 8–12-hour flying window. The operation we were planning was going to be a 24-hour war ... day and night (with the emphasis on the night). The peacetime planning did not work.

The first thing I figured out was that the two-hour long DCA CAP missions they tasked us for were way too short. It would take an hour each way to get to and from the CAP area. So, a two-hour mission was really a four-hour mission, but we would have to be launching new sorties in the middle of each CAP period just to replace the previous CAP on time with no gap in coverage. The two-hour CAP mission would therefore really be more like six hours for the pilot to brief / prep / preflight / start / taxi / take off / fly en route, CAP, and then RTB, land, debrief, eat, and repeat. In this case, each pilot would be tasked for about 14–16 hours a day. This might be OK for maybe a day or two, but after that our pilots would be run into the ground with fatigue. The 24-hour sortie generation requirement could also overwhelm our maintenance personnel and leave far fewer jets available to fly some of the OCA sorties we were also tasked for. Furthermore, if a single pilot flew a two-hour CAP mission, would he be available to immediately fly another one right after?

Something had to change and I figured out that it was the duration of the DCA CAPs. They had to be longer. Once I had that epiphany the solutions became very clear. If we could make the CAP durations run six hours long, then it would reduce sortie generation requirements, with the following benefits: each jet would fly only twice in a 24-hour period versus four or five times; it would provide a great deal more "turn" time (downtime) between sorties, so maintenance could have time to fix jets; and, pilots would be able to fly just one mission a day (although we still had a pilot shortage problem). So once I figured this out I had two groups of people to convince: our maintenance leadership at Tabuk and the combat planners in Riyadh.

The combat planners turned out to be the easy ones to convince. I explained the plan and reasons for using six-hour CAPs during DESERT STORM, and told them that the bonus part of this was that if we could do it this way, I would be able to *double* the number of OCA escort/sweep missions we could do. When they heard that, the combat planners were all for the longer CAP periods. Protecting the strike aircraft going north into Iraq was going to be a high priority and we were very short on assets and sorties to do that.

Convincing the maintenance leaders at Tabuk was going to be a little more difficult, I assumed.

The relationship between operational leadership (pilots) and maintenance leadership was always a balancing act and not always harmonious. Pilots wanted to fly the jets as much as possible, but maintenance needed to have a good deal of say over the availability of the aircraft, so they had time for both routine maintenance and inspections as well as fixing jets that broke. Crew chiefs and maintainers would always say, "We fix 'em, and you guys break 'em." Hah! That was pretty much the truth.

Fortunately, we had some great maintenance senior non-commissioned officers (SNCOs) in the Gorillas, and our Ops–Maintenance relationship was pretty sound.

Chief Master Sergeant José Matos was "the Man." He was the key enlisted leadership of our 58th TFS maintenance group at Tabuk, and he knew EVERYTHING. While Chief Matos was willing to listen to my ideas, still, for the same reasons that the planners had tasked us inefficiently, the maintainers initially looked at the very long sortie durations as bizarre and did not want to do it. But when I showed them the reduced sortie generation requirements and the enormous amount of time they would have for each jet on the ground to both prep and fix them, I turned them into converts.

We were ready to Rock 'n' Roll.

The result of this new concept for long-duration DCA CAPs had a multiplying effect. We had 24 PAAs. From that 24 PAAs, I asked our maintainers if they could provide 20 total "frontlines." That meant 20 F-15s ready to fly, or an 80% availability rate. That's a very high number for peacetime, but our maintainers assured us that, with our deployed squadrons high on the priority list for all the spare parts the Air Force could muster, they would be able to do this. And they did. For the entire DESERT STORM campaign, we maintained more than an 80% availability rate. I don't recall us *ever* missing a sortie for maintenance non-availability of jets. Amazing!

So, with 20 available airframes, my new six-hour CAP plan meant we only needed eight total F-15s to be able to provide 24-hour DCA coverage with a 4-ship on CAP the entire time. While four Eagles were on CAP, our maintainers would have 3–4 hours to get the next 4-ship ready. That was plenty of time, when you consider peacetime training turn times are normally 1.5–2 hours.

The other key element of my plan was to hold four F-15s on QRA alert posture. We did not really expect a "surprise" airfield attack by the IrAF, and by the time the war started we also had US Patriot and British Rapier missiles to protect the base. So the purpose of the four Eagles with four pilots on alert was to provide "back-fill" to any DCA aircraft that had to return early for maintenance or reload (if they became engaged), or to act as maintenance spare aircraft for the OCA mission requirements.

The end result was that we had eight F-15C Eagles available full time for as many sorties as they could support, to perform the critical OCA sweep/escort duties that the Riyadh planners so desperately needed. When I called Turk and told him what we could provide by using this planning methodology, I think he would have kissed me right through the phone if he could have.

The 58th TFS Gorillas had suddenly become the "darlings" of the combat plans staff in Riyadh. Every time they tried to get the Langley units to commit to more missions, the 1st Wing would say, "No ... not possible." And now here I was, not only offering them more sorties but actually asking them to give us more OCA missions. OCA is where the action is, and I knew we had the jets and the talent to kick ass.

As a side note—after DESERT STORM the long-duration CAP missions became the new standard for the Air Force. Why nobody had thought of it before, I don't know. Maybe it was because we had not fought a war for so long, and this was actually the very first 24-hour operations cycle (ops-cycle) conflict. If you asked anybody today where the idea to expand CAP times came from, I don't believe anybody could give you an answer. But I know it all started in that lonely little planning room in Tabuk, Saudi Arabia, with a yellow legal pad and a #2 pencil.

Now, for the pilot problem.

Once I knew we could support a much larger tasking order with the jet sorties, it was obvious we did not have enough pilots. It would take 16 pilots to fly the six-hour DCA CAPs (four pilots × four CAPs). Another four pilots would be on QRA scramble status. And we could be tasked for anywhere from 16–24 OCA missions in a 24-hour tasking cycle. That adds up to 36–44 pilots needed to fill a 24-hour tasking. We only had 30.

The first thing I did was go to Tonic and tell him we needed more pilots from Eglin to join us at Tabuk. The answer I got, and the answer I would get almost all the way up to the end of combat operations, was "No." This wasn't just Tonic being stubborn (although he could be at times), but HHQ was not approving requests for extra personnel. There were already tens of thousands of USAF personnel in theater and they did not want every swinging dick who wanted to fight a war to snivel their way over. In our case though, we really needed the extra pilots (I had requested six). So the next idea I had was to change the 24-hour clock to an 18-hour clock. If we had about 40 sorties every 24 hours, then in an 18-hr window we would have about 30 sorties. That's exactly how many pilots we had. Instead of every pilot being available to fly one long-duration sortie in a 24-hour period, he would be tasked to fly one sortie every 18 hours (approximately). For example, if somebody flew the 1200–1800 DCA CAP on Day 1, their next CAP sortie on Day 2 would start 6 hours earlier, 0600–1200, and so forth. This meant that every day, each pilot on average would wake up six hours earlier to "go to work." Imagine this in your own life. You wake up at 6am, work from 8am to 5pm, get to sleep as soon as you can, and then wake up at midnight, and then start the cycle again six hours earlier each day.

It was crazy, but we had to do it. It totally blew away our peacetime crew-rest requirements to have 12 full hours from the end of duty time to the start of the next duty time, with eight hours for uninterrupted sleep during that 12 hours. We were going to be lucky to get 4–5 hours of sleep every night, not to mention the constantly changing biorhythm of getting up six hours earlier each day. But this wasn't going to be "peacetime." This was going to be combat, and Tonic and Col Parsons approved the plan.

Tonic predicted after the first week or so of combat that we would gain air superiority and our mission requirements would decrease. He was right about the first part, but not the second. Our mission tasking actually went up (everybody wanted Eagles on their wings, protecting them) and the 18-hour duty cycle became exhausting. After two weeks most of us were walking around like zombies.

The other key player in this plan was Kory, our flight doc. Kory had been issued a truckload of amphetamines (specifically Dexedrine), or uppers, and the previously mentioned Restoril (downers), and he would be our acting "dealer." All pilots at some point in our careers had been tested with both pills to insure we did not have any unusual side effects (other than the desired or expected ones), but most of us had never actually experienced using either regularly. The Restoril was to make sure that we could get to sleep quickly and soundly for the small window of opportunity we would have each day between combat missions. The Dexadrine was intended to keep us alert (and in some cases from actually falling asleep) in the cockpit.

Normally, I would be sure I always had two or three uppers with me for the longer DCA CAPs. If I thought I needed one I would take it near the beginning of the mission and then maybe another half-way through. I didn't want to take one at the end of the mission to avoid the jitters when I came back to land, or when I was trying to get to sleep. The Restoril was always effective in canceling out the Dexedrine though.

It was funny, because even though Doc Cornum was being responsible and documenting our meds, he would sometimes drive up to us while we were walking to our jets and from a rolled-down window whisper, "Hey, hey, guys! Anybody need any ups or downs?" If he was on the streets of any US city he would have been arrested.

Some pilots did not want to use them, and there was no requirement to. Whether it was the stigma of drug use or they just felt they didn't need them, it was probably different for each pilot. But for me (and most of my flight members), I had no problem using anything that was potentially going to give me an edge, keep me alert, or help me to get some much-needed sleep.

After the war there was some backlash, with stories getting out in the news about pilots using the meds while flying. Even some generals (who did not have their butts strapped into a jet during these combat hops) complained about what was perceived as an over-reliance on the meds. But I can tell you this—for our squadron, Doc Cornum probably saved one or two lives and maybe a couple of jets with his diligent concern for our health, wellness, and combat preparedness.

**

Once I had finally put all the pieces in place, we had a solid plan for how the Gorillas were going to execute the ATO for the first three days of DESERT STORM. There were some changes in the missions along the way. For example, we picked up more mission commander responsibilities on the really big large-force missions because Langley did not feel comfortable leading some of these operations. No problem-o for the Gorillas though, with our extensive Pacific and European theater large-force exercise experience. Now it was just a matter of training and maintaining our proficiency while we waited out the seemingly endless desert "vacation."

The very first mission for us (as mentioned before) was going to be a night 8-ship sweep through western Iraq. I had to come up with a viable night tactic to execute this mission, because this is something we had never really practiced before in peacetime training. We spent a lot of time flying at night during the four-and-a-half-month DESERT SHIELD operations leading up to the war. Mostly it was the long duration DCA CAPs that gave my 4-ship and others in the squadron plenty of time to practice their night formations and learn flight management and execution techniques.

Up until that time in the Eagle community, except for very rare occasions on special exercises, the standard F-15 night formations consisted of 2-ship elements, normally flying with the wingman in a 2–5nm offset trail or echelone formation. This pretty much allowed the flight lead to maneuver wherever and whenever he wanted without worrying about a mid-air collision with the wingman.

As for the wingman, this was the easiest formation to maintain because almost always he could continuously monitor his flight lead's position on his own radar or while monitoring the Automated Airborne Interrogator (AAI) returns on the scope. (Note: The AAI allowed a friendly aircraft with the correct code to respond to another aircraft's electronic "query" regarding its position. If the response was within the other aircraft's radar scope field of regard, he could see the friendly reply on his radar scope, displayed as a diamond shape or circle. The system provided simple positional situation awareness and identification.) The only problem with this formation is that it was not very "offensively" oriented. With the wingmen in the back of the formation it was not possible to mass firepower on the enemy. "Massing of firepower" was a key element in F-15 tactics, which is why the classic daytime formation was a "wall of Eagles" or a 4-ship of F-15s spread out line abreast about 5 nm across.

I decided early on in our night training that my 4-ship element would attempt to practice and validate the ability fly a nighttime "wall" formation without night-vision goggles (NVGs) or Fighter Data Link (FDL). And we did. The basic formation was a little bit wider than a normal daytime formation just to assist with flight path deconfliction and to reduce the workload on the wingman spending time on formation management. About 5nm between #1 (flight lead) and #3 (element lead) with the wingman on the outside of the formation, about 2–3nm away from their respective flight leads. This doubled the total width of the formation from 5nm wide to about 10nm wide.

A standardized altitude deconfliction plan was also utilized based on a briefed "base" altitude for the flight lead. So, if the flight lead's "base" altitude was 25,000 feet, then #3 might be 2,000 feet below, and the wingmen would be 1,000–2,000 feet above their respective flight leads. Any time the "base" altitude changed, the flight members would flex to the new relative deconfliction altitudes. Having the wingman slightly above their flight leads also helped with visual mutual support for the wingmen. That's right … "visual" at night without NVGs.

We found that by using very low settings on our external lighting system, mostly our navigation or position lights (the little red/green/white lights on wingtips/tail) and our fluorescent formation lights, we could spot each other in most cases inside of 3–5 miles, depending on the nighttime conditions (very dark or moonlit). Positioning the wingman above their flight leads allowed them to look down on the flight lead against a mostly pitch black desert background versus looking up into the starlit night where the flight lead's aircraft lighting would blend into the stars. We also had contingency lighting options to quickly regain sight of each other by a communicated request or by whatever tactical action we were performing at the time. For example, a request to "Flash" meant for the other flight member to momentarily turn on their bright-red anti-collision lights, which could be seen from far away. Or a "burner" call meant that somebody had just engaged his afterburner, which was also very noticeable from far away. Use or calls of "Flare" or a shot call (Fox 1, or Fox 2) meant somebody had just dropped decoy flares or taken a missile shot respectively; that could be used both as a warning or to direct attention to somebody's position.

Those "contingency" lighting options were only to be used in the most extreme cases, because we knew they could easily expose our position to the enemy. Even the dimmer position/formation lights would be likely "strangled" (turned off) once we knew we were within 10 miles or so of the enemy. From that point, we would just rely on the "big sky theory" or good luck that we didn't hit each other.

Additional communication and flight formations standards were added to the mix, and within the span of just a few long night sorties we knew that the "Night Wall" was a viable Eagle employment formation. So, for Night #1 at the start of the war, that was the plan.

***

After about two months, the daily drudge of "peacetime" operations at Tabuk became a significant drain on everybody's moral. The lack of daily entertainment and distractions (including booze) made it necessary to find alternative outlets for our frustrations. Hitting the gym, Frisbee football, or whatever game we could make up, helped. We eventually ended up with a "movie tent" in the compound, where we would often gather in the evenings to watch some classic movie re-run for the hundredth time (reminiscent of the Korea alert tours, or the scenes in the *M.A.S.H.* TV series). Or, we immersed ourselves is some of the latest "new" technology ... hand-held computer gaming systems.

Cherry had a brand-new Nintendo Gameboy and he had no problem with my taking semi-ownership of the little box. Whether spending endless hours smoking cigarettes and drinking coffee in Cherry's room, or while on a 24-hour alert duty, it did not take me too long to become a master of Gameboy's "Super Mario Land." For me it was not important to complete the game to the final finish, but rather just how many "lives" I could retain at the end of play.

Back in the late summer of 1990, just prior to deployment to Tabuk, I learned that I had received another F-15 assignment back to Kadena. This was my dream, to return to Kadena as a weapons officer, and if possible, hopefully back to the Dirty Dozen. When it became obvious that we would deploy to Saudi Arabia, there was no way I wanted to miss an opportunity for combat, but I was also really worried about my Kadena assignment. I talked to Tonic at length about this and he assured me that he would do everything in his power to make sure I did not lose the assignment, going so far as to say that if nothing had happened at Tabuk after three months he would probably send me back to Eglin to out-process and head for Kadena. I was relieved by this, because Tonic and I both figured that if we were still sitting on our butts in three months (after the "emergency" efforts to get us to Saudi Arabia) there was going to be very little chance of a war kicking off. We were both wrong.

Around late October, Tonic and I talked again and he told me to plan to leave sometime in mid-November. I had mixed feeling about this. I wanted to get back to Sako and the baby, and get on to Kadena, but I also did not want to leave my squadron behind without me. Still, Tonic was so sure I was going home I told Sako to expect me home within a week or two. She was happy to hear that, because I had missed Sakura's first birthday and that was a hard time for everybody.

No kidding, within days of my proposed departure Tonic came to me and told me the return trip to Eglin had been shut off. I would have to stay in Tabuk for a full six months or longer if need be. I was livid! Not so much because I really wanted to leave, but I had already assured Sako I was coming home. I also thought now I was really going to lose the Kadena assignment, and for what? At that point the general consensus among all of us was that nothing was ever going to happen. As it turned out, we were all wrong and I would have kicked myself for ten thousand years if I had not hung on for another couple of months (and I still ended going to Kadena after all).

In the end I had to thank Tonic, although after a couple of days of stewing I came to the realization that it was not really his call. The pilots were not privy to the sensitive National Command Authority (NCA) decisions, but CENTAF leadership was, and they probably knew the intended timeline for Saddam to either comply with the Coalition's demand or the start of combat operations. That timeline was somewhere around the beginning of the New Year in January 1991. The other factor is that the Department of Defense was still urgently pouring more capabilities, equipment, and personnel into the theater. We had no intention of making this a "fair fight" and CENTCOM/CENTAF needed more assets. Logically they did not want anybody who was already in-country and prepared to execute the "Plan" to be leaving early … and for us, at that time, I *was* the Plan.

***

By early December, it became clear from daily news reporting and the "pounding of war drums" in Washington DC that we were on a likely path to war. From the very moment I returned from my first trip to Riyadh with "the Plan," I had been asking Tonic for permission to brief some of the key flight leads, those who would be mission commanders in the first three-days' ATO. I needed them to be able to plan their missions ahead of time and coordinate with other unit leads that would be integrated into the missions.

After months of "No, No, No … and, No," one day Tonic came to me and asked whom I wanted to brief. He told me, "OK, go ahead, but mission commanders only." I had already picked them out. As I mentioned before, I had already scheduled every single sortie and pilot for the three-day ATO. I knew whom I wanted to lead and fly in each and every mission. Key players were: myself; Capt Rob "Cheese" Graeter; Capt Jon "JB" Kelk (who was also #3 in my flight); Capt Rory "Hoser" Draeger;

and (USMC) Capt Chuck "Sly" Magill. These were all the key players who would lead the critical missions in the first three days of Operation DESERT STORM.

You might have noticed that everybody was a captain, which meant we were all "junior" officers with an average of 6–8 years' experience. Many other units would schedule their "field grade" or senior officers (mostly lieutenant colonels) as their flight leads and mission commanders, but for most of those cases it had to do more with rank and positions of authority rather than ability. My judgment was (and still is) that generally the most proficient and capable combat leaders are the captains. Fortunately, I had a squadron commander (Tonic) who agreed with me. Even Tonic stood back to give preference to the combat leaders in the squadron ... "the Captain's Mafia." I credit his wise determination on this issue as a key to our eventual outstanding success in aerial combat.

As the New Year rolled into 1991, things started moving faster. The first week of January, I was given permission to brief the entire squadron and key personnel. This was another "Objective Berlin"-style brief but in a much smaller venue—our intelligence/combat plans office. The room was packed with all the pilots and relevant personnel and my map was much smaller than the one I saw at Riyadh, but the impact of the Plan was the same: quiet awe at the complexity and genius of the mission planning objectives and our particular piece of the pie.

Pilots already knew what their 4-ship pairings were, and in this brief they would find out what missions they were tagged to perform. Some would be flying the OCA missions, and others the DCA CAPs and QRA back-fill missions similar to what we had already been doing. The 4-ship taskings gave the appearance of an "A-Team" and "B-Team" status for some of the flights, and although I denied that was the case, in reality it did have some elements of truth. The OCA teams had to be our very best 4-ships and mission commanders. Although there were a few young and inexperienced wingmen in some of these pairings, they were always surrounded by strong flight members. The DCA teams would not be expected to see as much action, and so for that reason I could pair some of the less-experienced flight members together. Even so, all of DCA CAP flights still had a very strong overall 4-ship flight lead to guide them around.

One such case was Capt Joe "Corn" Hruska. He was by far one of our most talented young flight leads (he would eventually go to Weapons School himself), and I would have preferred to have Corn in the OCA lineups, but I gave him responsibility to fly with and watch over one of our squadron leaders. Corn's job was to keep him alive. He was successful and he never complained about it. A real pro.

With the squadron briefed and all the pilots now focused on the expected task at hand, then it was only a matter of time. We had been in Tabuk long enough and everybody wanted to go home. The common saying now became, "The quickest way home is through Baghdad." We knew that the faster we could end this war, the sooner we would be home.

We did not know what day the war would start, but we knew that somebody knew. Actually, the preferred start date (we already knew the time: 0300) had probably been planned for months. Just like the D-Day invasion almost 47 years earlier, the date to start combat operations depended on the seasons and the phase of the moon. We wanted a near moonless night for the Tomahawks, F-117s, and other strike aircraft to do their work under the cover of almost total darkness. There were only so many of those days every month.

The final hint came when we were told to attend a pilot meeting for a special guest. When the meeting started, up stepped my old "friend" Buster. Brig Gen Glosson had come not to shake my hand (I'm sure he did not even remember me), but to give a last-minute pep talk to all the pilots (as he was doing for every single unit stationed in Saudi Arabia). Say what you might about Buster Glosson, but that "pre-game" pep talk was one of the best I had ever seen or heard. He got every single pilot fired-up and focused. It was perfect.

Two things that Buster said stuck with me. The first was, "There is no target or adversary worth dying for. If something doesn't look right, don't shoot and be sure to come back home alive." The second was his description of the "Buster Mission." (Yes, he had named it after himself ... and, why not? He was the head of the combat plans cell.) If we were airborne and we were given the codeword "Buster," it meant that they had located an aircraft with Saddam Hussein himself on-board that was likely trying to get out of the country.

I guess the US leadership assumed, when faced with the might of the USAF, that Saddam would probably prefer to flee rather than fight (We were all about 13 years off the mark on that one.) Our job would be to chase down Saddam's flight and shoot it out of the air (much as the Dirty Dozen had done in the Southwest Pacific in World War II, in finding and taking out Japan's Admiral Yamamoto). Buster went on to say, "Don't worry if you have to use all your gas to get him and can't make it home. We will find you and we will bring you back." That last part didn't sound like too much fun, but I think most in the room would have had no problem running the Buster Mission if they got the chance (and we almost did).

***

Now it was done. The wheels were turning. It seemed that the inertia was so enormous that nothing other than a complete and immediate pullout of Kuwait by Saddam would prevent this juggernaut from rolling. Even then, I am not sure we wouldn't have executed the three-day ATO anyway and just feigned ignorance.

A war machine is a dangerous thing. Once it is wound up tight like a clock spring, something has to give. The saying about releasing "the Dogs of War" is so true. You're never going to be able to round them up or call them back afterwards ... that decision is final. I know now that the war machine should only be unleashed in the most drastic cases of national emergency. I don't think on that particular day, though, that anybody questioned the decision.

The next day I was taking my flight on a four-hour DCA CAP that we assumed might be one of the final CAPs we would fly on a "peacetime" footing. The mission was routine and in fact included myself getting an instrument check-ride evaluation from JB (who was our squadron flight examiner at the time). Funny how even on the eve of war mundane everyday training requirements such as check-rides still had to be accomplished. I passed the check-ride.

We landed late afternoon at Tabuk and Tonic met me at my jet. I assumed it wasn't to congratulate me on passing my check-ride. He said, "Kluso ... we got the green light. It starts tonight. Get your guys together and let them know and then get whatever rest you can." I did the first, but there would be very little rest that night.

CHAPTER 8

DESERT STORM

I cannot remember if I even tried to sleep. I do recall carefully preparing what I was going to take with me: my "intel" pack, consisting of the wartime plastic-wrapped map and escape & evasion information (for if I was shot down), and the classic combat "blood chit" similar to what Doolittle's Raiders carried for when they hopefully landed in friendly Chinese territory after the first surprise US air attack on Japan in World War II. It was basically a waterproof document with an American flag on it and messages in several different regional languages, telling the person reading it that I was an American pilot and that my safe return to friendly forces would be greatly rewarded. In case that didn't work, I also carried some gold that I had purchased in the Tabuk marketplace, hoping to use that to barter for safe passage if needed.

I had my cigarettes too, of course.

I wasn't really worried about not coming back, though. My biggest fear was embodied in that fighter pilot mantra that Tom Wolfe's classic book *The Right Stuff* so eloquently stated, "Dear Lord, please don't let me fuck up."

I stopped into the movie tent about an hour before I had to meet up with my flight members for our mission brief, which was going to start around midnight. There were several pilots (those who didn't have missions until much later the next day) hanging out watching something. It was strange because nobody was really talking. And more unnerving was that nobody was talking to me at all. I am not sure if they didn't want to bother me, or if they were dealing with their own thoughts and trepidations, but it just did not feel right. Once I was together with my flight and the whole 8-ship of participants though, it was back to business as usual.

***

January 17, 1991. The mission brief went pretty smoothly. There actually was not much to go over because we had analyzed and pre-briefed this mission so many times in the last couple of weeks. We really just needed a quick review and to update the weather for that night. But it was actually the weather that generated some of the greatest concern.

After having had virtually clear weather and a million miles of visibility for the preceding 4½ months, suddenly NOW, on the night of all nights, our first combat mission, the weather decided to go to crap. The poor weather officer was not a real popular dude in our flight brief that night, not that it could possibly be his fault ... he was just the messenger. A cold front had moved in over Saudi Arabia and he told us we could expect clouds with embedded thunderstorms up to 35,000 feet all the way out to our air refueling tracks and the Iraqi border.

Embedded thunderstorms! Oh GREAT! There is absolutely nothing more terrifying to a fighter pilot than the thought of refueling off a tanker at night and in adverse weather. Another important fact was that of late some of the older KC-135 tankers had been ordered not to perform "auto-pilot" refueling operations because of recent malfunctions that had not been fixed. Trying to get into position for the air refueling boom to plug into the Eagle receptacle, while the KC-135 was flown hands-on (no auto-pilot), at night and in bad weather, was going to be like trying to mount a bucking bronco after it had already come out of the gate ... with a blindfold on.

The last concern brought up in the flight was the "roll-over" of our Mode 4 AAI. The Mode 4 was the most secure IFF interrogator mode we had. We relied on this system heavily to make sure we did not accidently fire on any friendly US aircraft. The normal standard worldwide policy was to change to the new Mode 4 code each day at the beginning of a new ZULU day, that is, at midnight Greenwich Mean Time (GMT). In Saudi Arabia, 0000 ZULU was at 0300 (3am), the time we would first be pushing across the Saudi–Iraqi border. Our concern was that if any of the friendly fighters, mostly the F-15Es that were going in ahead of us, would forget to roll their Mode 4 to the next ZULU day, then it would be possible that the one piece of information we needed to confirm a target on our radar was friendly (and not an enemy fighter) might be missing data.

One of the flight members was told to get a quick message off to Riyadh to tell the orbiting AWACS E-3 control aircraft to be sure to tell the earlier missions to change their Mode 4 code on time. We really had no idea if this message would get through, so stepping out the door to our jets I believe in the back of our minds we were going to go to extraordinary efforts to make sure we did not "Frat" somebody (fratricide, or friend-on-friend engagement).

***

My flight was driven out to our jets parked in "Death Valley," the parking area immediately next to the runway. The maintenance crews named this particular area Death Valley because there was absolutely nothing out there but a barren shack (no toilets or running water), spiders, and snakes, and four F-15C Eagles. Tonight we were using the call-sign PENNZOIL for my flight. I am not sure why the combat planners chose major petroleum corporation names for our F-15 missions. Normally those call-signs would have been the domain of the air refueling tankers, but these particular call-signs had a nice ring to them and were easy to say and hear in the heat of combat communications.

Across the way, on the other side of the runway in the area known as "Disneyland," Cheese Graeter gathered his jets as CITGO flight. Cheese was leading the second 4-ship flight in our mission (positions #5 through #8). He would take off first and proceed to the air refueling track, get topped off with gas for himself and his flight, and then wait for us in the approximate CAP area we had been using for the last several months.

As I was getting strapped into my jet with the help of my crew chief, Cheese's four Eagles started blasting off the runway right next to us in full afterburner, combat loaded, with a mighty roar. It was a stark reminder of what we were about to do. My crew chief looked me in the eye (almost like he thought he might not see me, or his jet, again) and said "Good luck, Sir. Come back safe." I just gave him a nod and said, "Thanks. I will."

About that time, as I pulled the handle to the jet fuel starter (JFS) to begin cranking up my Eagle, I said a Buddhist chant three times: "Nam Myoho Renge Kyo; Nam Myoho Renge Kyo; Nam Myoho Renge Kyo." I had become Buddhist when I married Sako (on her stipulation, but not reluctantly), but I had never really practiced it. Still I knew this is what they chanted: "Nam Myoho Renge Kyo"—Devotion to the Wonderful (Universal) Law of Cause and Effect through Sound and Motion. I did not know whether this would do any good, nor did I have any deep faith at this time in my life, but I thought ... what the hell, why not?

***

The takeoff and departure out of Tabuk was uneventful, just like it had been on many similar missions over the last several months. Only this time, the objective was different.

I decided to reform the formation to a close visual spacing, even though we expected some weather in front of us. Normally in bad weather I would rather leave the flight members strung out in a long trail formation, allowing each jet to maintain 1–2nm separation using their radars; it's called a radar-trail departure. Tonight was different because we were operating under emissions control (EMCON) procedures, which meant minimum use of radios and radars. We wanted to mask the number of aircraft we were launching out to our orbits for the night.

The plan was first to go to our air refueling tracks, which were far enough to the south that we would be out of sight of Iraq's long-range air defense surveillance radars. After air-to-air refueling, we would then move north up to an area where we had been flying our DCA CAPs for the last four-plus months; in other words, we wanted it to look to the Iraqis like just another day (or night) of routine Coalition air operations.

Closing the 4-ship into a visual night "fingertip" formation allowed us to navigate with a minimum of communications between flight members and with most everybody's radars turned off to mitigate passive detection by the Iraqis. This meant sticking together while flying through some nasty weather though, and I am sure it was not fun for Cherry, JB, and Willie, but those guys did a great job. The embedded thunderstorms that the weather officer forecasted were not evident to me, but a phenomenon that I did not expect turned the night into a specter of possible things to come—St. Elmo's fire started to dance its way across all of our jets.

I had heard of St. Elmo's fire before, but in all my years of flying I can honestly say I had only experienced it once, momentarily while flying at Eglin (never at Kadena) and it was a mild case compared to what I was witnessing now. First, I started to notice my flight members' jets beginning to radiate a greenish-blue glow, something like how old 1950s B-movies would portray flying saucers or UFOs in space. Then, my own jet also started to glow, as streaks of static discharge flew in ribbons from the front of my forward windscreen straight back over the top of my canopy. It was both a bit unnerving and disorienting. I would have some more "fun" as I approached our refueling tanker.

It did not take too long to find our air refueling rendezvous location and our tanker in its orbit, with Cheese's flight already on the wings of the KC-135 getting their pre-mission fuel top-off. As I brought my flight to a position about 1 mile behind the tanker, the most unusual optical illusion started to occur. We were flying in what is often described as a "milk bowl" effect; we were in a hazy cloud layer that allowed us to see out to maybe a mile or less, but nothing could be seen distinctly. So, while all of the maneuvering of Cheese's flight on the tanker was occurring, I could only see the position lights of the fighters and the tankers floating in the black murkiness of the night.

The illusion that occurred was that it seemed like either my own jet, or the tanker in front of us, was in some kind of barrel-roll spiraling maneuver, and that me and my flight were "falling" into the tanker and closing the distance faster and faster. In fact, none of this was happening and I was really flying in a level, stable position directly behind the tanker and Cheese's flight. It took all of my willpower and flying experience to concentrate solely on my flight instruments and ignore the horrific visual illusions until my mind re-caged itself and I could continue with the rendezvous.

What I was later able to deduce as the cause of this illusion was the normal formation movement of Cheese's flight around the tanker. As each jet finished refueling from directly behind and below the tanker, it would move to a position near one of the tanker's wingtips, and the F-15 on the opposite wingtip of the tanker would move down and to the center position of the tanker in preparation to receive gas. It made it appear that the KC-135 was rolling wingtip over wingtip.

As Cheese's flight cleared off the tanker, he let me know they were going to head off to their orbit area and look for some better weather. I told Cheese I would contact him on the radio when my flight was done refueling. From this point, I moved myself into the "pre-contact" position directly centered and slightly underneath the refueling boom that was jutting out the back of the KC-135, as the rest of PENNZOIL flight moved up to the wing positions. Now it was time for some more fun.

If I thought the St. Elmo's fire and the spiraling tunnel effect were bad enough, nothing was like the roller coaster ride that I was about to experience. This tanker definitely had its auto-pilot feature turned off. I am not sure if it was the pilot or co-pilot flying, but his or her attempts to keep the airplane level and on altitude resulted in more of an erratic up and down porpoise-like pitching, with a little "Dutch roll" (spiral tail-wagging) thrown in for good measure. It was impossible for me to maintain a constant position to allow the poor Boomer (refueling boom operator) to "plug me."

After multiple attempts, I finally had to break radio silence and tell the tanker pilot, "If you don't fly a little smoother we are not going to be able to get our gas, and we won't be able to complete our mission." I don't know what happened (if the pilot engaged the auto-pilot, or decided to not try so hard to maintain correct altitude), but right after that the KC-135 flight path smoothed out and we were quickly able to complete our air refueling. As the last wingman (Willie in PENNZOIL 64) moved off the boom, I changed the flight over to our AWACs check-in radio frequency ... and it seemed that all hell broke loose.

***

"The Plan" on Night 1 was for an initial multi-pronged attack across Iraq's air defense network. The attack portion of that plan in our sector was to be executed by Tomahawk land-attack cruise missiles and the F-117 stealth attack aircraft over Baghdad, and a mission of F-15E Strike Eagles attacking the western H-2/H-3 airfield complex. Preceding and supporting this initial "surprise" attack would be helicopter gunships. They would fly in at very low altitude, guided by Special Ops helicopters with night-vision and specialized navigation equipment, to destroy the picket line of Iraqi early-warning radar sites along the Saudi border. Another very "ballsy" event was a couple of EF-111 electronic attack jamming aircraft also going in early at very low altitude, with absolutely no supporting fighter escort. The EF-111s would pop-up and start jamming to blind and confuse Iraqi surveillance and air defense radars, to assist the F-117s' undetected ingress. Contrary to popular belief, stealth technology did not mean that the F-117s were invisible to radars, just low observable.

The H-hour for the first targets to be hit was 0300. Once cruise missiles arrived, and the F-117s and F-15Es dropped their bombs on their intended targets (and possibly even before that), the element of surprise would be over. Immediately after dropping their bombs, all the initial attack and support aircraft were supposed to head south out of Iraq and clear the way for our massive Eagle sweep north into enemy airspace, designed to take out the Iraqi fighters that responded to the initial warnings and attack.

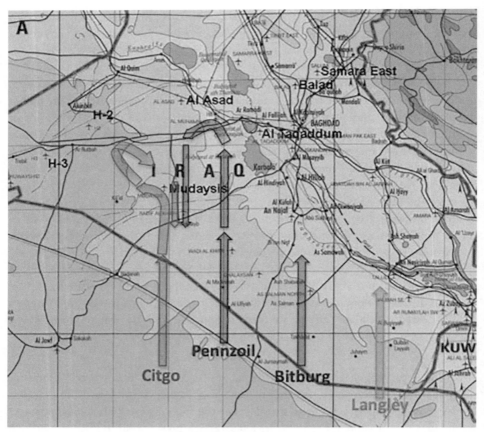

A map showing the mission flow for DESERT STORM, Night One/H-Hour (0300), 17 Jan 1991. It displays the generic ingress direction of the 4 × F-15C 4-ship fighter sweeps at H-Hour (left to right): 58TFS/CITGO (Graeter, Lead), 58TFS/PENNZOIL (Tollini/Lead-Mission Commander), Bitburg F-15Cs, Langley F-15Cs. Specific ingress/egress flow direction is shown for both Eglin 58TFS 4-ships as indicated. PENNZOIL engagement/shoot of IrAF MiG-29 by Kelk in approximate location at the tip of the first arrow/north of Wadi Al Khirr. CITGO engagement/shoot down of 2 IrAF F-1 Mirage by Graeter just south of Mudaysis Air Base.

The absence of friendly aircraft in Iraq was intended to give all the Eagles a free field of fire to shoot beyond visual range (BVR) against targets coming south, using highly liberal rules of engagement (ROE) and identification (ID) criteria. To insure that all the friendly aircraft were out of Iraq, our initial Eagle "push" time (starting time to leave our orbit and proceed on our attack) was supposed to be at 0315.

When I checked-in PENNZOIL flight on our primary air-to-air radio frequency with our E-3 AWACs controller, it was right at 0300 and he already sounded a bit frantic. The E-3 controller was requesting that we "PUSH NOW!", almost 15 minutes early. I was extremely hesitant to commit to the attack this early, however, because of the obvious conflict to the planned flow and because of the possibility that friendly aircraft would be in our field of fire. My first response to AWACs was "Negative" and I asked to him explain why he was requesting an early Push. Our controller quickly explained that they had indications of Iraqi fighters scrambling from the southern airfields, and this would put them right in the path of the Strike Eagles that had just hit H-2/H-3 airfields and were egressing at low altitude to the southeast. This information stuck in my craw, and I flashbacked to the planning meeting I had with the F-15E squadron a couple months before.

While I was visiting the E-model squadron to coordinate the final timing and routes to insure deconfliction, I noticed that their exit route would take them just a few miles south of Mudaysis airfield in south-central Iraq. Mudaysis was a forward-operating Iraqi fighter base and we knew from intelligence that the IrAF always had several fighters on alert-scramble status there. I pointed this out to the F-15E mission commander and I suggested he should exit Iraq due south and across the Saudi border, before turning southeast to RTB. He told me they didn't have the gas to do that, and although I had plotted it out as the same time and distance to cover, I did not want to second-guess him. I also had no authority over his mission planning. Now, as it turned out, my concerns were well founded.

I checked in Cheese and his CITGO flight and found out they were about 60nm south of the Push point. Cheese had taken his flight farther south to find some clear weather and had planned to turn north in a few more minutes to hit his Push point on time. Now, we didn't have the time.

I made a command decision (screw it!): "OK ... PENNZOIL, CITGO Fence In! ... we're pushing now!"

We quickly set up our avionics systems for combat (fence check) and "armed-hot," i.e., selected our master arm switch into the "hot" mode, so all weapons could now be fired; it was kind of like taking the safety off on a gun. PENNZOIL and CITGO flight headed north into a situation that would now be totally different to that originally planned.

First, all eight of our Gorilla Eagles were supposed to be spread out line abreast, but instead, because of Cheese's position to the south, my flight was about 50nm in front and offset to the east. That was not the biggest problem, though. As I looked on my radar scope to the north, I saw a slew of little round circles stretching from left-to-right across my scope about 40nm in front of us. These little round circles were the friendly Mode 4 interrogation replies of the F-15Es as they flew from the west to the southeast, and sure enough they were passing right by Mudaysis airfield. At least the F-15Es had rolled their Mode 4 codes at 0300, or this would have been even more disconcerting.

We also had to be concerned about the EF-111s that would be exiting to the south as well, because if they were jamming it might mask their own friendly AAI interrogations on our radars; they could possibly appear as enemy radar contacts to us. The EF-111s were supposed to be at very low altitude, which was listed as a "safe" altitude block in the Airspace Control Order (ACO); so long as they followed that plan, we would not shoot at them. But you never know what's going to happen in combat and they might have a reason (like low fuel or being chased by an Iraqi fighter) to climb out of the low altitude safe block.

I wasn't too worried about the F-117s. We did not expect to see them, even on our radars. Our worst fear was accidently hitting one, but I knew their ingress/egress altitude and we would be well above them.

Well, this was the hand we'd been dealt, so we were just going to have to take it as it came.

I told Cheese about the F-15E "paints" (friendly AAI responses), since he was still too far away to see them yet. Mudaysis was directly in front of CITGO's ingress route (our PENNZOIL ingress route was a little farther east between Mudaysis and Baghdad), so I knew Cheese and his CITGO flight were going to be the ones dealing with the F-15E identification conflict.

As our PENNZOIL flight continued to climb above 30,000 feet, and at a place that I approximated as crossing the Saudi–Iraqi border, suddenly we broke out through the top of the clouds into beautiful clear, dark skies. I sure did welcome the sight of all those stars and as I looked forward I could see lights across the entire southern portion of Iraq. There were no clouds at all in Iraq. I deployed PENNZOIL into our night 4-ship wall formation, just like we had practiced so many times before in our DESERT SHIELD CAPs.

This time it was for real, and we were ready to Rock 'n' Roll.

Cherry was my #2 (wingman) on my left (west) side, while JB (#3) and his wingman Willie (#4) were on my right (east) side. I immediately started picking up unknown (bogey) contacts on my radar and confirmed with the AWACs controller that these were likely Iraqi fighters. Most of the contacts we locked with our radars would turn and run away, whether aware of their potential demise or just to their good fortune.

Part of my first experience of combat was the spectacular display of antiaircraft artillery (AAA) and surface-to-air missiles (SAMs) firing into the night sky. Both the Baghdad and H-2/H-3 areas were lit up like huge multicolored (mostly red and orange) fountains. The CNN ground-level news video of the start of the war could not do justice to what we could see from 30,000 feet at night. I could only imagine what it was like for the strike aircraft to fly over or through that field of fire as they tried to concentrate on delivering their bombs on target.

I did not have long to enjoy the view before I picked up a contact on my radar, slightly to the right of my nose. It was a fast-moving aircraft that was on a rapid climb from 12,000 feet, coming straight toward us.

At first I thought it could be one of the EF-111s heading south and possibly climbing out of his safe zone. Since the bogey was to the right side of our formation,

I let JB know about the contact and handed off targeting responsibility to him. When JB confirmed he had locked the target, I broke my radar lock and reverted back to a search mode looking for any other nearby targets while I monitored JB's progress.

JB was having a hard time determining if this was a friendly or Iraqi fighter. I'm sure he had the same concerns as I about the whereabouts of the EF-111s, and he was not receiving either friendly electronic replies or enemy ID indications. Several times JB requested a "declaration" from the AWACs controller on whether this was Friend or Foe, but neither response was forthcoming.

It began to get tense for JB and the rest of the flight, as the unknown fighter continued climbing and approached inside 15nm. At this point JB was within range to take a BVR AIM-7 Sparrow missile shot. If this was an Iraqi fighter (such as a MiG-29 Fulcrum) carrying a similar AA-10A Alamo missile, then JB and most of the rest of our flight was in range of the enemy's weapon as well. Within seconds JB's, his wingman Willie's, and my own radar warning receiver (RWR) scope lights and audio tones came on, indicating that an aircraft had locked its fire-control radar onto our jets. The symbology of the RWR indication was that it was most likely an enemy radar lock and probably from an Iraqi MiG-29.

That last bit of warning was enough for JB and he fired what he believed was his first AIM-7 shot, but on his weapon status panel indicator it showed the missile was still on board his jet. JB had also momentarily closed his eyes to avoid some expected flash blindness from the night missile shot, so he never got a chance to confirm visually that his missile had fired.

JB and I could both plainly see the "dot" of a missile rocket plume dancing through the black night sky, but couldn't tell if it was JB's missile heading toward its target or a missile the Iraqi fighter had fired at us. None of us waited around much longer, however, as we started defensive maneuvering. JB called out that he was turning toward the east (the preferred way for him to go to deconflict with me and Cherry) and Willie calls "Notch East" also, indicating a 90-degree descending maneuver to the east to break the enemy radar lock. I call out "PENNZOIL 61, Notch West" and start a similar maneuver as Willie, but in the opposite direction (or so I think).

I also attempt to dispense some "chaff" (packages of fine aluminum strips used to confuse enemy radars and missiles), but having changed our countermeasure dispenser (CMD) from what we used in training to a different mode in combat, I accidently dispense a couple of huge MJU-10 flares, used to decoy infrared (IR) heat-seeking missiles. At night the MJU-10 flares appear almost as an explosion, and Cherry, looking over in my direction (immediately after my defensive maneuver call) believed that I might have blown up.

Cherry's concern was eased as I confessed my mistake over the radio. Also, my RWR threat indication stopped flashing its visual and aural warning, so I was successful in either defeating the MiG-29 radar or for some reason he was no longer locked on to me.

As I turned back quickly to the north to re-establish our flow direction, I noticed off in the distance what looked like a small 4th of July sparkler descending across the night sky. I had no idea what this was at the time, but JB saw the same thing. No sooner did I turn back north, when I picked up a radar contact *very* close, inside 5nm, below my nose and crossing right-to-left. This radar contact approximated the last location at which I had seen the Iraqi fighter, now accounting for my defensive maneuver. I locked the target and saw it was pointing in my direction. I have just seconds to decide if its hostile or friendly. I am smack in the heart of an enemy missile zone if this unknown fighter should choose to shoot at me.

Shoot? Don't Shoot? Shoot? ... DON'T SHOOT!!! I cannot take a chance, and I just hope I don't take an enemy missile right in my face. I hold my shot ... and fortunately I don't see any missiles coming my way. It is a pitch-black night, but I rolled up my wing anyway to look down on the unidentified jet traveling quickly under my nose. As I do this, we are very close, and I could see into the cockpit of the unknown fighter. I recognized the interior cockpit lighting of another F-15 Eagle. It turned out this "bogey" is actually Willie (JB's wingman). He had called out earlier that he was maneuvering east for his defensive reaction, when in actuality he had turned west, right towards my flight path. I would never have forgiven myself (nor would have Willie) if I had shot him down. Training and adherence to ROE (and maybe a little luck) staved off a disaster.

Our radar scopes were now "clean" where the Iraqi fighter used to be. When JB and I talked about it later on the ground, and confirmed that his missile did actually come off his jet, JB reported this action as a likely shoot down of an Iraqi MiG-29 fighter. I don't know how they found out, but by early the next day JB's "Kill" was confirmed.

JB's engagement would turn out to be the first aerial kill of DESERT STORM, although for some reason CNN would report that the 1st Fighter Wing's Capt Steve "Tater" Tate had the first shoot-down. Because of our early push across the border, JB's kill came a good 15–20 minutes ahead of Tater's. In fact, our mission would get two more confirmed kills before anybody else that night.

Shortly after JB's engagement, I found a couple of targets over Mudaysis. It would have been easy from my position to turn Cherry and myself to the west to engage these targets, but I knew from so many large-force missions that remaining disciplined and sticking with planned flow and areas of responsibility was critical. If I flew west to engage, I would fly directly across Cheese's CITGO flight path and create a confusing and dangerous situation. Also, I had my own responsibility to lead my flight to the north to sweep the western Baghdad corridor. I couldn't just drop that responsibility and leave JB and Willie on their own, so I told Cheese about the Mudaysis contacts and handed them off to his CITGO flight.

It was not long after that we started to hear Cheese and his flight on the radio coordinating their attack and taking Fox 1 (AIM-7 Sparrow) shots against the Iraqi fighters. Cheese had significant problems sorting out the Iraqi F-1 Mirage fighters that had scrambled right over the top of the low-altitude egressing F-15Es. He did a great job holding his fire until absolutely sure of whom he was shooting. When Cheese's AIM-7 missile hit the first Iraqi F-1, it exploded into a huge fireball that was probably accentuated by the deep nighttime darkness, and we heard an excited "SPLASH, SPLASH!!" on the radio.

To this day, I still don't know why Cheese said the word "Splash." We immediately knew it meant he had shot down his target, but until then nobody that I knew of had ever used the word "Splash." In training, we always called out "Kill" if we assessed a satisfactory simulated weapons shot that would have been successful in downing the training aircraft. "Kill" was what we expected to use and hear ... but "Splash?" It was actually the perfect word to use (like we had heard in old World War II movies), and it became the standard for the rest of the war.

When I heard that "Splash" call I was elated, probably as much as if I had shot that Mirage fighter down myself. It meant our mission was starting off successfully, in spite of the challenges of the change in plans. Soon after, Cheese called another "Splash." Wow! Splash two, already (and JB's, which we didn't know for sure about yet). It turned out, though, that Cheese did not actually shoot at the second Iraqi F-1. Nobody knows for sure, but I assume this poor Iraqi pilot, who likely was following his leader (the first F-1 that Cheese shot down), had either became disoriented or had enough of the war (and ejected) after seeing his flight lead demise. Whatever the reason, his F-1 became a tumbling inferno as it crashed into the nighttime desert floor. Cheese rightfully got credit for his second "kill" of the night.

For the rest of the mission, we would occasionally lock up a few more targets, but all of them would basically run away from us. We continued on our planned route and soon were heading south for Saudi airspace and to avoid conflicting with follow-on waves of hundreds more fighters and bombers.

When I knew that PENNZOIL and CITGO flights were safely across the border in friendly territory, I called for everybody to turn on all their exterior lights to a bright/flash mode. I was amazed as I looked out across the night sky to see my flight still in perfect formation, and right alongside to the west was Cheese and his CITGO flight. We came out in the perfect line-abreast 8-ship formation.

There was a lot of excitement as we landed, still at night, back at Tabuk. Maintenance and weapons troops already knew about the missile expenditures and the possibility of aerial victories. We had just a little bit of time to debrief and get the details of Cheese's exciting engagement and also discuss JB's shot and the likely kill of his target. We headed straight back to our rooms to get some much-needed sleep ... my 4-ship was going on a large-force daytime OCA mission in just a few short hours. OBJECTIVE—BAGHDAD!

***

The first full daytime missions of DESERT STORM were about to begin, and I was going to be in on one of the *big* ones. This was a large-force strike mission of two squadrons of F-16 Falcons and all the OCA support they needed to accomplish their mission; F-4 Wild Weasels to suppress enemy SAMs; EF-111s to provide electronic jamming support; and 20 Eagles from the Gorillas and Langley's 1st Fighter Wing. This is one of those missions Langley gave up in deference to our experience in the Gorillas and we had overall charge of the air-to-air pre-strike sweep and escort duties. I wasn't the mission commander though; I had chosen Chuck "Sly" Magill, our USMC exchange pilot in the 58th to lead this one.

Sly was an experienced fighter pilot, but was new to the Eagle. He wore the recognizable Top Gun School patch he had earned from his duties as a Marine F-18 Hornet driver. I had helped put Sly through his Instructor Upgrade in the Gorillas and watched him gain experience in leading large-force missions during many Nellis and RED FLAG trips. So I felt he could do this one, and just to be sure I would fly as the lead of his other 4-ship at the leading edge of the pre-strike sweep. I had some other significant missions, for which I needed Cheese Graeter, JB Kelk, and Hoser Draeger to lead, so I thought I could kill two birds with Sly leading this one and my being there to watch over his planning and execution.

The overall plan was pretty straightforward, a classic "Alpha strike" type of package (as they called it in the Navy). Our 8-ship of Eglin Eagles would sweep about 25–30nm ahead of the main body of the strike package to take out any airborne Iraqi fighter CAPs. Strung out along the flanks immediately in front, to the side and rear of the massive train of F-16s would be the F-4 Wild Weasels, EF-111s, and the three separate 4-ships of Langley Eagles to prevent Iraqi fighters from getting too close or swinging around the back end of the long train of strikers.

For our 8-ship sweep, Sly came up with a very solid and simple plan. His 4-ship would be on the west (left) side and would sweep all the way to the northwest side of Baghdad near Al Asad, one of Iraq's major fighter airfields and a likely source of enemy fighter activity. After his 4-ship had completed their sweep, Sly would take them to the southwest to look for any fighters coming from the west side of Iraq trying to end-run the strike package. My 4-ship would be on the east (right) side and we would sweep toward the other major airbase, Al Taqaddum, and then flow to the southwestern border of Baghdad's extensive SAM defense zone. From there our job was to flow quickly to the west to get out of the line of fire of the huge strike package coming up behind us. This flow plan was important to avoid the possibility of fratricide and not impact the strike package ingress route.

We had great weather that day and everything was running like clockwork. All the participants were in synch and getting their pre-mission air refueling, meeting up in our rendezvous pre-strike orbits, and then "pushing" on time. It was a juggernaut that was on a mission and it would not be stopped ... and out in front of this massive display of USAF air power were ... two lonely Iraqi MiG-29 Fulcrums.

Those poor Fulcrum pilots had to be the unluckiest guys ever to strap on a fighter jet. I doubt they had any idea of what they were up against or what was coming their way, but if they had even an inkling of the approaching tsunami wave of Air Force fighters, then I would say they were probably the bravest pilots in the air that day.

The radio call about the MiG CAP came from our AWACS controller fairly early on, and he had already identified them as "BANDITS" (enemy fighters). The MiG-29s' CAP location was smack in the middle of the area of responsibility for my 4-ship, just southeast of Al Taqaddum and presently outside of the Baghdad SAM rings. I was already anticipating another engagement for my 4-ship and a chance to add a couple more Iraqi fighters to the Gorillas' scoreboard. Figuring this time it would be my turn to get a missile off of my jet, I started to lean my 4-ship more and more to the east, as a lined us up to be in position for long-range BVR AIM-7 shots and then a quick exit to the west to deconflict with the strikers behind us.

As the enemy CAP started to show up as contacts (small brick-shaped blips) on our radars I got a call from Sly to the west. Sly directed a sudden change in plans and told me he was going to engage the Iraqi Fulcrums with his 4-ship. Almost before I could say anything, I watched as Sly's 4-ship of Eagles cut across our nose and flowed to the northeast to engage the lone 2-ship of Iraqi Fulcrums.

Wow. At the time, I could not really say anything. I'm sure JB (my #3) and the rest of my flight was wondering the same thing as I … "What the hell just happened?" But, Sly was the mission commander and it was within his authority to change the flow of the mission if he thought he needed to. My biggest concern at this point was not who was going to engage the MiG-29s, but that with Sly's flight diverting to the northeast, the western flank of the strike package ingress route was totally exposed. I suggested to Sly that I pick up his original routing, and Sly concurred and cleared my flight to reestablish a new course toward Al Asad. The only thing we could do at this point was to embrace our new responsibility, turn our jets to the northwest, and start looking for any other Iraqi fighters in that direction.

And then a (not so) funny thing happened. As Sly (with Hoser Draeger as his #3) rushed headlong into their first combat engagement, we could hear their excited communications of radar locks and missile shots. We were rooting for them also, because that was our job … shoot down Iraqi fighters; it didn't really matter to me who got to do the shooting. But as Sly and Hoser's engagement progressed, my 4-ship started getting radio calls from our AWACS controller about Iraqi fighters in our vicinity and closing on us fast. IRAQI FIGHTERS?! Where had they come from? We had only seen the two Fulcrums that Sly and Hoser were in the process of dispatching. My 4-ship searched frantically on our radars in the direction the radar controller told us to look, but we were "clean" (no radar contacts).

The AWACS controller's voice became more and more anxious as he called out the MiG's position approaching 10nm, then 5nm … and then, the worst thing you can possibly hear without any situational awareness, "MERGED!" … meaning the bandits were within our formation. I immediately called for the 4-ship to "BREAK LEFT," starting max performance defensive turns with chaff and flares to decoy any undetected missiles from the unseen Iraqi fighters. After 180 degrees of break turn and no bandits in sight, I called for another defensive break turn. If there was an Iraqi fighter out there, one of us would surely see it inside the middle of one of our break turns, or at least see a smoke trail of his missile shots.

Instead, nothing was to be seen, and then … slowly … slowly… I started to figure out what had just happened.

I gave my AWACS controller my flight's position off of the "Bullseye": a geographic or latitude/longitude point we could use as a common reference via bearing and range to that position. I told him we were now out to the west, and we had exchanged flow plans with the other 4-ship. Suddenly the light bulb came on for our controller and the rest of my flight also. The "bandits" our controller was calling out were actually the MiG-29s that Sly and Hoser had gone to engage in the east. When Sly changed the flow plan mid-stream, nobody had bothered to mention to our AWACS about this, and our controller, of course, assumed my 4-ship was the one to the east engaging the MiGs. The "ghost" bandits we could not locate actually did not even exist.

My biggest fear was that I had somehow screwed up and led my whole flight into an ambush, but at this point I was just happy we had not stumbled into an unseen hornets' nest of Iraqi fighters. I reorganized my 4-ship and we continued on with our new flow plan, eventually sweeping out to the southwest uneventfully and heading on back home to Tabuk.

Sly and Hoser did what they were supposed to do with the MiGs. After the Fulcrums played a game of cat and mouse, staying in their CAP near their protective SAMs, at the last minute they turned directly face up with Sly's 4-ship and both Iraqi fighters went down in flames from BVR AIM-7 shots. I doubt they even knew what hit them.

The highlight of that mission for me actually came shortly after I landed back at Tabuk. After taxiing my jet out into the Death Valley parking area near the approach end of the runway, I climbed down the ladder and started to organize my gear to catch a ride back to our operations building. Col Rick Parsons (the wing commander) had come out to our spots, presumably because he had already heard of the engagement on this mission. As he walked up to me to ask what had happened out there, Sly's 4-ship came up initial and performed a standard overhead break turn over the top of the airfield in preparation for landing.

This was the first daytime mission where we had shot down some enemy aircraft, and in the back of my mind I just kind of wondered if Sly and Hoser were going to follow through with the traditional fighter-pilot method of demonstrating to the airfield they had just downed an adversary … an aileron roll over the runway … a "Victory Roll." We had talked about this among the pilots, but nobody ever committed to saying they would do it, mostly because we did not know what the repercussions would be. This was not "our fathers' Air Force," and in peacetime this type of action would likely result in a long-term grounding or even loss of one's wings.

As Col Parsons and I started to chat, I kept one eye on Sly as he came around his final turn with his landing gear down in what looked like an ordinary landing approach. But, just as he came in over the threshold of the runway, and right before his wheels touched down I watched, amazed, as Sly slapped his gear back up, plugged the jet into afterburner, pulled up the nose ... and performed a beautiful slow roll, right there in front of the whole world, and Col Parsons. I had a huge smile on my face, but when I looked over at Col Parsons I saw him with his jaw locked tight, turning five shades of red, and a laser beam stare penetrating Sly's Eagle. It didn't get any better when Hoser performed the exact same maneuver following Sly.

I thought, "Oh wow! Sly and Hoser are screwed!" But just then, the entire crowd of crew chiefs and weapons troops out in Death Valley (and all across the airfield) let out the biggest whooping and hollering we'd heard since the day we arrived in Tabuk. Those were "their" Eagles (us pilots, we merely borrowed them) that had just come back with weapons expended and a couple of Victory Rolls. I looked back at Col Parsons and he just shook his head and walked back to his car. That was his way of giving tacit (even if uninvited) approval for his boys to do Victory Rolls after any daytime kills. Cool.

I did not intend to relive the details of somebody else's MiG engagement in this book, but I felt it was necessary to do so in this case for a couple of reasons. No account of any individual's actions is ever going to be reiterated exactly the same when told from different and unique perspectives and with the passage of time. But, ever since that day, when I have read the accounts of this specific engagement in other books (written by somebody else from versions of the pilots involved), I have been perturbed by the imprecision of the account and by the possible intimation that my 4-ship had in some way performed in a less-than-gallant manner.

I don't know where those interpretations came from, and sometimes things can just be "lost in translation" when the events are retold by a third person, but I have to take this opportunity to clear this up and protect the reputation of my 4-ship and my own. Cherry, JB, Willie, and I performed in an outstanding and professional manner that day, even when the mission plan was changed airborne at the last minute.

I did not blame Sly one bit for his desire to be the one to engage the MiGs. When he first saw me on the ground, in fact, before I could congratulate him on the kills, he apologized for the change of plan and for the confusion that followed in the air. I was over it by then anyway, because we completed the mission and got all our Eagles and pilots back in one piece.

It wasn't until the next day that I learned of the greater problems created by the last-second change of flow plans. I received a call from one of the squadron weapons officers with the Langley Eagles, and then from the F-16 overall strike mission commander. They were both rather upset by what had happened.

Because of the extra distance and time Sly's 4-ship had to take to move over to our area in the east, the change significantly impacted the flow of the rest of the strike package and the ability for the Langley Eagles to protect them. With Sly's 4-ship in the middle of their ingress route, the F-16s had to deviate to the east and the next thing they knew they were being engaged (shot at) by Iraqi SAMs, which their original route would have avoided. The Langley Eagles could not be of much assistance either; they were now more worried about avoiding Sly's friendly 4-ship of Eagles, which was now in their line of fire anyway, if some other Iraqi fighters had happened to show up.

In the end, maybe it was just "No Harm, No Foul." In spite of the perturbations, the mission was completed, everybody got home safe, and we bagged two more MiGs. But to me, it reemphasized what I had learned over and over again at so many large-force FLAG exercises ... stick with the plan and cover your responsibilities! Don't ad lib unless there is a really good reason to do so.

I never told Sly about the calls and retribution I had to fend off. I assumed he already knew or expected some of the fallout. In a couple more days, it would not matter anyway. The entire character of the air war over Iraq was going to change drastically in a few brief moments of vicious contact with the enemy.

***

It was the morning of January 19, 1991, and we had been in a non-stop shooting war for the last 48-plus hours. Hundreds of targets had been hit and nine Iraqi fighters had already been shot down (five of them by the Gorillas). We had lost a couple of our own coalition fighters and crews to enemy SAMs and AAA, and we had yet to learn that the US Navy had lost one or two aircraft to Iraqi fighters on the first night. (After the writing of this book I discovered from authors Douglas Dildy and Tom Cooper, that the US Navy SEAD mission that came in to the fight immediately after our egress on Night One would lose Navy Lt Cmdr Scott Speicher in his F-18 Hornet. Lt Cmdr Speicher's loss was a mystery for many years and he was MIA, presumed to possibly be a hidden POW under Saddam Hussein. It would later be confirmed that Lt Cmdr Speicher would perish that night after he was ambushed by Iraqi ace Lt Zuhair Dawoud in his lone MiG-25 attack that night.)

Some of us were on our fourth or fifth combat missions, with precious little sleep in between.

JB Kelk had the lead of our 4-ship this morning (I was #3), as well as overall lead as the air-to-air mission commander role for another big-strike push up north to Baghdad. I had complete faith in JB and I knew we would not have any issues with flow plans or mission management. JB was a seasoned mission commander, but unfortunately on this day he would not have a chance to demonstrate that. We got a call for a mission scrub (cancellation) due to poor weather in the target area while we were still in our airborne orbit waiting to head north. There was a low undercast of solid clouds stretching from the Saudi border as far north as we could see toward Baghdad. The F-16 strike aircraft were carrying "dumb" bombs that day, i.e. regular unguided bombs not much different to those dropped from B-17s during World War II. The F-16s needed to be able to see their targets to hit them, and it wasn't going to happen today. The entire mission of more than 70 fighters was told to RTB and we figured we would try it another day.

Everybody except for JB's 4-ship that is. We were directed to an orbiting KC-135 tanker and told to get gas and wait there for another mission tasking. When JB queried the controller about the possible tasking we were told, "Standby for possible Buster Mission."

BUSTER MISSION! This was it! A chance to take out Saddam Hussein himself and end this war today. So we waited … and waited … got more gas … and waited. Finally, we were told to disregard the Buster Mission and RTB to Tabuk. Damn!

We never did figure out what prompted the Buster Mission call, but it was the only time during the war that I know of that the "Buster Mission" codeword was ever uttered. The nice thing about our landing at Tabuk that morning, however, was that we were going to have a little more time this day before our next mission. A chance to get something to eat, a hot shower, and maybe a full eight hours' sleep was in store.

That is, until I got the call from Riyadh.

On the phone was Capt Richard "Spad" McSpadden, my old friend from the Dirty Dozen during our golden days as Lieutenants at Kadena. Spad was working a non-flying job for the war in the Combat Operations cell in Riyadh. He oversaw all the daily F-15C missions and coordinated any changes.

Today he asked me straight up, "Kluso … I need four Eagles to fly a CAP in the vicinity of H-2/H-3 airfields (western Iraq). The Iraqis shot a bunch of SCUD [surface-to-surface] missiles at Israel last night and the Israelis are pissed. We're going to send up a bunch of strike aircraft to do some SCUD hunting [presumably to make sure we kept the Israelis out this war]. We need somebody out there in a couple of hours to fly a CAP to protect the strikers. Can you guys do it?"

My first reaction was going to be to tell Spad, "No." I knew our schedule like the back of my hand and all of our Eagles and pilots were already "booked" for other missions. We had no extras … except for the F-15s and pilots who had just landed. That would be us.

I told Spad I would call him right back and I quickly conferred with our maintenance chief (Matos) and the rest of the guys. Cherry, JB, and Willie were up for it, and maintenance said they would have no problem turning the jets to an add-on mission. I called Spad back and said we were a "GO." Then we hit the Tabuk flight-line kitchen for a pancake breakfast (more on that later), did a quick flight brief during the meal, and by time we were done eating our jets were ready for us to "kick the tires, and light the fires."

***

The value of the paired 4-ship concept and the continuous training and recent combat missions in those pairings paid off in spades. To be able to turn around and immediately execute what would normally be a complex and potentially hazardous mission was a force multiplier that our adversaries could not even come close to matching.

We carried the CITGO call-sign with us on this day (since nobody else was using it at the time). We first rendezvoused with our air refueling tanker to top off our tanks before proceeding to our planned orbit area. An uneventful tanker event finished, I had time for a quick smoke, and then we pushed north into western Iraq to set up a protective CAP and wait for the friendly strike aircraft we were supposed to protect. We really did not know what to expect but I assumed this would be a routine and uneventful mission for us.

We had barely arrived on station when I got a call from our AWACs controller. He advised us that there was a very large US Navy strike package that was going to be passing directly through our CAP area enroute to a target near Baghdad. Not wanting to be an obstacle to their flow (and not wanting to look like a potential "target" to any trigger-happy Tomcat pilot), I moved my flight farther west and we watched the Navy package drive on past us. I asked our controller to let us know when the Navy fighters were on their way out, and about 30 minutes later we got the call, "CITGO 21, we have your Navy package coming out southbound, and we also have bandits about 100 miles north. Bandits appear to be in pursuit."

It was the last part of that transmission that got my heart pumping a little bit faster. "Bandits? Airborne? ... in pursuit?" I knew we had a tasked mission to stay on orbit, but I still had to ask, "CITGO 21 copies. Let us know if you need us to commit [engage the enemy]." The response from AWACs was immediate, "CITGO 21, Commit!" WOW! From a routine mission to a commit against Iraqi fighters. Things were about to happen very quickly, with nothing to fall back on except teamwork and experience.

I quickly maneuvered the 4-ship due east and called for "Tapes On," to turn on our video tape recorders (to document what was about to happen); "Burners" (afterburners) to gain altitude; and "Combat One" to drop our two external wing fuel tanks for the extra speed to cut off the Iraqi fighters before they could run down the slower-moving Navy strike package. The due east heading would allow the Navy jets to pass by us north to south, and as we approached their 6 o'clock from the west we could turn north to engage the Iraqi fighters.

It played out just as planned. As soon as we turned north, I picked up two radar contacts about 50–60nm away. By this time, AWACs had identified the bandits by type and these were called out as MiG-29 Fulcrums. Hello again, Mr. Fulcrum.

As we turned north we throttled back to normal mil-power (military power) settings (the highest non-afterburner power), but maintained our altitude above 30,000 feet to increase the range of our first AIM-7 BVR shots. The MiG-29 carried the AA-10A Alamo missile, which had approximately the same range as our AIM-7s. By having an altitude advantage, it would also give a shot range advantage that I wanted use to get the kills before we entered into a merged visual dogfight, where some of our tactical advantage could be negated.

Cherry (#2) was on my right side (east) and JB (#3) was on the left side with Willie (#4) farther west of him. It was going to be four of us versus two Fulcrums … 4 vs. 2. I liked those odds, but quickly the complexion of the engagement started to change. As the bandits approached 30nm on our nose, the two Iraqi contacts maneuvered to the northeast and started heading in the direction of Baghdad. I had already seen too many Iraqi fighters turn away and disengage after our radars locked on and set off their radar warning receivers … now it appeared this was happening again. Unless they turned back towards us right away, there was no chance of being able to engage these Fulcrums. "Well," I thought, "at least we have done our jobs and chased them away from the Navy strike package," which was now flowing safely across the Saudi border. No sooner had this thought crossed my mind, when I got another call from AWACs, "Two more bandits airborne at low altitude [30nm farther north] ID MiG-29s." Two more Iraqi fighters airborne, a 4 vs. 4 … now this might be more of a fair fight.

What I saw in front of me on my radar looked very familiar. Through much study of both Soviet tactics and intelligence from the Iran–Iraq War, I recognized what I was seeing as a possible decoy maneuver by the Iraqi formation. By turning perpendicular away from my flight, the lead element of the Iraqi Fulcrums may have been trying to get us to follow them. If we flowed to the northeast to follow the first fighters, it would allow the new enemy aircraft, the ones that AWACs called out to the north, to outflank our left side and come around the corner to ambush us from behind. This was a very common Iraqi tactic, used with much success against Iranian F-14 Tomcats and F-4 Phantoms.

The difference today was that we were not Iranian fighter pilots and we weren't flying Tomcats and Phantoms. Both the F-14 and F-4 had problems with their radars in a "look-down" mode, trying to find targets down low below their own altitude. Thus they would often not see the trailing Iraqi fighters on their sensors and would "take the bait" and follow the decoys, to their eventual demise. But, the F-15's radar and missiles were designed as a "look down—shoot down" weapon systems, so on this day we could see all of the targets. The other factor in our favor was our intelligence on the Iraqi tactics, as well as many hours of experience gained against our own Aggressors and other simulated adversaries, who would test us against these types of tactics.

The pace of the engagement started to quicken. Once I had determined the likelihood of the lead-across decoy tactic, instead of following the decoys out to the northeast I did the opposite—I turned CITGO 21 flight hard back to the north to offset and stiff-arm the decoys and concentrate our radars and firepower on the trailing Iraqi fighters. Just like I had done back at Eglin with Mongo Robbins on our 2 vs. 4 ride against the F-16s, the plan was to feint, maneuver, stiff-arm, engage and get out before a merge, while maintaining the superior odds of a 4 vs. 2 engagement.

JB (#3) and I now took charge of the radios to communicate our radar targeting picture to the flight and AWACs. At that point, the AWACs controller and our wingman remained silent, only to speak up if they saw something we were missing. I took my first radar lock on the lead bandit and JB locked the other radar contact about 5nm in trail. Before we could make our final radar locks, however, the second group of bandits also started to maneuver: first a turn to the west and then a turn due north away from us. Once again, I thought it might be all for naught and the airborne Iraqi fighters might simply decide to go home and fight another day. But then the second (north) group quickly turned another 180 degrees right back to south, flying head-on to our flight.

We would normally take locks in most cases around 15nm, but today JB and I locked "long" at 25–30nm in anticipation of long-range AIM-7 Sparrow shots, maybe also just because the anticipation was too much and we couldn't wait any longer. This time, to our surprise, the Iraqi fighters didn't flinch and continued to press on straight ahead at very low altitude (about 3,000 feet) and very high speed (about 700–800 KIAS). The next surprise I got was an updated identification of the targets from my own aircraft's Non-Cooperative Target Recognition (NCTR) capabilities. The ID was not a Fulcrum … it was a MiG-25 Foxbat!

I don't recall updating the ID to my flight over the radio. At the time, I am not really sure it mattered to me—Foxbat or Fulcrum—because both were hostile enemy aircraft and our ROE allowed us to fire BVR. Now all JB and I had to do was wait patiently for the next 30–40 seconds, as our high rate of closure brought the two Foxbats into optimum shot range for our AIM-7s. With my radar and JB's radar locked on to these individual targets, we could not continue searching for any other enemy contacts, so I directed Cherry (#2) to "look low" with his radar and told Willie (#4) to look high with his radar. In this way, just in case we had missed anybody the wingmen had the flight "covered" with their radar search patterns.

As the lead target continued to slide inside 20nm, I gently placed my right thumb over the "pickle button" on the control stick handle. This button would commence the launch signal to the AIM-7 missile I had selected next in priority to fire. I also pushed the nose of my Eagle down to start a gradual descent and take some extra speed to help the missile velocity as it came off the airplane. The rest of CITGO flight followed.

It was generally advantageous to be higher than our targets. Sometimes, however, you can be too high, and this can cause problems as the radar antennae starts to reach the limits of how far it can travel to maintain a lock in any general direction.

Within seconds the lead Foxbat was inside 15nm and I slowly started to feel the firmness of the pickle button under my thumb as I increased the pressure and the words "Fox 1" were now forming on my lips ... and then, something totally unexpected happened.

The Foxbat started to make an apparent counter-radar missile defensive turn to the east; it was much the same radar defensive turn I had made against the Iraqi Fulcrum on the first-night mission. This was too much! Whether this Iraqi Foxbat pilot was the luckiest guy in the world, or he had skills well beyond what I expected from the Iraqis, his timing and execution were perfect. We had not observed any such defensive maneuvering from our adversaries up to this point, and our intelligence had not assessed such a high level of training for Iraqi fighter pilots.

Were these really Iraqis flying these Foxbats? But the proof was right in front of me on my radar scope, and as the small green radar target on my scope quickly traveled from left to right, changing aspect from head-on to a right 90-degree beam aspect, my high-tech F-15C pulse-doppler radar did exactly what is was supposed to do—it "broke lock" (lost the radar contact).

Just like that, the Foxbat disappeared off my radar scope, and not coincidentally JB's target performed the same maneuver and JB also lost lock of his target. And if that was not enough, about this same time the AWACs controller warned us that the original two Fulcrums that had maneuvered off to the northeast had turned around and were heading back in our direction.

SHIT! This was not going as planned. We went from a 4 vs. 2 BVR engagement to a low situational awareness (low-SA) intercept, with possibly up to four Iraqi fighters out there somewhere. I quickly told JB to look for the Fulcrums out to the northeast, hoping he could provide some information or engage them before they interrupted our fight, but I don't think this request ever really made it through to JB. In the meantime, I adjusted my radar to an extreme low look-down angle and patiently waited for the Foxbat to come out of his defensive maneuver.

While a target travels perpendicular to another fighter's radar, it is in a region known as the "Doppler notch." The target's speed toward the other fighter is no different than the ground speed of that host radar, so there is no Doppler speed factor for the radar to sense. The target's Doppler speed appears as the same speed as the ground itself, which presents a huge flood of useless radar ground return to the host radar. So, pulse-doppler radars like that on the F-15 "blank" out targets that are in a beam aspect at lower altitudes.

To simplify, it's a known radar "blind zone," and these Foxbats were apparently taking advantage of that.

Having observed this same adversary defensive maneuver many times while training, I knew the answer was to place my radar where I expected the Foxbats to reappear, and be patient. Sure enough, about 10 or 15 seconds later (although it seemed an eternity), as the lead Foxbat maneuvered in a right-hand turn back to south, he exited the radar notch blind zone and reappeared on my radar about 6–7nm in front of us. Fortunately, Cherry had stayed disciplined with his radar search, looking low as I had told him to do earlier, and he found the trailing Foxbat as it also turned "hot" right towards us.

We were back in business! But regrettably—because of the closer range, high closing rate, and our extreme altitude difference—both Cherry and I could not take early AIM-7 shots in the face. It was just too tight, and it became obvious we were going to end up in a situation I was trying to avoid—a visual merge with two living, breathing Iraqi fighter pilots and their jets.

Here we go!

I rolled to my right and started to pull my nose downhill in one last attempt to see if I could get a shot on the lead Foxbat and also to gain a Tally-Ho (visual sighting) of the bandit. My weapons display indicated a "no zone" shot, which meant I could shoot a missile but it would have virtually no chance of arriving on target ... this guy was just way too low and way too fast.

About 1nm in front of me and 20,000ft below me, I see the lead Foxbat skimming over the tops of the low undercast cloud desk. He was absolutely smoking fast, heading south in a straight line. I considered trying to convert to his 6 o'clock, but I knew that he would be long gone by the time I got around the corner and accelerated to his speed (if I can even do that). My decision was made for me, though, when about the same time I heard Cherry call "Tally-Ho! Engaged!" as the trailing Foxbat reached us and started a wide, high-speed turn right underneath us.

As I continued my descending right turn in Cherry's direction and began to cross behind him, I saw Cherry roll his jet over and perform a vertical split-S maneuver, like the second half of a loop starting from upside down and pulling the nose from high to low toward the ground. All I could say to Cherry was "GO!", although the proper element communication from me would have been to say "Press," which meant that #2 (Cherry) now had the lead and I would follow and support him. "GO!" just seemed more appropriate at the time.

Everything was a blur for the next five or six seconds as Cherry and I max-performed our jets in a high-G screaming-ass dive toward the ground and to an offensive position behind Foxbat #2. During this time, JB and Willie must have been watching the rapid sequence of events and Willie (#4) had the wherewithal to blurt out over the radio, "Combat Two!", recommending that we drop our last remaining external centerline fuel tank in order to lighten our load and give the highest level of performance for the coming maneuvering fight. Cherry and I followed that plan and punched off our tanks in the middle of our split-S dive.

Cherry and I were now "clean" Eagles. Nothing extra on our jets to create any additional drag other than the missiles we carried on our wing and fuselage stations. I can say from experience that an F-15C, with Pratt & Whitney 220 engines, at low altitude and low fuel weight, is an absolute beast of a machine. I am not really sure there was any jet out there at the time that could match up with the turn and energy performance of our Eagles.

If that Foxbat pilot had any idea of where we were prior to the merge, he must have been dumbfounded at how quickly Cherry and I arrived at such a highly offensive position behind him. I watched as Cherry pulled maximum Gs to pull out at the bottom of his split-S maneuver; he would tell me later that he totally "over-G'd" the jet, i.e., exceeded the maximum allowable G-limit of the Eagle, well over 9-Gs. In the meantime, my descent path was not quite as vertical as Cherry's, and I was able to ease my way through the bottom half of the turn with 6- or 7-Gs, arriving about 2nm away from the Foxbat, on his right side in his 3 o'clock position, as I pointed my nose at him from across his turn circle. Cherry arrived close to the MiG-25's dead 6 o'clock and within a second or two I saw missiles coming off of Cherry's jet in rapid sequence ... Fox 2 [an AIM-9M heat seeking missile]... Fox 1[an AIM-7 Sparrow radar missile] ... Fox 2 [another AIM-9M] ... Fox 1 [fourth missile, AIM-7 again]. He was like a freakin' Roman candle. The only problem was, Cherry's shots were not hitting his target.

As I watched from across the circle, I noticed the Foxbat in a shallow but very fast 2–3-G right-hand turn, and putting out a well-timed series of countermeasures. Chaff (the aluminum strips to decoy radars and AIM-7 missiles) ... flares (to decoy AIM-9 heat seeking missiles) ... chaff ... flares ... more chaff ... more flares. It seemed his supply was almost endless and I didn't know who was going run out first; Cherry's missiles or Mr. Foxbat's chaff and flares.

Cherry's first AIM-9M (-9 Mike) shot was an obvious miss. I saw the missile come off of Cherry's jet, but about a second later the Foxbat dropped a big load of flares, and Cherry's missile bit-off on the flares and flew away into nowhere. We knew the version of -9 Mike missiles we carried at that time had a big problem against Soviet flares, which was fixed in later versions of the missile, but that was no help on this day. The cheap Soviet flares did their job.

Cherry's next shot (AIM-7 Sparrow) came off his jet. I watched as the motor lit off and the "big white" missile lumbered in the direction of the MiG (AIM-7s were fast missiles, but being larger and heavier they took a little bit longer than the skinny AIM-9 to accelerate). As I watched the missile pull away from Cherry's jet, it made a sudden vertical turn straight down toward the ground. I could only conjecture what had happened; maybe a control fin had fallen off the missile (which seldom, but sometimes happened) or the AIM-7 seeker decoyed itself on the Foxbat's chaff or an erroneous radar return off of the ground itself, since we were so close to the ground. It didn't really matter, because immediately after that came Cherry's third shot—another AIM-9M that was once again decoyed by timely flares.

At this point I had had about enough of this Foxbat. This whole time (it had probably been only 10 or 15 seconds since Cherry's first shot), I had been sitting in a perfect position and weapons parameters with an AIM-9M locked on and tracking

Cherry's MiG. I figured from the angle I was sitting at that any flares from the Foxbat were likely going to be less effective, so I decided to take back the lead of the flight and I radioed to Cherry, "CITGO Two, Come off!" This was intended to tell Cherry to break off his attack and become the supporting fighter to me, so I could pursue and hopefully finish off the Foxbat that was giving his missiles such a hard time.

Cherry never heard my directive call (he would tell me later). Most likely, at the same time I was telling him to "Come off" he was probably saying "Fox 1" in his radio as he took his final (fourth) shot. Simultaneously I let loose with my first missile shot of the war, as I called "Fox 2" and fired my AIM-9 at the Foxbat.

At some point in all this, Foxbat #2's pilot had probably had enough. It appeared he was now (finally) out of chaff and flares, because nothing more was coming out of his jet. He probably could not see Cherry, because Cherry was positioned at his deep 6 o'clock position and that was a known blind spot for the Foxbat, although he may have seen the smoke trails from the multitude of Cherry's missile shots.

In all likelihood the MiG driver saw me out the right side of his canopy, with my nose pointing straight at him and an AIM-9 heat-seeker on its way, pulling lead to intercept him in his turn. Cherry's Sparrow, however, guided sure and smooth this time, as it cozied up to the tail section of the Foxbat and the warhead went off. I was expecting a big fireball, but instead I just saw the warhead detonate and maybe a few small pieces of the MiG's tail sparkle and come off as the jet continued to fly on. Shortly afterwards my AIM-9M arrived at the Foxbat's tail with similar results as Cherry's AIM-7.

Somewhere during our final shots and hits, Cherry (he would tell me later) saw the Foxbat pilot eject from his stricken jet. It must have been a very dangerous, low-altitude and high-speed ejection (which often results in extreme injury to the pilot), but obviously better than the alternative. Cherry called "Splash!" upon seeing the pilot eject, but for me all I saw was a Foxbat that appeared to still be flying.

I changed my weapons selection to guns, because if our missiles were not going to stop him I was going to close to gun range and take out the Foxbat with my Eagle's 20mm cannon. But as I approached the slowing Iraqi fighter inside 2,000 feet, I noticed his afterburners were no longer lit. He appeared as a "dead" airplane as I passed just a few hundred feet behind his darkened afterburner "cans" and I observed Foxbat #2 slip into the low cloud deck and disappear like a sinking ship. Much later, as I left the area, I would see black smoke from his eventual ground impact, rising above the bright sunlit clouds.

No time to admire our work though; there was another Foxbat unaccounted for out there, and maybe those other MiG-29s that AWACs had warned us about could still be returning. I was still fast. I had never deselected burner from the time I rolled out across from Cherry's Foxbat, and now I was close to 700 KIAS at about 3,000 feet, skimming just above the low cloud deck and rather close to the ground. I wanted to get turned around in a hurry, so I continued in my right-hand turn and pulled more than 9-Gs over-G'ing my jet just as Cherry had done. I did this without even realizing it, until I would review my video tape of the event later and hearing the "Bitching-Betty" voice warning telling me "Over-G, Over-G, Over-G."

Another thing I would not hear or know until post-mission (actually about a week later, when I had time to go over the video tape and audio) was that our AWACs controller made a great heads-up call to Cherry and I, "Threat, 8 miles south, inbound." If I had heard that, I would've known immediately that Foxbat #1 (who had left the fight when we first merged) had done his best to get his fast-but-lumbering fighter turned around and back into our fight to help his wingman. Problem was, he was already too late. Fortunately for me, because I had selected "guns" mode just before flying past Foxbat #2 as he dove into the clouds, while I made my high-G right-hand turn back toward the south my radar was still slewed to the right (where it had been when it last broke lock) and in an auto-sweep/auto-lock type mode. So, as I came around the corner to the south ... Ba-Ding! My radar locked up the other Iraqi fighter as he tried to sneak back into the fight.

About this time, Cherry also saw what was happening and called out on the radio, "Lead, you got one on your nose!" "Thank you very much, Cherry" I thought, as I picked up the Tally-Ho on the target and watched him fly from left to right across my nose, as I continued my high-G turn and rolled out about 1nm right behind him. Once again, if Mr Foxbat saw me at all, it must have made his eyes water how fast my Eagle could get its nose around, and how fast he found himself in a defensive predicament. But, I had a predicament too.

At the time, I had no way of knowing whether this was the original Iraqi Foxbat #1, or whether it was an enemy aircraft at all. Cherry and I had been very preoccupied in shooting down his bandit, and there was no way to keep sight of the other Foxbat that whole time. I had no idea where JB and Willie had gone, and it possibly could be one of them, or maybe an F-14 Tomcat from the original Navy package had decided to come back and join the party. In any case, the airplane that was immediately in front of me at relatively close range could be any one of those possibilities, since the planform of all those aircraft I mentioned (both enemy and friendly) can look very similar.

I did not have all day to sit back there and decide if I should shoot this aircraft or not, however, so I had to think of something quickly. The first thing I noticed, even though it was a bright, sunlit day, was I could see two huge afterburner plumes coming out the back of this twin-tail, twin-engine fighter. I thought if I could eliminate the possibility that it was one of my 4-ship flight members, then I could be more confident that this was an enemy fighter. So over our discrete radio frequency I called out, "CITGO flight ... anybody in burner?" and after not hearing a positive reply from anybody I called out, "CITGO, EVERYBODY OUT OF BURNER!"

My assumption was that if my flight members insured they were not using their burners, then the only logical conclusion would be that this was in all likelihood a hostile aircraft, i.e., Foxbat #1. In retrospect, that was probably not going to be a 100% foolproof method of ID, so fortunately by the time I had gone through this complex communication query, I had already figured out what type of airplane was in front of me. I noticed the fighter had two wing-pylon (weapons/store) stations sticking out under each wing. F-15s and F-14s only had one such pylon under each wing, but I also remembered Foxbats carried double pylons on their wing stations. This must be Foxbat #1 and I quickly followed that revelation with a "Fox 1" (AIM-7 Sparrow).

I hit the pickle button and waited to see the big AIM-7 missile thunder out in front of me, but nothing happened. I heard the "clunk," of the missile being ejected from the fuselage weapon station, but the missile motor apparently never fired, and it fell to earth like a stupid bomb. I didn't hesitate to change my weapon select to an AIM-9 and shot the heat-seeking missile within heart-of-the-envelope shot parameters, the heat-seeker tone just screaming at the huge infrared heat signature from the Foxbat's burners. Immediately after I shot my AIM-9, I observed what looked to be a single flare come out of the back end of the Foxbat in front of me. Not a whole string of flares like I saw from Cherry's Foxbat, just one single flare. I thought, "Damn! I don't think my AIM-9 is going to work!" But as I watched, the AIM-9 did not decoy on the flare and appeared to track properly toward the target.

Still, as the AIM-9M arrived at the tail end of the Foxbat, it seemed to miss just slightly behind the burner plumes of the Foxbat and the warhead never detonated … CRAP!

OK, another AIM-7, here we go … I watched mesmerized and seemingly in slow motion. I heard the train-like rumble of the Sparrow's rocket motor light-off, and soon the missile appeared out in front of me and started a smooth and rapid acceleration toward the target. An AIM-9 heat-seeker would normally pull a lot of lead to fly on a predicted intercept path to the target, much like a bird hunter puts his shotgun in front of his target to let the bird fly into the path of his shot. But the AIM-7 instead flew this beautiful arcing turn from the outside of the Foxbat's own turn circle, almost like it had its own conscious mind and was trying to mimic the flight path of the MiG-25 in front. The AIM-7 was so much faster at this range (less than a mile now) that it rapidly caught up with its target.

While this engagement was happening, in my cockpit I was encountering two phenomena I had never experienced before (to this extreme anyway), and which I would never experience again—intense temporal distortion and tunnel vision/hearing. The temporal distortion created this bizarre slow-motion effect. Things that would normally be over in an instant stretched out now to what seemed like tens of seconds or even minutes. From Cherry's fight and "splash" through the whole ID sequence of events with the "afterburner" communication, to each individual missile shot, and its results. The tunnel vision/hearing just seemed to block out almost everything but my own breathing and the radio communication between me and my flight. I could not hear my jet's engines roaring anymore, nor the normal loud high-speed rush of air over the canopy. The rest of the world went to silent and the focus of my sight was almost solely on my target of interest … the Foxbat in front of me.

The only way I could explain this to somebody else is when I saw something similar about 10 years later that reminded of this episode. When I watched the opening sequence of *Saving Private Ryan* (the invasion of Omaha Beach scene), my heart started to race just like it did that day over Iraq, and I started to grip the arms of my chair in the movie theater. Tom Hanks's character goes into a daze after a nearby explosion, a strange slow-motion trance, then suddenly snaps out of it. It was like that.

The Sparrow arced faster and faster toward the target and to my relief it guided all the way to right underneath the Foxbat's belly and then … nothing? I saw the smoke and the missile arrive at its target, disappearing as it flew just under the belly side of the Foxbat. But where was the detonation of the warhead? Then unexpectedly … KA-BOOOOOM! And just as suddenly, I snapped out of the trance.

The missile had arrived on target, and in all likelihood instead of the proximity fuse of the warhead going off, the missile flew right up inside the fuselage of the big Russian fighter and detonated with the backup contact fuse. The delay of this happening was probably a couple of milliseconds, but it seemed like an eternity until I saw the results. What was once 70,000lb of steel and jet fuel became a huge fireball mixed with thousands of minute bits and pieces. This was nothing like Cherry's shoot-down of his Foxbat, or anything like I had ever seen before or after. One second there was a MiG-25 in front of me and the next it just evaporated.

There was a common saying by US fighter pilots that when a jet takes a hit from a large blast-frag warhead on a missile like the AIM-7, all that is left is "hair, teeth, and eyeballs." We used to laugh at that saying, but I wasn't laughing now. I had no idea if that Iraqi pilot had remained in his jet or had at some time ejected from his doomed fighter. All I did know was that if he was still in that Foxbat when the Sparrow arrived, then there was absolutely no chance he could have survived. I only had time much later to think about that though, because at this moment, my heart leapt out of my throat, the sky went from tunnel dark to ultra-bright sunlight, and I could hear myself screaming on the radio, "SPLASH, SPLASH! Everybody out westbound!"

And then the next thing I said, as I realized all of sudden that I was totally and utterly alone, "Where are you guys?" I knew where Cherry was, because I had already directed him out of the fight shortly after his engagement, and he was at the time about 8 or 9nm south of me, heading for the border. To this day, though, I still have no clue of what JB and Willie were doing during our engagement and where they went afterwards. I always assumed they cleared out of the area once Cherry and I started turning-'n'-burning down low. Being anywhere near a "fur-ball" was not a safe place to be, because big fighters, chaff/flares, and missile shots tend to attract a lot of unwanted attention. Regardless, Cherry and I would not meet up with Willie and JB until a little bit later.

The big issue right now for me, and mostly for Cherry, was our dire fuel state. We had used afterburner for quite a while on the initial commit to the intercept, jettisoned some of our extra fuel that was still in our external drop tanks, and then used more afterburner during the actual low-altitude fight with the Foxbats. At low altitude and full afterburner an F-15 can gulp jet fuel at a rate of 2,000lb per minute or more, and we only carried about 13,000lb in our internal fuel tanks. During the middle of our engagement I heard my "BINGO" warning going off (a little transmission from Betty, "BINGO FUEL ... BINGO FUEL"), telling me I had reached a preset fuel state, which normally meant I had only enough gas to make it home or to my airborne aerial tanker. Cherry and I both continued flying and fighting right past our BINGO settings. I had about 3,000lb of gas, but Cherry was in an "Emergency Fuel" state with about 1,500lb of gas, and we were both still over enemy territory. Not only did we not have enough gas to fight anymore, we did not have enough to make it all the way back to Tabuk.

The only options were to get to a KC-135 tanker ASAP or divert to an emergency landing field just south of the Saudi–Iraqi border called Al Jouf. It was a Special Ops base, and we had been told we could use it for emergency refueling operations. The first thing I did was contact my AWACs controller and asked him to send the nearest airborne tanker north to rendezvous with us. The controller replied with a "Standby," to which I impatiently replied, "I don't want to hear 'STANDBY'! I want to hear that you have a tanker heading north, RIGHT NOW!" Even though I knew the controller was doing everything he could, Cherry still reminds me how good that made him feel when I yelled out those orders to the AWACs over the radio. It wasn't long before I got a response from the controller and confirmation that a tanker was indeed heading northbound. Great! Now the question was if Cherry had enough gas to make it.

I couldn't relax just yet, not until we got our gas and made it back into friendly territory, but I was starting to breathe just a little bit easier ... and then, one of those very strange "fog of war" kind of things happened that I will never forget.

As I pulled back my power and continued to climb to preserve precious fuel, I noticed a radar contact that was about 9 or 10nm on my nose start to move north toward me. I had confirmed earlier through radio contact and electronic ID means that a contact in this area was Cherry's Eagle heading south. But now, the radar contact was moving north. I wondered, "What is Cherry doing coming north?" since I knew he did not have enough gas to come back to rejoin with me, although I applauded the dedication to element mutual support.

I was about to lock the radar contact in order to direct Cherry to a turn back to south, but I noticed there were now two radar contacts on my scope—one at about

5nm coming toward me, and another still at about 9nm heading south? What the hell? Which one of these is Cherry and who is the other contact?

About that time I looked up at my left 11 o'clock, level, and got a Tally-Ho on a fighter coming my way. I didn't know what it was, but I did know it was not an Eagle. I almost held my breath as the "speck" that was a fighter sprouted wings and tail surfaces as it grew larger in its approach, now towards my left side at about 2nm. I quickly locked up the target and slaved one of my remaining AIM-9M missiles on him just in case.

As I watched, the fighter continued straight ahead. As he started to pass abeam my jet at my left 9 o'clock, I quickly recognized the planform—it was an Iraqi F-1 Mirage.

At first I instinctively flinched, and I very nearly started a hard left bank to pull max Gs to turn and shoot the enemy fighter, but I stopped and continued straight ahead. This was not the time to be a hero and notch another aerial victory. I was low on gas, I was low on missiles, and my wingman needed my help to get to the tanker and get back home. Most important, I was all alone with nobody else to help me if I got in trouble. The price of exchanging an Iraqi Mirage versus a USAF F-15C (and its pilot, namely me) was not worth it.

Caution being the better part of virtue, I let the Iraqi Mirage continue on his way while I kept a wary eye on him to make sure he did not have any of his own ideas of grandeur to engage an Eagle. I don't know if that Iraqi pilot ever actually saw me, but I assume if he did he was probably thinking the same thing I was … "Whew! That was close!"

I managed to catch up with Cherry, as he throttled way back to preserve fuel and allow the tanker to come up north to meet us. As I made contact with the tanker on the "boomer" frequency; the boomer is the enlisted airman who actually operates the refueling probe, or boom, and manages the refueling process and gives you the gas. I saw that there were already two other F-15s on this tanker in refueling position.

I had no idea of who the other F-15s were, I just knew that Cherry needed gas … immediately! I told the boomer to get those F-15s off of the boom so Cherry could get gas … and bless him, he did exactly that. The boomer disconnected the refueling probe from the other F-15 and stowed it in the up position, which was the communication-out signal that "You're not getting any more gas."

When the F-15 moved forward again in apparent attempt to get still more gas, the boomer retracted the probe one more time, and the other Eagles started to get the hint that maybe we needed gas more than they did. I made a radio call on guard also (the common emergency frequency that all aircraft would monitor) to describe in the best way I could that whoever was on the tanker with two other Eagles needed to move off the boom to the tanker's wing position. The other Eagles complied and Cherry swooped down and got his gas. Just enough to get us home

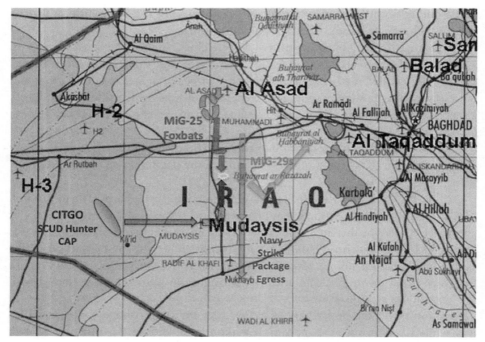

A cropped version of original enhanced map of Iraqi air bases, with the mission flow of the 2 Foxbat shoot downs by Tollini/Pitts, January 19, 1991. Arrows indicate the southbound flow of the USN strike package egress, 2 IrAF MiG-29s, chasing the USN package, then eventually turning northeast toward Baghdad, then the path/arrival of the 2 IrAF MiG-25 Foxbats and eventual merge with Tollini/Pitts as described in text.

to Tabuk, and then I followed right after. As soon as we departed the tanker, the other Eagles resumed their refueling operations.

I did not know it at the time, and not until I got on the ground, but the other two F-15s were Cesar "Rico" Rodriguez and his wingman, Craig "Mole" Underhill, and they were also a bit low on gas. Rico and Mole had just come fresh from their own engagement and shoot down of two Iraqi MiG-29s, not too far from where Cherry and I engaged the Foxbats. When Rico and I met up on the ground back at Tabuk later in the day, he was none too happy with the tanker incident, but after I explained Cherry's fuel situation he understood the priority to get Cherry on the boom.

I never found out who the tanker aircraft commander and boomer were, but the crew on the KC-135 that came north to pick us up and give us an emergency load of gas took the initiative and executed a very courageous mission. We did not have "air superiority" over Iraq at this point (evident by the melee and the number of Iraqi fighters we had just encountered) and the tanker missions had been told to stay south of the Iraqi border under the protection of our defensive CAPs in those areas. This pilot and crew had decided to break the rules and proceed north, even though they had no idea of what they were heading into and if Iraqi fighters might attack them. If the Iraqis had found our -135 before we got there, the tanker and its crew would have been toast. I will always hold a special debt of gratitude to the tanker crews and boomers, and also to our AWACs controller that day, who did such a fantastic job.

JB and Willie had met up with us at the refueling point and, having more gas, they flew defensive cover while the rest of us all took turns sipping gas from the tanker, like a couple of gazelles drinking at a watering hole, hoping no predators showed up. From there we made our way back to Tabuk, reporting into our operations about our missile expenditures (eight total missiles expended between Cherry and I, to take out the two Foxbats), so they knew we were probably coming back with some confirmed kills.

This time when we got into the pattern, probably every able body was out on the field watching to see if we did some victory rolls. Cherry and I did not disappoint them. When Cherry and I taxied into our parking spots next to each other in the Disneyland shelters, the maintenance and weapons troops were going wild, jumping up and down with "thumbs up" signs. As my crew chief helped me unstrap from the jet, he asked me "How many?" and I held up one finger and one for Cherry's. The weapons crews were pulling the spent missile umbilicals off the weapons stations and keeping them as souvenirs (they gave me one of the AIM-9 parts, and I kept that for years, eventually passing it along to my father).

Cherry and I ran up to each other for a big "bro-hug" and slaps on the back, spewing out our mutual stories and filling in what we were both thinking throughout the fight and the return home. It was almost like the scene in *Top Gun* at the end of the movie with the celebration on the deck of the carrier ... actually, it was exactly like that, except without the corny Tom Cruise / Val Kilmer dialogue.

It was done now.

Over the course of my young career, I had wondered if I would ever see combat. And then, over the course of the previous few days, I had wondered if I would get a chance to defeat an enemy fighter in the air. I had already passed up several opportunities to engage the enemy by delegating those targets to other flight members, but this time a kill was mine.

I had fulfilled a desire in the depths of my soul, one that had started as a small spark or ember, but over the course of my career and several intimate combat missions had become a raging inferno. Now I wondered if I could extinguish those flames. It was a dark place and I didn't really want to look at what was inside there.

I had another mission later that night and, because of the extra daytime mission we had scrambled to take on, there was precious little time to sleep. But I needed sleep. My whole flight needed sleep. I took a Restoril in the hope I could get three or four hours of shuteye, but none was to be had. It wasn't just the traces of adrenaline that were probably still coursing through my veins, it was the thoughts of the Foxbat pilot I had just downed. Who was he? What did he look like? Was he a father like me, with small children at home? Why was he a fighter pilot, and did he have the same love of flying I had?

These thoughts rolled over and over in my head and I could not get rid of them. I did not expect this and I was trying to find a way to deal with it. I mean, this is what fighter pilots do, right? Especially air-superiority fighter pilots. We shoot down "MiGs." We "kill MiGs." But nobody ever mentions that there are other human beings in those airplanes. What do we call that? And then, I found a way … a way to "justify" my actions and the results. It was him or me, and dammit, I was glad it was him. There!

Now back to war.

***

We didn't know it at the time, but if we didn't have air superiority before January 19, we definitely had established it after. What we had seen and experienced that day was the first time the IrAF had come out in the daylight to fight, to take on the greatest air force in the world. They lost. They lost big time.

It may seem that to lose four or five jet fighters in a day (among the hundreds of frontline fighters available to the Iraqis) would not be a big deal, but in modern warfare I believe it's different. It is more about the way it happens and the impact on the psyche of the pilots, squadrons, and command elements involved. When you throw your best pilots and best game plan out there, and it doesn't even come close to being successful, the moral of a unit and an air force can be destroyed. Not that they weren't brave aviators; just to strap on a jet you probably know is inferior and to tangle with pilots you probably know are better trained is an extreme act of courage.

I don't really know what happened inside the IrAF, but after that day—the day Cherry, Rico, Mole, and I smacked down four topline Iraqi fighters in a matter of minutes—the IrAF stood down (meaning not generating any combat sorties), a stand down that lasted over a week. Nothing flew. Not a thing.

We continued flying both defensive CAPs and offensive sweep and escort missions for a while, but they seemed pretty pointless. So it wasn't too long before we started performing a mission we had never trained for: area denial.

We moved our fighters and even our support assets (tankers, AWACs, reconnaissance) farther north, and basically just took over all Iraqi airspace, except for the heart of Baghdad metro and its active SAM rings (we still avoided that area). We roved the general area across the western, southern, eastern, and northern portions of Iraq (just to the north of Baghdad) looking for anything that moved. And still, for a long time, nothing moved.

It wasn't until the Coalition started dropping precision-guided bombs on IrAF hardened shelters, which turned out to be not so "hardened" after all, that the

IrAF probably figured it was better to run for it than to lose most of their modern aircraft as they sat on the ground. At the beginning of this phase, when Iraqi fighters, often untouched, started fleeing into Iran, it became a newsworthy story. CNN was asking, "Where were our Coalition fighters? And why were we letting the Iraqi fighters escape?"

Escape? Hell, they were just trying to save their ass. I figured the more that went to Iran and Syria the better, because they were never going to come back, and it might just end this war sooner than later. But apparently the big brass in Riyadh didn't see it that way. So, somebody (and I swore if I ever found out who I would kick 'em in the balls) came up with something called the CINDY CAP.

In deference to anybody reading this by the name of Cindy (or if your mom, sister, or better half is named Cindy), please realize that "Cindy" was just the code name for this particular CAP orbit location. All of our airspace orbits and tracks had codenames so they were easy to remember. This one just happened to be called CINDY.

***

The bad thing about it was the location. The CAP was wedged between the eastern outskirts of the Baghdad metropolitan area and the western border of Iran. For a fighter CAP, it was a terribly small strip of airspace, only about 30nm wide. It was the closest approach of airspace between Baghdad and the Iranian border, and where some wise guy in the planning cell (or above) figured the Iraqis were most likely to jump across the line into Iran.

So Riyadh started tasking us and the other F-15 squadrons to CAP in CINDY every day and night.

It sucked and it did not work, because the Iraqis knew we were there. The IrAF, therefore, would just go find another place to cross the border, and instead they would park SAMs and large-caliber AAA directly underneath the CINDY CAP and take pot shots at us.

We were lucky we never lost an Eagle there, but a Langley jet almost got hit one night right after I had transferred control to them. I alerted them that AWACs had warned us of an enemy height-finder radar active in the area, a sure-fire hint they were about ready to launch something. The Iraqis wanted to know the altitude of our fighters, and sure enough they did.

Fight a war for long enough, and people (mostly generals and politicians) will start coming up with stupid things to do. The CINDY CAP was the best example for us, but I told our pilots *not* to CAP or orbit there, but just to pass through the region momentarily and then go on to other areas along the border in a random fashion. Once we started doing this, the Iraqis never knew exactly where we were going to be or where we were going next. So, occasionally we were able to catch some Iraqi fighters by surprise as they tried to get out of town. It was at this time that the Gorillas and other Coalition fighter units were able to take down more Iraqi fighters. It was like shooting ducks in a barrel, as the saying goes.

***

Endless hours over barren desert, in a combat-loaded Eagle, and guys start looking for something, anything, to shoot at. It started one day with Cheese Graeter and his wingman Capt Scott "Papa" Maw flying in the area of Mudaysis. The F-15 radar is so good that it can sometimes lock-up vehicles on the highway, if they are traveling fast enough. And sure enough, Cheese and Papa started to run an intercept on a target down low, which they suspected could be an Iraqi helicopter because after the Iraqi stand-down, those were about the only things we would see flying.

By the time Cheese and Papa arrived at their target, they were disappointed to see it was just a truck, but not just any truck. It was obviously an Iraqi military vehicle, and when the occupants observed two F-15s buzzing their truck they pulled off to the side of the road, got out, and ran for a nearby ditch. Cheese observed this and reported it to AWACs, and then decided this was a valid military target, so why not strafe it with the Eagle's 20mm cannon?

As Cheese would retell the story to us later, what commenced at that point was a somewhat hilarious attempt by two Eagle drivers, who had never strafed before, to hit a small stationary target on a desert highway in Iraq. On each attempt, Cheese and Papa would miss, and miss so badly, that the poor Iraqi military occupants hiding in the ditch likely feared for their lives. Cheese said that every time he and Papa completed another pass, Cheese would see the Iraqis get up and scramble to another ditch farther away.

Finally one of the passes was successful, and Cheese and Papa left with a burning Iraqi truck on the road and hundreds of rounds of 20mm cannon ammunition expended. What they got for their effort though was grounded.

Grounded! When Col Parsons found out what they had done, he grounded Cheese and Papa, for almost a week as I remember. This was crazy! Cheese was one of our most experienced mission commanders and weapons officers, and we needed him in the air, but so be it.

After that incident, Col Parsons gave out very strict orders that there would be no more unsolicited strafe missions, unless we were directed by the Airborne Command Element (ACE), the senior mission director on board the AWACs aircraft. Period. We all understood and nobody else wanted to get grounded.

It would only be a few days later, while Cheese and Papa were coming to the end their punishment, that the question of strafing would come up in my flight briefing.

Mongo Robbins, my old Weapons School mentor from my early Gorilla days, was visiting our squadron and had permission to fly combat missions with us. He had been sent to Saudi Arabia with the task of gathering all the information he could about the air war—our results and lessons learned—and compile an extensive

"Baron" report, or after-action report. Flying with the best unit in the theater was going to help him do it, and I could not help but feel a sense of pride that Mongo would be flying as #3 in my 4-ship on this day.

Mongo asked, "What if we do get permission from the ACE to strafe? How do we do it?" I had been fortunate enough during my first tour with the Dirty Dozen to fly with Maj "Uncle Budge" Wilson. He had flown A-7 strike fighters before, and he told me that the gun sight and the gun position in the Eagle were exactly like it was in the A-7. Budge said if I ever needed to strafe, I should set up the F-15 radar for ranging to the ground (which we could still do at that time), dial in the gun reticle (aiming circle) to a 30-mil depression angle, come in at a 20-degree nose-low dive angle, hit the trigger at 6,000 feet slant range, and come off by 3,000 feet.

I actually got to try this method one day over the water at Eglin AFB, while we were practicing gun passes at a towed target in preparation for the William Tell competition. We shot the plywood and aluminum target off the tow plane and it ended up in the ocean below us. Having lots of bullets still left in our guns, we decided to strafe the now floating target. I used Uncle Budge's method and it worked! I was the only one able to hit the stationary target in the water. I told Mongo and my flight members exactly how to do this, but what were the chances somebody would ever tell us to go strafe something in Iraq?

We were on another midday area denial mission over the entire central area of Iraq that day, and there really was not much going on. I decided to take the 4-ship across the area just north of Baghdad, head toward the Iranian border, and then head back around Baghdad in a counter-clockwise flow to join up with our airborne tanker (one of several typical refuelings during these six-hour missions).

About the only action we got most of the day was some random large-caliber AAA coming up to around 25,000 feet and leaving sizeable black clouds of shrapnel patterns in the sky. I moved the flight up above 30,000 feet just to make sure some Iraqi gunner did not have a lucky day.

As we were heading east, I think it was actually Mongo who spotted a large Iraqi transport aircraft sitting by itself on a lonely airfield just northeast of Baghdad (I would later determine through some map study that this base was likely Samarra East). I decided to drop down a little closer and use my Eagle Eye rifle scope to get a closer look at the airplane. Sure enough, it was Russian-made IL-76 Candid transport, much the same as our USAF medium-lift C-141 Starlifter.

The Candid had been parked on a ramp, and it had a circle of sandbags or some other kind of temporary barrier built up around it. That alone made it look like an important target. We had been told at the start of the war to be on the lookout for these large-type cargo aircraft. They would be what Saddam would likely use if he decided to leave the country. The Iraqis had also been known to load chemical weapons on these aircraft and use them as toxic "crop dusters" to spray extensive areas with deadly chemicals like Sarin nerve gas.

Based on those operational uses, the Candid was considered a high-priority target, so I reported the sighting to our AWACs controller. I added that if they could scramble some F-16s up north to take out the lonesome Candid, I would hold our 4-ship on station to help protect the strike aircraft. AWACs acknowledged my report and suggestion and told me he would let me know as soon as he could get some Vipers up there to take out this target. So we went on about our business, and eventually returned to our tanker for a refueling.

It was about an hour or two later that we were back up in the same area again, and as we flew by the airfield we saw the same IL-76 on the ground, apparently untouched. I asked our controller if he was going to be able to get some F-16s up there, and he responded by saying that there were none available for the extra tasking. I thought, "That's strange," but not as strange as what he asked me next. "Can your flight strafe it?"

What?! Did he just say that? I initially did not know how to respond, as I quickly rewound Col Parsons previous verbal orders: "Absolutely no strafing … unless directed by the ACE." I sheepishly parroted the wing commander's orders to our AWACs controller, "Ummm, well, we are not allowed to strafe unless the ACE directs us to strafe," fully expecting that to be last we heard about strafing. There was a long pause from our AWACs controller and then he offered up, "Roger. ACE directs you strafe the Candid."

HOLY CRAP! Did he just say that? I couldn't believe it, but before they could change their mind I quickly responded, "Copy! Cleared to strafe!" And from that point I came up with the plan for the 4-ship.

This was Mongo's chance to get into the war and get some ordnance off of his jet (even if it was just bullets), so I told him to go in hot and take #4 (E.T. Murphy) with him, while Cherry and I held high as top cover. It was always good to have somebody else watching from above to make sure there were no MiGs floating around that might jump us, or more likely to call out if we observed any SAMs or AAA to the strafing fighters. When strafing a ground target pretty much 100% of your concentration is on the target and setting up the gun pass, so having a couple of sets of "eyeballs" to call out dangers is important.

Cherry and I watched as Mongo rolled in, performed a beautiful diving pass, with cautionary defensive chaff and flares spewing from his Eagle, and got a perfect hit on the Candid's right wing, which exploded into a little ball of fire. Mongo would later relate to us back at Tabuk that as he sighted up the target he noticed a bunch of people sitting near the Candid. Apparently they saw Mongo pointing his Eagle right at them, and Mongo watched as, he said, they scattered like a bunch of ants surprised at a summer picnic.

That was unexpectedly easy and successful and we reported our results back to AWACs.

Our long day was almost over, and we only had to swing back to the northwest around Baghdad, hand over our orbit to the next 4-ship, and head on home to Tabuk with the notch of a ground kill under our belts. But we were in for one more surprise.

While we were on our way back to Samarra East after our previous refueling (and before the strafe), I had seen some more transport aircraft at another Iraqi base just on the northern outskirts of Baghdad. This was a big airfield with lots of taxiways and hardened aircraft shelters, and I recognized it as Balad (an airfield that would eventually become the USAF's major operating base after Operation IRAQI FREEDOM).

I had seen and reported at least three AN-12 Cub turboprop transports (like our C-130 Hercules transports) sitting in the open between some of the shelters. Comparable to the Candid, these were also high priority targets.

As I told our controller we were going to RTB, he once again surprised me with a request, "Are you guys able to strafe those Cubs on Balad?" I replied, "Sure. If ACE directs." His immediate response was, "ACE directs strafe."

OK, here we go again.

This time I told the 4-ship we were going to swap roles, and Cherry and I would strafe while #3 and #4 (Mongo and E.T. respectively) were to hold high as top cover. I thought that based on the size and apparent importance of this airbase, it might be a little more sporty going in there, and I did not want to give the Iraqi air defense time to react to an initial surprise attack. Historically, being the last man (#4) across a defended target is the most dangerous place to be. They will always wait to shoot the final fighter.

I rolled in first from north to south, lined up the first of three AN-12s sitting in a row, and did my best to apply the approved "Uncle" Budge strafe technique. In retrospect I probably got a little greedy, as I tried to sweep my sights through the path of all three targets instead of concentrating only on the first one.

The result was I never saw if I hit anything at all, but I probably scared the crap out of any gunners or personnel on the ground as I sprayed 20mm cannon rounds over a wide swath of the Balad parking area.

I made a hard pull off to the left and back around to north and was able to observe Cherry's gun pass as he did a much better job than me, and got a direct hit on one of the closer Cubs. I felt we had done what AWACs wanted us to do and now we just had to rejoin the flight and head home.

Then I heard, "Four's in." What? It was E.T. Murphy and he was going in on a gun pass! That was not what I wanted to have happen, and then, "Three's in." There goes Mongo! It was too late to say anything, as they were both already screaming down the chute.

I heard E.T. call "Off" target, and then I heard Mongo yell out, "Three's, MUD SPIKE, Roland—CLOSE!" The hairs on the back of my neck stood on end, because

Mongo was saying he had just been locked-up by an Iraqi close-range Roland SAM that was likely defending the airfield—"SPIKE" meant an aural and visible radar warning receiver indication that he was being targeted and probably shot at.

Immediately after Mongo's call, I also received a Roland spike at my close 6 o'clock position. I was not too worried about myself, because I felt I was far enough away from the airfield that the shorter-range Roland missile could not chase me down. I directed the flight to "push it up!" (to go into afterburner and attain speed and altitude) and get away from Balad airbase as quick as possible.

I had not heard any more from Mongo after his initial spike call, so I waited as long as I could (maybe 10 seconds) and then attempted to "check-in" the flight on the radio to confirm everybody was OK. The response I got was, "Two" (Cherry), a long pause ... then "Four" (E.T.). My heart sunk as I thought, "We just lost Mongo." I was almost afraid to do it, but I waited about another 10 seconds and then tried the check-in again and this time, "Two" (Cherry), a slight pause then a wavering "Three" (Mongo), and "Four" (E.T.) Whew! Mongo was still with us.

We did not have much time to talk about what had happened over Balad while we were still airborne, but I reported back to AWACs not to send anybody else over Balad. I gathered everybody up and we made it all the way back home to Tabuk. Later, Mongo would tell us the story of how he actually saw the Iraqi Roland missile as it fired off its launcher, and the reason he could not respond to the first radio check-in call was because he was still down at almost ground level, jinking his F-15 left and right around the hardened shelters attempting to dodge the aggressive SAM that was locked on to his jet. Fortunately Mongo's defensive maneuvering was successful, and he acknowledged he should have held high like I had told them to do. But at least we had a day for all of us to remember, and Mongo had a "There I was" story he could tell his grandkids someday.

***

I mentioned something about "pancakes" earlier in the book, so now it's time to fill in that gap.

There really wasn't much good to eat around Tabuk. We had our chow hall on base; it was OK, but basically served the same meals day in and day out. Sometimes we could get off base to eat, but there wasn't much in the way of Western-style cuisine there either, and roasted chicken and shawarmas (pita-style fare) was about the best of the local food we could find.

BUT! ... on the Tabuk flight-line there was a small restaurant (usually known as a flight-line kitchen in Air Force slang) that was there to serve all ranks and workers. It was run by a bunch of Pakistani expats and open 24-hours a day. While they also did not have much to cook, and made possibly the worst hamburgers known to mankind, there was one menu item at which they excelled ... pancake.

I say pancake in the singular because you never ordered more than one at a time. They were HUGE ... the size of a large dinner plate and about ¾ inch thick. The only thing they had to put on them was butter and blueberry syrup (no maple), but they were the most delicious pancakes I have ever eaten then or now.

It did not take long for the popularity of the Tabuk flight-line kitchen to grow, and soon there were long lines of customers, even in the dead of night. That's where this story begins.

My flight and I had just returned to base around 0200 from one of our very long CINDY CAP missions (almost 10 hours long with transit time included). We were tired and we were hungry. So, we all decided to grab a pancake before we hit the sack. There was another long line, and we had to wait about 30 minutes, but finally we made it to the front. Just as I said to the guy taking orders, "One pancake, please," the air raid siren went off. There was a loud groan from the crowd while the clerk taking my order, plus all the cooks, grabbed their gas masks and went running for a nearby shelter outside. Reluctantly, the rest of the military customers standing in line did the same thing.

I looked at my guys and I said, "We are not going anywhere." The Iraqis had been shooting SCUD missiles on a regular basis for most of the war. They had never shot anything at Tabuk, but nevertheless we had a Patriot battery there to protect us. But, unfortunately, whenever the Iraqis would shoot a SCUD at Israel, it would set off the warnings for Tabuk too, since we were out to the west in the same direction as Israel.

We'd had so many false alarms that it had reached the point where I figured that if we heard our own Patriots launching, then we'd really know the SCUD was coming our way and we'd take cover and don our gas masks. But today, we were finally first in line for pancake and dammit, I was not giving up my spot. Sure enough, about 15 minutes later, the all-clear siren sounded. The line reformed behind us, the cooks returned, and as the order-taker stood once again in front of me and removed his gas mask, I said (holding up my index finger), "One pancake, please."

***

My days in Tabuk were running short. I had been sitting on my Kadena return assignment since the previous summer, and Gorilla's commander, Tonic Thiel, kept telling me that as soon as things slowed down a bit he was sending me home to depart to my new assignment. The funny thing is ... it just never seemed to slow down.

Even though we had established air superiority weeks prior, strike units were still requesting more and more Eagle sorties to protect them. That was really a testament to our success, not only for the Gorillas but for the entire F-15C air superiority community as a whole. We had shaken off the subpar air combat performance demonstrated during most of the Vietnam conflict, and we had totally exposed the so-called news media "experts" who were predicting high Coalition losses against an adversary that had modern fourth-generation fighters available to them. Combat experience really validated our day-to-day training, as did the exceptional FLAG-type exercise program and the USAF Fighter Weapons School, which had overseen the mentoring of tactical and operational expertise. The Air Force did what it was designed to do.

Finally, one day near the end of February, when my 4-ship had a vanilla DCA CAP mission scheduled, Tonic came up to me and told me this would be my last mission at Tabuk. Tonic said that after this mission I should pack my stuff, wait for the next airlift mission that was heading westbound, and get on it.

We all knew the ground war was going to start in just a few days. It was not as much of a "big secret" as the start of the air war had been.

The Iraqi ground troops had been pounded mercilessly and the IrAF pretty much no longer existed as a viable fighting force. Once the ground war started, all available strike aircraft would be dedicated to close air support (CAS) missions to our own ground forces, and there would be little need for as much Eagle air support ... finally!

I had mixed feelings. I really wanted to get home to Sako and the baby, and I really wanted to move on to Kadena again, but I felt like this was "my" squadron. These were "my" guys, whom I had trained and watched over for the last year. I was extremely proud of them for everything they did and how well they did it. With few exceptions, everybody was willing to fly whatever was asked, regardless of how tired they were or what the mission was.

The Gorillas ended up with 16 aerial victories, the most by any squadron during DESERT STORM. More important than that was the fact that we did not lose a single US aircraft on any of the missions that we were involved in, as offensive sweep and escort duties. And finally, I had met my personal goal—making sure that every Gorilla pilot came home to his family. That's all I really needed to feel accomplished.

For my last mission, I scheduled myself to fly with my original 4-ship: me, Cherry, JB, and Willie. We flew the mission "straight up," of course, since it was a combat mission after all. But, for the landing back at Tabuk, I had something special planned.

We had a British RAF Tornado squadron at Tabuk also, and I had spent the last four or five months watching the Brits perform their unique "battle breaks" when they came back to land. The RAF battle break was when they would come in at low altitude right over the approach end of the runway, then pull up and turn (break) in a beautiful sequential order that looked like a fan unfolding. This was way more cool than the standard USAF overhead break, where we would fly over the field level at 1,800 feet and wait four or five seconds as each jet took its turn to break over the runway to land ... boring!

So, I briefed the flight that we would replicate the RAF battle break when we got back to Tabuk ... and we did. We flew low, right over the Patriot missile battery, lined up with the runway centerline, and then as we flew over the numbers at the runway threshold, we started our fan break up and to the left, came back around and landed.

I was hoping the maintenance folks and other Gorilla pilots had seen our break, because I was doing it as much as a salute to them and their efforts. But everybody I asked on the ground, "Hey, did you see our battle break?" would say "No." Everybody was so busy doing their everyday job and tasks that nobody had time to watch our effort to entertain … nobody apparently except Col Parsons.

As I walked towards our operations building at Tabuk for the last time, I happened to cross paths with Tonic, who apparently had probably just been chewed out by Col Parsons. The conversation went something like this:

(me) "Hey, Sir. How ya' doing?"

(Tonic) "Hey Kluso. I'm good. You're grounded."

(me) "Yes, Sir."

It was more of a "symbolic" grounding, because Tonic had already told me that it was going to be my last sortie and to pack up and leave. But it just seemed, I don't know … perfect.

Another funny (in hindsight) turn of irony occurred shortly after this, maybe the same night, at dinner in the chow hall. After grabbing one of my (hopefully) last chowline meals and sitting down with other Gorilla pilots, I was slowly making my way through some kind of mystery meat stew, which was typically like chewing on shoe leather. Tonic was sitting directly across from me and we were chatting, and he asked me something like, "Well, Kluso … you ready to get back home?"

Before I could get the words "Yes, Sir!" out, my wind stopped cold as I felt a partially chewed piece of something lodge itself firmly in my throat. An initial attempt to re-swallow only lodged in further, and in my attempt to cough it back out I had no air to push it with. My face started to turn red and I felt like my eyes might bulge out of my head … as Tonic looked at me rather calmly and said, "Kluso … are you choking?"

I could barely get a nod of affirmation completed when I felt somebody lift me from behind with arms wrapped in front and I was on the receiving end of a firm Heimlich maneuver that quickly ejected the evil piece of meat back onto my plate exactly where it had started from. My hero was Lt Col Mike "Crowman" Crowe, a reserved but dependable field grade officer who was part of the Gorillas' combat contingent, and fortunately that night he was sitting right next to me. To think, I had made it through almost two months of combat operations and I almost died at a chow hall table choking on a chunk of mystery meat. On the infrequent times I have met up with Crowman since then, or chatted on email, I still feel the need to thank him for saving my life that night. I am not joking about this one.

After a couple of days of waiting around the operations area, a C-141 that was bound for Ramstein AB in Germany finally landed at Tabuk. Germany was "west" enough for me, and I knew I could probably catch another hop from there back to the US east coast and then work my way home to Eglin. So, I grabbed my A-3 bag, which had everything I had lived with for almost six months jammed into it, jumped on the Starlifter, and headed toward home.

I was the only passenger on board and the crew was great. They asked me if I wanted to sit up front on the flight deck with pilot/co-pilot, and though I actually wanted to get some sleep I told them there were two things I wanted to see: the moment we exited Saudi airspace and the moment we were going to touch down in Germany. I figured that if I saw both of those I would know I was really going home.

It did not take long for the first event, as we turned northwest after takeoff from Tabuk, hit the coastline of the Red Sea, and turned north toward Europe, out of the Kingdom. It seemed like it was only a few minutes (rather than hours) later that the loadmaster woke me up and said, "Sir, we're about to land in Ramstein." I shook off the cobwebs and quickly climbed up into the flight deck just in time to see us on final approach into Ramstein.

It was almost sunset, the sky was beautifully lit, but the night shadows darkened the landscape, which was now sparkling with the lights of homes, cottages, and churches attempting to delay twilight's calling. It was one of the most beautiful sights I had ever seen.

When I got into the Ramstein base operations, the first thing I did was check for the next flight to the United States. There was one in about four hours. Great! The next thing I did was go to the Army & Air Force Exchange Service (AAFES) snack bar and order an American cheeseburger, fries, and two beers. That was the best cheeseburger I think I had ever eaten ... and the beers? Oh My GOD!

Another long flight to the east coast and then a commercial puddle-jumper to Fort Walton Beach airport, and I was back home. Sako was there to meet me, with Sakura, who no longer recognized me and cried at the strange man who was kissing her mama. But it did not take too long for us to be a family again.

I thought the Gorillas as a group would be back before I left for Kadena, but it didn't work out that way. Even though the war officially ended a couple of days after I got back to Eglin, the 58th TFS got stuck waiting their turn for the massive exodus of troops and equipment that took more than four months to send over there.

After five or six weeks, Sako and I packed up our household goods and returned across the Pacific, back to the place I considered my "home"—Kadena AB, where I would be assigned once again to the 12th TFS Dirty Dozen. This time, instead of being the brand-new 2nd lieutenant, I was the combat experienced weapons officer ... and I had work to do.

CHAPTER 9

Return to the Dozen

Author's note: This next chapter and portions of the remainder of this book are going to cover material that may seem somewhat disconnected from the topical and chronological story-telling up to this point. For others, it may seem to have a less than positive tone, but I felt compelled to cover this territory for several reasons. First, for my own life story it involves how the past, present, and future are intertwined and led to where I am today and where I might end up. Second, I felt compelled to raise the flag of caution to my fellow warriors, some of whom I still help train, to the potential dangers that lay ahead for the air superiority community if we continue on the slippery path of becoming dependent on technology versus hard-earned expertise in tactics and operations. Third, I believe there is a message here for us all as individuals, families, communities, societies, and the world in general. Subtle change over years and decades can create imperceptible momentum that at some point can be difficult, if not impossible, to reverse. There are examples throughout history, whether in business, politics, culture, or world affairs ... or in this case, the US Air Force, where the "fall" is not perceived until we actually hit rock bottom. With this in mind, I offer my counsel.

***

The return to Kadena and the Dirty Dozen was everything I thought it would be. Shortly after arriving I took over the 12th FS Weapons and Tactics shop. (The unit title Tactical Fighter Squadron / TFS was expunged from the Air Force unit designations in the 1990s and became just Fighter Squadron / FS.) I went to work training a new squadron how to prepare for war, but something was a little bit different. We had a new weapon: the AIM-120 Advanced Medium Range Air-to-Air Missile ... the AMRAAM.

The AIM-120 was actually first fielded, probably ill advisedly, near the end of DESERT STORM. I think it was more of a ploy to try to get the military's newest "toy" some exposure to combat and maybe even to shoot down an enemy aircraft. What actually happened was that the pilots (who were mostly against the idea) found that the new F-15 software for the weapon system, including its radar, had some big glitches that had not been totally fixed before it was hastily made operational.

The other issue was that this was an entirely new generation of AAM, and it can take months or even years of extensive training and experience to understand how to best utilize and integrate new technology. You don't really want to do that in the middle of a shooting war, unless there is some extreme need to do so, and our AIM-7M missiles had been doing their job just fine in most cases.

So, my job in coming to Kadena was to help create a level of operational expertise and viable tactics for use of the new AMRAAM. We were really the first MSIP F-15C squadron on Kadena to have the AMRAAM capability in our jets, and the first in the entire Air Force that had the time and ability to start developing new operational tactics.

From experience growing up as an "Eagle Baby," I had watched the struggles to overcome the inertia of the "we've always done it this way" philosophy, and so I made an effort to take the opposite approach. I found a three- or four-month period in our training plan where I instructed the squadron to come up with a consensus on how to best employ the AIM-120 in Eagle tactics, but what I actually asked the squadron pilots to do was to throw out everything we already knew and start over again. Nothing was off limits. I really didn't care what hair-brained or crazy tactics our guys came up with. I wanted to see and experience it all. And, in the end that was the best thing I could have ever done.

The Dozen pilots tried all kinds of tactics. They included single-ship Eagles lined up in a long lead-trail formation, taking turns at shooting and then leaving to let the next F-15 take over. Or wall formations that were 20nm wide, or, stacked high-to-low with extreme altitude differences. Whatever … you name it. What we found was that even though we had a new weapon that would allow us to launch it and leave before we ever saw the results, the old tried-and-true intercept tactics that we had developed in the Eagle community still worked the best: 4-ship wall formations whenever possible; element visual mutual support; establishing a position of advantage on intercepts and not just pointing at the adversary; and being able to defend oneself when things didn't go as planned.

We were able to test out our new tactics and operational standards at a FLAG exercise the following year, in the summer of '92 at COPE THUNDER in Alaska (as mentioned previously, the Philippines COPE THUNDER exercises ended in 1991 after Mount Pinatubo erupted and closed Clark AB for good). The large-force employment training in traditional OCA and DCA missions was perfect to demonstrate both the advantages and the limitations to our new weapon, as well as to help validate and improve on what we felt we had established as sound tactics.

The other thing we found, which was to be expected, was that our training adversaries could quickly learn our tactics and adopt effective counter-tactics. So we could not always fly the same standard tactics and game plans every mission. Over a two-week exercise the learning curve was steep, just as it would be in combat when an adversary will either adapt or die.

The problem that began to occur in the mid-90s and beyond is that the core elements of the Eagle community, supported in part by the very Weapons School that had been the genesis of the F-15's success, began to rely more and more on technology and basic standardized tactics. Over time, greater dependence on technology over tactics would lead to the creation of technicians instead of tacticians, and focus on replacing expertise via experience with mediocrity via process. I know these are harsh claims and might possibly be disputed by today's Air Force and the Air Superiority (F-15C / F-22) communities, but let me take you back to where it all started.

***

Not too long after DESERT STORM ended, an election took place in the United States, and along with it came a vision of an extended period of peace falling over the world, especially after our first post-Cold War conflict had been won relatively easily. As I am sure happened after World War II, the Korean War, and the Vietnam War, it seemed like maybe we had more capability and manpower than we really needed in the US armed forces. A drawdown therefore began, and with it we threw the baby out with the bathwater.

In reality Mr. Reagan's Air Force, as I label it, required a couple of decades to build; it was only "his" air force because it mostly came to fruition during his tenure and with Reagan's emphasis on undermining the Soviet Union. But over the next couple of years, some momentous manpower, policy, and weapons acquisition decisions would have significant detrimental effects, which continue to ripple through the air superiority community even today.

One of the first blunders in manpower management was the total devastation of the mid-level NCO core in most of the essential Air Force technical skill levels, and particularly for the aviation maintenance personnel. These were not only the critical "worker bees" for aircraft maintenance, but they were the ones who trained the younger airmen, and would eventually be the SNCO leadership that would take the lessons we learned coming into and out of DESERT STORM through to the next generation. They were gone … most of them … and almost overnight. The result of the NCO cuts would be felt in aircraft readiness and sortie generation for years to come. This would have a direct impact on the ability to fly and train the fighter pilots who needed those jets and sorties to be available.

Another poor decision occurred in rated aviator (mostly pilot) management. For many years, one of the core principles for rated officer/fighter-pilot management was to maintain a solid and consistent surplus of highly skilled and trained fighter pilots, especially at the higher level of experience, such as operational instructor pilots. Having this surplus of experienced instructors is what in World War II made the difference between us and our adversaries—the pilots of the German Luftwaffe, and Japanese Imperial Navy and Army. By the end of the war in both theaters, the Axis countries still had plenty (if not more than before) of frontline and advanced fighter aircraft to fly. What they didn't have were enough well-trained pilots to fly them.

Over the course of a long war, Germany and Japan kept many of their experienced combat pilots on the frontlines, and eventually almost all of them were lost, and therefore could never pass on their experience to follow-on cadres of younger pilots. If they did manage to get enough airplanes in the air, they were getting their ass kicked by US pilots who had been taught by combat-experienced veterans sent back to the Unites States to train them. This philosophy of trying to keep a core of experienced, combat veteran pilots to instruct and improve the fighter community was essential. It helped immensely as the United States became involved in the Korean conflict and maybe in some part Vietnam.

As mentioned before, in Vietnam there was a significant drop off in capability that may have mirrored what we saw after DESERT STORM, where a loss of the core World War II/Korean War experience and a greater dependence on technology versus tactics were to blame. But that period was short lived, and over the course of the 70s and 80s, and with maturation of the Eagle community and Fighter Weapons School, we witnessed again the buildup of a surplus of experienced and talented instructors.

In attempting to micro-manage what was "perceived" as a glut of fighter pilots post-DESERT STORM, the manpower machine went through extreme variations of stopping and starting the "pipeline" for pilots—UPT and the fighter pilot replacement training units, the Formal Training Units (FTUs). This was instead of allowing the pilot surplus to attrite slowly at the senior experience level (those retiring or voluntarily leaving the Air Force). This aggressive sine wave of starting and stopping pilot training at the front end would create even greater ripple effects, impacting on the ability to develop and manage the experienced operational and training instructor levels for many years afterwards.

It can take generally two or more fighter assignments (or about four to eight years) of advanced-level training to become a really effective instructor. If you have heard of the "10,000-hour rule" (i.e., it takes 10,000 hours of effort in any endeavor to become a professional-level expert at it), then that would be about the time and effort expended by a fighter pilot to reach instructor status—not just flying time, but the daily activities of briefing, debriefing, study, etc..

Another event that had an adverse major impact, in my opinion, is when the Air Force changed how and by whom young F-15 pilots received their initial training at FTU. In the early 90s, a major reorganization within the US Air Force moved fighter pilot training (including F-15 training) out from under Air Combat Command (ACC)—the operational command structure for fighter aircraft and pilots/ crews—and placed it under Air Education & Training Command (AETC). AETC was the command that traditionally ran the undergraduate/entry level training such as UPT. There was nothing technically wrong or inferior about AETC, but since it was a separate command structure to ACC, it established the situation where ACC's product (a trained fighter pilot) was being produced by another command. Therefore ACC could not precisely direct how AETC trained the new fighter pilots, and therefore it did not have full control over the product (trained F-15 pilots) they were given.

That alone may not have been such a big deal if it wasn't for the *coup de grâce*. For years (at least during my time as an Eagle pilot to that point, but I am sure well before also), there had been a standing policy that only operational F-15 pilots with established IP credentials were eligible to receive assignments as FTU instructors. This harks back to the idea of sending the most experienced frontline pilots to teach the new/young generation of fighter pilots. That policy had worked for years and was one of the other reasons that the Eagle community had risen so quickly to such a high level of expertise by the time DESERT STORM came around.

Partly because of the aforementioned mismanagement of the rated fighter pilot personnel, it was becoming more and more difficult to find authentic instructor-rated operational F-15 pilots. There were already too few in the actual operational squadrons, and not enough to go around for new assignments as FTU instructors. So, whether at the request of AETC or ACC (or maybe both), they dropped the requisite requirement from IP to 4-ship flight lead. To the lay observer this may not seem significant, but it would be like accepting a high-school graduate as a valid candidate to teach courses at a university level. Somebody like that does not possess the knowledge, skills, or experience to teach at that level. Some may be talented enough to overcome their lack of experience, but for the others it would mean either failure or the need to reduce the standards of what was an acceptable consequence or product. And this is what happened.

As more and more operational 4-ship flight leads were sent to be IPs at AETC's F-15C FTU, they were having a much harder time just passing the FTU Instructor Upgrade course. Rather than "flunk" these desperately needed IP candidates, the FTU eventually had to reduce its own standards of acceptable instructor performance, which would also mean that it would have to accept lower-level standards of performance for the students as well.

Now multiply this continuous cycle of events over years and years, and what is the result? A slow and almost imperceptible deterioration of air superiority expertise began to occur. It not only affected AETC and the FTU, but affected the operational units also, and eventually I believe it affected the "School House" itself, the bastion of air superiority expertise, the USAF Fighter Weapons School. And, I submit to the reader, this has not only affected the F-15 (and maybe F-16) community, but since that is where most of the initial F-22 Raptor pilots came from, then it has likely become like a zombie virus just lurking under the surface.

What happens when an organization loses practical experience in its core elements? Normally it will attempt to replace experience with "process" or method. And this is what I believe has happened in the air superiority community. Strict adherence to "tactical standards" has become the mantra of the F-15 community. The previous mantra in my time—"flexibility is the key to airpower"—has gone the way of the dinosaur, replaced by the tactical "bible," the classified 3-1 ("Three dash-One") fighter employment, tactics and procedures.

Now, we have always had a 3-1 tactics manual, but it was mostly used as a historical guide to fighter tactics, and not a strict "how-to" book as it has become today. I can understand that today, if there is not a high-enough level of instructional expertise, then who can theoretically define on any given day or mission what is correct, incorrect, or a better way of employment?

Wait! Did I just say that?

Actually, that *is* the responsibility an experienced fighter IP and it is his *job*: to identify both correct and incorrect employment methods, provide a multitude of options and techniques to fix problems, and constantly look for new and improved tactics, techniques, and procedures. Those are not things found in a book, and it seems that the present-day Air Force air superiority community has lost sight of this. The result is a lack of fundamental fighter pilot skills and core combat values, along with tactical resources and tools, all of which are essential to foresee and resolve the complex multi-dimensional problems that arise during training and especially in combat operations.

A well-trained and experienced fighter pilot is more akin to a great artist than anything else I can think of. It takes both physical capacity and technique-oriented training, but also the ability to grasp the deepest philosophical elements of warfare. If it is made into a "paint by numbers" effort, then the results may appear reasonable or acceptable, but in the end it will not only be inferior but also lacking in perception and imagination. If you have read Sun Tzu's *The Art of War*, then you will know what I am talking about.

Just as I found out during my failed Weapons School Dissimilar BFM sortie, if you become reliant on performing the same moves and counters each time because of perceived previous success, some day you will meet an adversary that does something different that you aren't prepared for. This concept of inadequate experience (or tools) to deal with complex and fluid environments was expounded in a theory called "The Law of the Instrument," from Abraham Kaplan's *The Conduct of Inquiry: Methodology for Behavioral Science* (1964). Redefined as "Maslow's Hammer" by Abraham H. Maslow in *The Psychology of Science* (1966), Maslow stated, "If all you have is a hammer, everything looks like a nail."

This is the difference between a method-based approach (where it is the employed method that is most important regardless of what the problem is), versus a problem-based approach where it's the problem itself that is most important and it takes a multitude of "tools" (based on experience and instinctive courage) to win. In other words, attempts to formulate fixed or standard solutions to complex problems may provide temporary success, but over the course of time will ultimately end in failure. Tactical and operational problem-solving must be intuitive rather than rehearsed. The desired end result is something called "intuitive expertise."

Now, let me say this. There is absolutely nothing wrong with the individual personal quality of the fighter pilots we have flying in the US Air Force today. They are just as motivated and intelligent (maybe even more so) than the fighter pilots of my day and, in some areas, they may even have more skills since they were raised in the technology age. But they cannot know what they don't know, and they cannot improve if they are not allowed to innovate.

Based on the previously mentioned manpower and doctrinal *faux pas* of the 1990s, the fact that over the last 20 years the air superiority community has not progressed to the point (in my opinion) where they *should* be is not entirely their fault. But the fact that they have not come to recognize this and take strong corrective actions, that's a different story. Unfortunately, since there has been a couple of generations of "devolution" the new reality may appear to be perfectly fine and normal. And frankly, I don't think anybody will ever know the difference, unless ... unless there is another war, but this time against a peer competitor, and one that lasts more than a few weeks.

I sincerely hope I am wrong about this point.

***

I once read a great book while I was still a young fighter pilot, *My Secret War* by Richard S. Drury. In the book, the author recounts tales of his experience as an A-1 Skyraider pilot during the Vietnam War. As well as the tales of his combat experience, he also recalls his disenchantment with the upper-echelon leadership, in particular with the careerists who seemed to put their own personal aspirations above those who they were supposed to lead and take care of.

I have to assume it has always been that way in the military, and it will probably always be that way. My own experience, in particular after having seen good and bad leaders come and go, slowly evolved into that same disappointment. In fact, I believe amongst my peers we all had similar thoughts and concerns; why would some of our best and brightest leave the Air Force, while the less capable and egocentric would stick around and get promoted?

The other common notion amongst us, though, was that a war (or combat) would change all that. That under the stress and demands of combat, the cream (of the leadership) would rise to the top and dregs (the "managers") would fall by the wayside.

We were wrong.

It was somewhere in the middle of my second assignment at Kadena (third F-15 assignment) that my discouragement reached a point where I had pretty much decided I was going to get out, that is, separate from the Air Force. I began to see that nothing had really changed in the areas of leadership and policy as they continued swinging from good to bad, like a pendulum with much of the weight leaning toward the bad.

In 1989 the US Air Force instituted the Aviation Continuation Program (ACP), more commonly known as the "Pilot Bonus." Maj Brian E.A. Maue wrote in the *Air & Space Power Journal* (Winter 2008): "Enacted in 1989, ACP was designed to slow the exodus of military pilots to civilian airlines—an industry that offered 'an alternative lifestyle, better retirement and benefits, and shorter work weeks.' Congress's establishment of the ACP sought to increase the retention rates of full-time Air Force pilots by making their compensation competitive with that of civilian-airline pilots. The Air Force offered its pilots an ACP contract of five annual payments of $25,000 for agreeing to serve an additional five years."

The "Bonus" was looked upon with suspicion by many fighter pilots at the time, myself included.

For one thing, most of us did not fly fighters for the money to begin with, so why pay us more? Second, we had some apprehension about whether the details of the program would be changed at a later time to meet the Air Force's requirements, or worse, that a decision to decline the ACP bonus (and its service commitment extension) would negatively impact our flying careers? Our leaders and the manpower gurus assured us at the time those things would *never* happen. They lied.

Well, maybe "lie" is a harsh word. I am sure they were sincere at the beginning, but in fact as time goes by in the Air Force, people and policy are constantly changing and promises are forgotten. It's the only thing you can ever really be sure of. Promises that pilots who took the ACP bonus could abandon the program at any time, just by re-paying the bonus money they had already received, turned out to be totally false. Unfortunately, none of us read the "fine print" in the bonus contract.

The broken promise of "non-retribution" for not signing up for the ACP bonus would take a couple of more years to come about, but it did happen. In the early 90s, during the massive Reduction In Force (RIF), drawdown post-DESERT STORM, the selection or non-selection of the ACP bonus became a discriminating factor whether to allow fighter pilots to continue to fly and maintain their currency and flight status. It was called "Feet on the Ramp" policy (at least by us pilots), and the rated officers who declined the ACP bonus were immediately grounded. At one point, whether or not a pilot had accepted the ACP bonus could also be observed in his professional records when eligible for promotion boards, and when receiving promotion recommendations from their superiors. It was not hard to imagine that a pilot/officer who had committed to a longer stay in the Air Force (via the ACP bonus) would be looked upon more favorably than one who had not.

What fighter pilots wanted was not more money, although many of us took it when it was thrown our way ... including myself, but more flying time, better training, and less of the daily BS that detracted from those priorities. Instead we received the bonus, and leather jackets (the World War II-style aviator jackets were brought back after more than 40 years) as a morale-boosting measure. That effort failed, but they were nice jackets.

It was in the light of all these issues, and many more professional and personal considerations, that I had decided I was done. My first ACP bonus commitment was almost over and I could leave the Air Force when I reached the end of my second Kadena assignment. Then, something changed that. The USAF Fighter Weapons School at Nellis AFB contacted me and asked that I come back to be a Weapons School instructor.

I had already been asked to do that once before, at the same time I received my second Kadena assignment. I turned down the offer the first time because I really wanted to stay in an operational unit and not at the schoolhouse. Having turned it down once, I was surprised to get another offer. So I changed course and decided to stick it out and go to Nellis. I felt it was something I needed to do to pass along my operational (and specifically combat) experience.

Once I made that commitment, I saw a different path and objective for me. If I was going to stay in three more years, then I might as well stay in for a full 20 years (or more). That would allow me to reach the minimum active duty retirement criteria, which would be great for me and my family, but more important, it would allow me an opportunity to pay back a debt of gratitude I felt I owed the Air Force. Let me say that again, and clearly—I wanted to pay back a debt of gratitude I felt towards the Air Force, and especially to the people who had assisted and mentored me, and to those I could help along the way.

While my disillusionment with leadership and policy may have tarnished my overall attitude toward the Air Force as an institution, I could never forget all the great people who had done so much for me along the way. If I did leave early, I would never be able to pass along the things I had learned, or be able to help others.

My primary goal now was to be a squadron commander someday, not just to be promoted or to wear that badge on my uniform, but to use the position to help others as I'd had done for me. That was my decision. On to 20 years. But then … my follow-on "dream" assignment to Weapons School evaporated overnight. I was selected to attend Air Command & Staff College (ACSC) at Maxwell AFB, Montgomery, Alabama.

Oh, well.

CHAPTER 10

The Long and Winding Road

In the summer of 1994, Sako and I packed up the kids and moved to Montgomery, Alabama, for a one-year diversion at the USAF's Air Command & Staff College (ACSC). It was a good year off from the grind of being an operational weapons officer and instructor pilot. Not that I was happy to be away from flying (I wasn't), but the overseas operational environment was all consuming. Workdays were typically 12–16 hours long, without much idle time in that length of day.

Even when not officially occupied, the work environment constantly surrounds you. Normally all social contacts and even family life are intricately woven around the unit ... around the squadron. Your neighbors and most of your friends are all squadron mates or other officers with close connections to each other professionally and personally.

Some of those same connections, or re-acquaintances, were also present at ACSC but on a much smaller scale. One thing I noticed while attending this Air Force-wide school is how small the fighter pilot community (or any kind of pilot or aircrew cadre) is compared to all the other Air Force specialties.

The rated aviator represents only about 20% of the Air Force officer corps, and the fighter pilot portion is about 5% of that total officer corps. So if we felt "special," it might seem appropriate based on the limited opportunity to achieve fighter pilot status. Also, it made me realize that there was a huge organization of professional officers and enlisted personnel who made it possible to get a single F-15 into the air to train or engage in combat.

Most of our stint at ACSC was a matter of biding our time until we could finish and get our follow-on staff (desk) job. Virtually no graduates of this mid-level professional school would return to flying right away. The "curse" of going to school was not just the "school" part of it, but knowing that an additional 2–4 years would be spent afterwards out of the cockpit. The other concern was what kind of staff job I could find and where it would be, and would it lead back to the F-15 cockpit and a chance at being a commander afterwards. Plus, there was competition for a limited quantity of premier staff positions, with a large number of officers all graduating at the same time and looking for similar jobs.

I was hoping I had an "ace in the hole" when I first departed for ACSC for a possible opening at the Special Programs Office at Headquarters, Pacific Air Forces (PACAF) Hickam AFB, Hawaii. Known at that time by the office symbol PACAF/DOQB, the Special Programs branch had oversight of all fighter aircraft requisition programs. All the newest "toys" for the F-15 would be reviewed and defined by the fighter pilots who worked in this office and similar ones across the Combat Air Force (CAF) command structure. If I couldn't fly for a couple of years, there was nothing else I would rather do than to help secure the newest and best equipment and weapons for the air superiority fighter community.

Before leaving for ACSC, PACAF/DOQB had told me they would like to "hire" me following my school, if they had a position open. That was the problem. Even though I continued to check back with the branch chief in Hawaii, they told me that they did not have any jobs coming open when I graduated. That was a bummer. Things started looking pretty bleak for me as we approached graduation and I watched my fighter pilot peers picking up great follow-on staff jobs. I was starting to get worried, and I decided to set my sights lower on a stateside staff position that would probably not be as rewarding as the DOQB opportunity.

Sako would not hear of this, though. She had her sights set on us going to Hawaii, and no matter how impossible it looked for us to get that assignment, she continued to tell me (and other people) that we were going to Hawaii next. I thought she was crazy. What Sako told me was that she was doing her Buddhist chanting (prayers) for us to get the Hawaii assignment. She would chant the same "Nam Myoho Renge Kyo" chant as I had done just before I took off on my first combat mission, but instead of just saying it three times and quitting, Sako would chant for hours on end. She had faith and confidence that her chanting would reach across the universe to align all the forces necessary for the smallest things to fall into place and that we would be in Hawaii that Fall. I just had to laugh, but I told Sako, "OK, go ahead and chant, but I'm telling you, there aren't any jobs for me in Hawaii."

It was actually down to the very last day, and I had to call another branch chief at ACC at Langley AFB, Virginia, to accept a job he had been holding for me to come to the ACC staff. I appreciated his efforts but in reality it wasn't really the place or job I wanted. I was going to be just another staff officer cog in a huge headquarters staff agency, but either way I needed to call him and accept the position.

Before I made the call though, Sako encouraged me to call Hawaii one more time ... what could it hurt?

So, I made the call expecting to hear the same thing I had heard for the last 10 months, "Sorry Kluso, no job openings yet." But, when I heard the phone pick up on the other end and I greeted them with the now customary, "Hey, this is Kluso," I received an unexpected response. The DOQB branch chief told me one of their officers had just received notification that day that he would be attending the following year's ACSC class, and they asked me (like they had to?), "You still want the Special Programs job?" HELL, YES!

Even though Sako had been practicing her Buddhism for a long time, this was the first time I had seen her declare with such confidence what the results would be. And, this time, it made me start to think, "Hmmmm ... maybe there is something to this chanting thing."

***

What a great staff tour Hawaii turned out to be. It validated my decision to stick around for a few more years, and also to direct my efforts to work for others, and ... it was in a tropical paradise.

I worked with a great group of professionals and just tried my best to follow in their footsteps. I was able to promote and garner support for critical F-15C upgrade and modification programs that would help maintain the classic jet as a premier air-to-air fighter for decades to come. I was also able to gain access to future programs and help shape forthcoming missile and advanced fighter programs like the F-22.

Hickam AFB was a great place to live, with all its history, and it was also a wonderful environment for our kids as they grew into the first school-age years.

There were frustrations with the job, as can be expected, and most of those involved decisions on procurement programs emanating from the highest levels of the Air Force and our government. Probably the biggest mistake that myself and my F-15 staff peers witnessed during the mid-90s was the Air Force's hopeless effort to support a buy of more than 700 F-22 Raptors to replace the F-15C. Even the most inexperienced young staff officer knew this hardline stand by the Air Force leadership was like "pissing into the wind." The end of the Cold War and the overwhelming annihilation of the IrAF had already resulted in a significant drawdown of fighter units and capabilities across the CAF.

The other factor was that there was no clear air superiority "peer" competitor to the USAF and to the F-15. As much as some "experts" tried to slant China as a near-term peer competitor, the facts and reality just did not support that. The eventual loser in all of this spin by the Air Force leadership was some of the critical F-15 upgrade programs that lost funding for one simple reason—if the F-15 received these upgrades, it would compete directly against the Air Force's prized F-22 program and the 700-plus airframe buy.

A better option in the mid-90s would have been to cut the F-22 buy in half (to about 350, which was a number that Congress had already offered to the Air Force) and divert some of the savings to the F-15 programs, which would give the Air Force two very complimentary and impressive airframes for the air superiority mission for the next 30-plus years. In the end, the Air Force went all in with the plan for 750 Raptors ... and nearly lost it all. Not only did we get fewer than the 750 Raptors, indeed fewer than 350 Raptors, but the Air Force ended up with about one-fourth of the original F-22 buy (187 total) and delayed the Raptors' procurement by many years. It also found that the F-15 would need to be around for much longer, but now it was missing some critical upgrades that had been unfunded. And while all of this went down, a bunch of "iron majors" on staffs around the world just sat there, shaking our heads, watching in disbelief.

***

I returned to the Dirty Dozen for the third and last time in July of 1998. After the four-year layoff from flying the Eagle, I attended the "TX" refresher training course for experienced F-15 pilots at Tyndall AFB, Florida. I was actually a bit surprised how fast my previous skills and experience came back to me. From there it was back to Kadena.

During my last year on the PACAF staff in Hawaii, I had already been offered follow-on F-15 assignments and sponsorship for squadron commander positions at Elmendorf AFB in Alaska and Mountain Home AFB in Idaho, but I had turned them down. Some people thought I wanted to go back to Okinawa because of Sako, but actually that was not the case at all; Sako really wanted me to get an assignment in Europe, but there weren't any available. I wanted to go back to Kadena to have one last opportunity to pay back the wing and the organization there for everything they had done for me. I knew that Kadena was still the best place to train young fighter pilots, and I wanted to be one of the leaders there who had the opportunity to do that. Unfortunately, I did not have a sponsor (normally a general officer who will insure your placement in a squadron commander position) at Kadena, so there was no guarantee I would ever get a fighter squadron command there. To me, though, it was worth the risk just to have an opportunity … any opportunity.

By good graces, and at the request of some leaders at Kadena who already knew me, I was "drafted" back into the 12th FS, initially as assistant operations officer (ADO) then finally to the prized position as 12 FS/DO—I was the Dirty Dozen operations officer, or OpsO.

The DO position in a fighter squadron, in many ways, is about as good as it gets (if not the commander) because of the responsibility for oversight of all pilot flying operations and training. I had a glorious one-year stint as Dozen OpsO—raising young fighter pilots; traveling all over the Pacific for training exercises; watching the kids grow up in a place they loved, surrounded by family, good friends, and neighbors. It was almost too good to be true. I felt sure I would receive one of the three upcoming fighter squadron command positions after I finished my DO tour. I was one of three fighter squadron DOs, and we had three fighter squadrons at Kadena (12th, 44th, and 67th), so naturally we all thought we would each move up a step when the time came.

But not too long after I took over as 12th FS/DO, we got some bad news in the Dozen: the continuing drawdown of fighter units across the Air Force had finally arrived at Kadena. There was going to be a restructuring of the squadrons from three 18 Primary Assigned Aircraft (PAA) squadrons to two 24 PAA squadrons. They were going to make two slightly bigger F-15 squadrons out of the three F-15 squadrons at Kadena. The 12th FS Dirty Dozen was going to deactivate (close down).

It was a shock to everybody in the squadron, and many across the Air Force who had been members of the squadron. The history of the Dirty Dozen was rich, going back to World War II and before, and having a distinction of always being overseas. But the way the Air Force decides to close down a squadron is by looking at all the accomplishments of individual units and attempting to preserve those with the most history and mission accomplishments. At Kadena, over the many years and wars, the Dirty Dozen fell slightly short of the other two squadrons.

We made the best of it over the coming months, flying our asses off and finishing the tour with a one-month deployment to Australia in October 1999. Fittingly, I led the last 6-ship of Eagles from Australia all the way back to Kadena. When we landed, we shut down the jets for the last time, and "folded the flag."

Before most of the airmen and pilots departed or moved to the other squadrons, we had one last huge bash to close down the Dozen. It included an "auction" of much of the squadron memorabilia (because the Air Force would retain very little) in order to preserve the history and the memories. Former Dozen members from all over the world participated by e-mail, phone-in, letter, or in person.

It was a bittersweet ending to a great fighter squadron. I am sure everybody feels like their first fighter squadron was "the best!" But in the case of The Dozen, it definitely embodied a unique status. It was a phenomenon that rarely occurs in professional organizations—an inimitable collection of talented and motivated individuals who create an environment of excellence that somehow sustains itself over many generations.

It turned out I was personally the "Last of the Dozen." Tasked with overseeing the final paperwork and distribution of 12th FS heritage, I worked from my office for several months, alone in the darkened and rather haunted squadron building. I was also waiting for the upcoming announcements about who would be the next fighter squadron commanders, and even though there were three presumed candidates, there were now only two fighter squadrons at Kadena. Everybody told me I would surely get one of the fighter commands, and I had no reason not to believe that. We were all wrong.

***

The command of the 44th and 67th fighter squadrons went to the two other operations officers. They were both nice enough guys, but in this case it was more about the politics of leadership positions than experience and ability. I was not the wing commander's "boy" and they were. Fair enough. I knew how it worked, and I had been warned about it before I ever came back to Kadena. Still, I was a bit shocked by the announcement and to say the least, and not happy about it.

In the end though, this was one of the best things ever to happen to me, for a couple of reasons.

I did receive a squadron commander position, and it was for the 18th Operations Support Squadron (18th OSS). The 18th OSS is a "non-flying" unit that oversees all operational flight functions, such as airfield operations, air traffic control, scheduling and airspace management, intelligence, weapons & tactics, combat plans, and several more similar operations areas. It was a big squadron, made up of many more Air Force personnel and specialties than a regular fighter squadron. The OSS did not have the glamor of a fighter squadron command, but it had many more opportunities to use my leadership and management skills than I would have had in a fighter squadron. Actually, I already knew how to run a fighter squadron. I wasn't quite sure what I needed to know or learn in running an OSS, in fact, the largest OSS in the US Air Force.

It turned out to be a great command opportunity, and I will never regret that assignment. The other benefit of receiving the OSS command was that it made me reflect on my Air Force career, mostly on the future of that career. The fighter squadron commands created an obvious path to promotion to colonel (O-6) and often general officer positions: group commander, then wing commander, and so on. Receiving a "non-flying" command appeared to put me on a sub-track. Promotion to colonel was likely, but it would be an uphill battle to go much beyond that. I understood that, and promotions had never really been the main focus of my goals the entire time I was in the Air Force. My goals were instead based on trying to create opportunities for positions where I could do my best and contribute the most to the "mission"; promotions just came along as part of that process.

The one thing I did know I wanted to do was to command. It was the primary reason I had stayed in the Air Force when I had had serious doubts earlier in my career. It was part of the "paying back the debt of gratitude" I had toward the service and the community. I wanted to be able to do something for other people, the airmen who would serve under me.

I talked with my group commander at the time, Col Doug "Roach" Cochran. He was a great guy and a great leader. Roach knew that I was extremely disappointed initially at not receiving a fighter squadron command, and he told me that if it had been up to him, he surely would have given me one … but it wasn't. I did, however, ask Roach at least to give me two full years as the 18th OSS commander, so I could really do my job, create a great organization, and help the young officers and airmen in the unit.

Roach knew that it was typical for squadron commanders to be in the position for only a single year. It was a strange policy (and still is, it seems), but the institution of "The Air Force" often seems to treat squadron command positions as more of a "square-filler" for promotion, rather than an essential cog in the efficient function of the Air Force and, in this case, the combat mission. Therefore, often about the time a squadron commander was just figuring out how to run the unit and achieving some goals and progress, he or she would be sent to Senior Service School (SSS), the service schools for officers promotable to full colonel. Then ... "next man [or woman] up"!

I was hoping I could stave off the inevitability of selection to SSS and actually achieve something as the 18th OSS commander. Roach said that he would do everything he could to keep me in the commander position for a full two years.

Unfortunately, as a full colonel, Roach probably had even less control over his own ability to stay at Kadena, and six months later he was gone and replaced by another group commander. My "deal-maker" was gone and not too long after that, sure enough, I was selected to attend USAF Air War College, the SSS back at Maxwell AFB again. A BIG decision was looming over me, one that would forever change the course of my life ... for the better and for eternity.

CHAPTER 11

The Buddha and The Fighter Pilot

There is probably no bigger or more agonizing decision for a fighter pilot than when it's time to leave.

The Air Force (and the military in general) is an extremely demanding profession, and to make it a career and stay there for 20 years or more takes a great deal of commitment. But the opposite side of that coin is that it becomes a very comfortable place to be.

I don't mean comfort like watching-football-on-Sundays-in-an-easy-chair type of comfort, but more of the comfort that comes from familiarity—familiarity in knowing the job and the people, and the likely path of your future. There are not a lot of big decisions that need to be made while you're in the military. Somebody else will decide when and where you are going next. Somebody else will decide when you're ready for the next job, or promotion, or responsibility. The military lifestyle and social architecture provides everything you think you might ever need, and it eventually becomes a crutch or safety net. It is all-consuming of your life and your life condition.

The decision to leave is different for everybody and it's never because of any one thing in particular. It tends to happen when the balance of the pros versus cons starts to weigh increasingly to the "leave" side of the scales. The love of the profession becomes tarnished with influences that are increasingly negative, and I had my share of all of those.

For the most part for me, though, it came down to family and my own life.

I did not want to drag my family through more and more short assignments and locations, just chasing that next job and promotion. They had stuck with me without complaints, and even though I knew Sako was sometimes the object of certain prejudices toward Asian (or foreign-born) spouses of officers, she had always been supportive of my career and me. I had no reason to expect anything different if I decided to stay.

The big issue then was what, and who, I would be if I came out on the other end of a 30-plus year career?

I had achieved so much in the previous 18–19 years in the Air Force. I had grown as a fighter pilot and as a leader, but the one thing I could not quantify was if I had grown at all as a human being.

The world of the officer, and especially of the fighter pilot, is a very small world. You are insulated in a cocoon of professionalism and social interaction that almost totally excludes the rest of society, and in some cases the rest of the Air Force. It is special partly because of that, but it does not allow much of a vector for personal growth. I was not really sure that I liked my metamorphosis over the years. I was increasingly becoming an over-bearing, type-A personality, and that had never been me before all of this. I justified this because I had come to put "the mission" above everything else. I felt my job was to produce the best fighter pilots in the world and nothing else was really important.

The OSS command allowed me to reflect on this, and I started to realize that it was really people who were important, and if I took care of them, they would take care of the mission. It's cliché, but I found this held true. When I reflect back, every decision I made that was for the good of the person turned out to be the right decision ... and most every decision I made for "the good of the Air Force" was almost always doomed to failure or regret. But in the end, I did not know or trust who would take care of me. This is when I began a profound change in my life and a new journey.

Sako knew I was struggling mightily with this decision ... should I stay or go? I am sure I was pretty stressed out and likely taking it out on her and the kids. After 13 years of marriage, therefore, while she patiently waited for a critical moment in my life to come to a head, Sako encouraged me finally to try the Buddhist practice I had agreed to join when I married her, a practice that had sat dormant in my life for all that time.

Surprisingly, I decided, "Why not?"

Practicing Nichiren Buddhism under the guidelines of the Soka Gakkai International (SGI) involves twice daily recitations of sections of the Lotus Sutra and chanting the words "Nam Myoho Renge Kyo" while seated in front of the *Gohonzon*—a scroll inscribed with a combination of Chinese and Sanskrit characters that are unrecognizable to laymen and even most scholars, but represent the deepest reality of life and a true reflection of our own life condition. I began to chant at least once a day, for about 10–20 minutes, and then eventually started chanting twice a day (morning and early evening). It was a struggle at first because even the Lotus Sutra recitations were in Japanese phonetics of Chinese characters, but after having done it over a couple of months, it became as natural as breathing. I also began to attend SGI meetings (often held in members' homes, not temples or churches) and studying the doctrines of the Buddha's teachings (sutras) and those of Nichiren Daishonin (the *Gosho*).

The study, daily practice, and activities began to have an effect. Doubts and even fears (from my Christian upbringing of being struck by a lightning bolt) soon started to fade away, and the feeling of a life "rhythm" started to take over. Very quickly a sense of clarity to my life also began to emerge in my consciousness, almost as if a fog or haze was lifting and I could finally see the landscape and a clear, correct, and "middle" path to take. The fear of leaving the comfort of the Air Force no longer concerned me, and I regained a confidence that I had an identity and value to my life that was not just attached to my rank and position.

***

From this new perspective, the first thing I had to do was tell the new operations group commander (the "OG," my direct supervisor) that I was going to decline attending the following year at SSS. Actually, the correct Air Force term for this is "Declined with Prejudice." It's a harsh term, and the words imply the treatment likely to follow somebody who dares to utter them. I made this decision with full knowledge of what to expect. I would likely be branded as no longer a "team player," and that I had basically declared my desire the leave the Air Force, although I had not fully made that determination yet—I was still looking for a safety net.

I had a staff meeting with the OSS flight commanders, senior enlisted troops, and my secretary and office staff. When I told them all what I had declared to the OG, the officers almost audibly gasped, while the rest of the office looked a bit confused. The officers understood perfectly that I had pretty much signed my own "death warrant." I had to explain to the rest of the staff that it meant I could expect to be promptly removed as the OSS commander and would likely have to suffer with an unwanted assignment or be shuffled off to a meaningless and inconsequential job somewhere else on the base. It was a very subdued staff meeting from that point on.

Things started to move fairly quickly from there. As predicted, I was quickly removed from my command position. This was going to happen by that summer anyway, if I had continued on the path to school, but leaving a couple months early and in the manner in which it was done was an obvious sign of displeasure from my leadership. I was happy to find a savior, though, in the wing Inspector General (IG) office.

The acting wing IG, Col David "Meat" Mintz, was always looking for strong officers to man his shop, because it was not the type of place or job most fighter pilots wanted to end up in. When he heard I was going to be available for an undetermined amount of time, he quickly snapped me up, and soon I was working on the opposite side of the base, at Wing IG.

I was extremely grateful for Meat's compassion for an unwanted fighter pilot, and I did everything I could to repay my debt of gratitude and give him the best of my talents during the time I had remaining.

During this time, another savior came along to cushion the blows I was just beginning to receive. Col "Roach" Cochran, the previous OG when I first took over the OSS, was now in charge of rated officer assignments at Air Force Personnel Center (AFPC) headquarters. When he heard about my predicament, he told me that he would try to get me a decent assignment, or, if I wanted he could just leave me at Kadena until I was eligible to retire.

I could not really believe what I was hearing. I had a little more than 18 months' commitment remaining to be able to stay in the Air Force until "retirement eligible," and to finish the payback of time in service for the final pilot ACP bonus I had accepted a few years prior. AFPC would normally never allow somebody who is assignment eligible with more than one year commitment remaining to remain on station (and I had about a year and a half still). When offered a chance to remain at Kadena until the end, I didn't really have to think about it. It was an instant, "Yes, Sir!" I will be forever grateful to Roach for doing that for my family and me.

And then the pendulum swung.

Shortly after I had been told I would be able to move over to the IG office and start working there, the OG sent his deputy over to my temporary desk in the 44th FS to talk with me. I kind of knew what was coming, but not exactly how it would be delivered. The colonel told me I was being "grounded" (could no longer fly) and that my last flight would be later that week. I pretty much expected this, although it seemed incongruous to the mission of the Air Force and the Operations Group, because I was by far the most experienced F-15 IP at Kadena (and possibly in the Air Force) at that time. Millions of dollars of taxpayers' money that had gone into my training, plus the experience that money couldn't buy, and now I was going to be "feet on the ramp," that most horrible of fighter pilot terms. But that was not really the *coup de grâce* ... it was when the deputy operations group commander told me that they did not want to even see me anywhere around the fighter squadrons because I was ... how did he say it? ... "a negative influence on the young fighter pilots."

I am not sure the colonel could even believe those words came out of his own mouth, any more than I could. Actually, I felt kind of bad for the guy because, first, he was just the messenger, and second, he was not a very big guy and I think he thought I might come right out from behind the desk and throttle him. But I didn't, although I was extremely disappointed. Disappointed that after almost 20 years of giving everything to the F-15 fighter pilot community, and in particular for almost 10 years of that at Kadena, I could somehow be labeled as a "negative influence" to the young fighter pilots. Unbelievable.

In the end, though, this was absolutely the best thing to happen to me. In fact, through my Buddhist practice, I learned to recognize these colonels as "good friends." Instead of holding on to resentment for their treatment of me, I could recognize their own humanity and appreciate that they had just provided me a reason to chant even more. Chant for my future happiness *and* for theirs also.

This was a revolutionary concept that I soon grasped as the path to my own enlightenment. To recognize the common humanity and life conditions we all share and that all life inherently possesses the Buddha nature within. To hate, resent, or disrespect another human does not create value in one's life and only brings about more of the same to oneself … the strict Law of Cause and Effect. From this point on I could move forward, but I had one more obstacle to overcome.

I had never really dealt with the end results of my engagement over Iraq … the violent shoot-down of the MiG-25 Foxbat and its occupant more than 10 years previously. As I had said earlier in this book, I had found a way in my mind to justify my actions on that day. But the darker side of this was that in the process I had somehow dehumanized the brave Foxbat pilot who had come out to face me that day. I had (and have) been asked to tell the shoot-down story many, many times and early on, I was happy to do so with great enthusiasm. Whatever the audience, I knew they wanted to hear about the "glory" part of aerial warfare and I tried not to disappoint them … but, that is a pretty thin veneer that soon gets rubbed raw.

One incident that I recall I would really rather not even repeat, but I feel I need to, not least to describe the depths that we can go to rationalize our actions, if nothing else. It was not long after DESERT STORM and I was back in my hometown of Stockton, California, for some leave and a visit. I was with my best friend Bradley, and we were out for the day together catching a late lunch, then to one of his favorite bars for some afternoon drinks. Behind the bar was a friend of Brad's and he was a pretty rough-looking dude—California biker type, with the long hair, scraggly beard, lots of tattoos, and a few real scars.

So, Bradley tells his bartender friend, "Yeah, Ricky here [Brad still calls me Ricky] shot down an airplane during the war."

Biker Bartender says "Oh yeah? Tell me about it." So, I gave him a condensed (non-fighter pilot) version of the engagement and the results, and he seemed duly impressed. Then Biker Bartender asked me a question I had not heard from anybody that I had told this story to … yet, or since. He said, "So, what's it feel like to kill another human being?" I thought to myself, "What!? … KILL another human being?" Nobody is supposed to ask me that question.

I was taken aback, embarrassed and at a loss for words. I panicked for just a moment, and then feigning nonchalance and mocking false bravado, I blurted out, "Oh, he was just a Rag-head." As soon as those words came out of my mouth, I wanted to grab them in mid-air and stuff them right back in my throat and choke on them. I could not believe I had just said that, and in fact, rough-and-tough Biker Bartender even had an expression of semi-shock on his face, a "wow, that's pretty cold dude" kind of look.

I have always regretted that I said those words and I would never say anything like that ever again. But also, I could never take them back. I realized this was something I would have to live with, and it wasn't until later, after I started my

Buddhist practice, I understood that a dark little seed had been planted deep inside my heart. This seed would only grow in time, much like a small black hole out in the universe can slowly pull in more and more dark matter.

Having seen and read many reports since that time about Post-Traumatic Stress Disorder (PTSD), I could empathize and associate with those who have experienced the results of combat, especially when directly or indirectly involved in the death or injury of others (friends, enemy, or innocents alike). Burying the responsibility deep inside denies one of the opportunity to deal with it, and that's when that "black hole" begins to grow.

In my Buddhist practice, besides our recitations of the Lotus Sutra and chanting of "Nam Myoho Renge Kyo," at the end of each session we have an opportunity to offer silent (meditative) prayers. One of those prayers is to those who have passed on from this lifetime—family, friends, or whoever we feel the need to pray for. When I started this practice, I soon realized I needed to include the Iraqi Foxbat pilot in my daily silent prayers, even though I still did not know if he survived or not. I also recalled that my hero, Saburo Sakai, had turned to Buddhism himself after his wartime experiences, and wondered if he did not also pray for all those he had shot down in combat.

Once I began this process, it was like opening up a window shade to shine a bright and penetrating light on the dark force inside my heart. The act or cause would not disappear, but I would no longer add any more negativity to it either. I would still experience karmic retribution, but that effect could be lessened by living out a more noble life for myself, and for anybody, or anything I had harmed in the past. This was a revolution for me ... a human revolution.

My mind started to move in different directions than it had ever done before. As I chanted more and learned deeper Buddhist concepts, the futility and utter failure of war became clear. If the Law of Cause and Effect is pure and unadulterated ... if we were all truly connected as one big micro/macrocosm of the universe, then how could the act of war and violence create any kind of positive outcome?

Now, most people would think, "How can you be a fighter pilot, or soldier, or whatever, and be Buddhist also?" Actually, there is no disconnect between our daily lives and chosen path (or profession in this case) and Buddhism. In fact, one of the most noble paths a person can take is to serve in the duty to one's sovereign country, and make a selfless sacrifice for society as a whole. The reality of life is that violence and war do exist, and because of our inherent human condition it is something that will never totally disappear from the face of the Earth. For that reason, there will always be a need for some type of military or police force to deal with the darker aspects of human nature. Then the issue becomes, is there a better way to deal with or prevent human conflict?

This difference lies solely in what is in our hearts. If we harbor the desire to kill or harm based on secular or even religious justifications, then our hearts move closer to that of a sociopath, doing so without conscious thought. The first step in this process is when we find a way to dehumanize the other party, see their needs as less noble than our own, or raise the fear of others to a point of hysteria. If you look at any conflict, from the most basic 1-on-1 human relationships to the great global wars that continue to this day, this is the common theme and thread of discord.

If we are instead able look at all human beings as our brothers, sisters, mothers, and fathers, then would it not be better to deal with the root causes of conflict before it occurs, and not wait until conflict is unavoidable? If we can see that in the end we only harm ourselves when we choose to harm others, then why not spend more time and resources on prevention versus the tremendous weight of the "cure"?

These might seem like relatively simple philosophical choices, but in actuality they are the most difficult to put into practice. When we view life and the world from our own individual perspective, we naturally blind ourselves to the true interconnected nature of life. So, let's try to look at it from a different (Buddhist) perspective.

There is a Buddhist principle known as *Esho Funi* (in Japanese language). The literal translation of the term is "life and environment are two, but not two." In this case, "environment" does not mean only the natural environment, but society and the world itself, even down to our individual relationships.

Buddhism is the polar opposite of the western concepts of dualism, or in modern socio-political terms, objectivism. In this case, the non-dualistic aspect of *Esho Funi* means that not only do the person and the environment affect each other, but in actuality they are a single entity and mutually possessive, in other words the classic Buddhist cliché of "one with the universe." As individuals, not only are we part of the universe (which might be somewhat comprehensible), but simultaneously that same universe exists within us and within all life. Now if you find that is difficult to wrap your head around, then it is no wonder that mankind lives in a daily delusion that we can somehow by will or force move the universe in a direction of our personal liking without suffering any consequences.

Taken on a grander scale, this concept applies not only to the individual, but also to the greater society and culture the individuals inhabit, indeed all humanity, life, and the Earth itself. Both the beauty and the dark turmoil of life are an assimilated reflection of the participants ... all of the participants, not just "the other guys."

Another way to view this is as the body and its shadow. If the individual or society is the body, and the world or environment is the shadow, then as the body bends so does the shadow. Everything is a reflection and true manifestation of our thoughts, words, and deeds. From *SGI Quarterly* (April 1988): "As Nichiren (Daishonin) wrote, 'If the minds of the people are impure, their land is also impure, but if their minds are pure, so is their land. There are not two lands, pure and impure in themselves. The difference lies solely in the good or evil of our minds.' ("Evil" means self-centered and shortsighted tendencies based on greed, arrogance, fear, and aggression.)

The single most positive action we can make for society and the land is to transform our own lives, so that they are no longer dominated by anger, greed, and fear. When we manifest wisdom, generosity, and integrity, we naturally make more valuable choices, and we will find that our surroundings are nurturing and supportive. Often we cannot foresee the long-term results of our actions, and it is hard to believe that one individual's choices can really affect the state of the world, but Buddhism teaches that through the oneness of self and environment, everything is interconnected.

So, if our "enemy" is actually our "shadow," then if we can change our own hearts and minds, over time we can actually change the darker side of our environment and the world. If we bow in respect to our enemy, then the shadow will naturally bow back to us also. In this case, "respect" would mean that we start to deal with our problems through education, culture, dialogue, and compassion for others, well before succumbing to the easy choice to draw a blade. This obviously is a profoundly difficult path to follow, but it's actually the foundation of the fundamental purpose of faith and religion to begin with … to move us towards peaceful coexistence.

As my own personal human revolution progressed, I began to see this new reality all very clearly. At this moment, my new "mission" now became to help others to perceive this within themselves.

***

My days of active duty in the US Air Force were quickly moving to a close. I worked hard in my last year for Col Mintz, and the IG team at Kadena, with the objective of helping the wing achieve an "Excellent" rating on its next major inspection. The 18th Wing had not done so well on its most recent evaluations by higher headquarters. Even though many of the leaders in the wing were those who had come down hard on me, I still felt a debt of gratitude to the organization itself and the people as a whole, and I wanted them to be able to show what a great service they were providing to their country and the Air Force.

With the help of other officers and enlisted staff in the IG office, we pushed an aggressive agenda of self-inspection and staff assistance leading up to the real inspection. When the higher headquarters inspectors arrived and evaluated the wing, the overall grade of "Excellent" was achieved, with many units receiving "Outstanding" ratings. Myself and several other members of our IG office were also recognized as "Outstanding Performers" for our work in preparing the 18th Wing for this inspection.

I felt vindicated. I had not been defeated by self-pity, nor by resentment toward others who may have treated me harshly. I had put my Buddhist practice to the test and come out victorious. It was time to move on.

***

I loved my time in the US Air Force and as a fighter pilot, and everything positive and negative that came with it. I would never trade that experience for anything in the world. Connecting all the dots—the life events that I had jotted down on a notepad, and all the days in between—everything now had an obvious place and purpose, bringing me to where I currently stood. It was not a goal or an end state, but part of the continuing "flow" of life, like a great river meandering and changing the landscape on its eternal journey.

During my last remaining days in the Air Force, I had more time on my hands than I ever had before, so I began to reconnect with my passion for music.

I was never a formally "trained" musician, but I had once been a drummer, and by now I had also become fairly proficient at playing guitar. I began to write songs, which gave me an outlet for my ever-growing observations and wonderment about life. People ask me now (all the time, actually), "Don't you miss it?" (the flying, they mean), and I honestly say to them, "No. I don't." The challenges of songwriting and thrill of performing have replaced much of what drove me as a fighter pilot.

But I do miss the camaraderie. You will never feel as closely connected to most people (sometimes even your own family) than you do to those with whom you fly and train, and in particular those you fly with in combat. I am sure most military members, regardless of their service or duty, would say the same.

I had a career—the Air Force—but that career is over. Today I have a job. And I continue my love of life and music. After all ... I Am the Music Man.

Epilogue

I wish I could explain the culture of the fighter pilot in more explicit terms, but it's something you have to "be" and experience firsthand to really understand it. But, as I was writing this memoir, one of my old Dirty Dozen OpsOs (Lt Col "Budman" Bennett) forwarded this email to me, so I will provide it (exactly as sent) for your own judgments:

From "Budman" Bennett—I think this represents the way a lot of us feel about each other. And I believe in this context it applies to the "Fighter Pilot as a Character Trait" and not simply one who flies fighters. In my view, it applies to most military aviators and those associated with them. Sent to me by Johnny Johnson, one of the best—if you flew an F16, you owe him for his Test Pilot work at Edwards. Cheers! Budman sends.

MILITARY AVIATOR TRIBUTE

As we get older and we experience the loss of old friends, we begin to realize that maybe we bullet proof Fighter Pilots won't live forever, not so bullet proof anymore. We ponder … if I was gone tomorrow did I say what I wanted to my Brothers. The answer was no! Hence, the following few random thoughts.

When people ask me if I miss flying, I always say something like—"Yes! I miss the flying because when you are flying, you are totally focused on the task at hand. It's like nothing else you will ever do (almost)." But then I always say "However, I miss the Squadron and the guys even more than I miss the flying." "Why?" you might ask. They were a bunch of aggressive, wise ass, cocky, insulting, sarcastic bastards in smelly flight suits who thought a funny thing to do was to fart and see if they could clear a room. They drank too much, they chased women, they flew when they shouldn't, they laughed too loud and thought they owned the sky, the Bar, and generally thought they could do everything better than the next guy. Nothing was funnier than trying to screw with a buddy and see how pissed off they would get. They flew planes and helos that leaked, that smoked, that broke, that couldn't turn, that burned fuel too fast, that never had auto pilots or radars, and with systems that were archaic next to today's new generation aircraft. All true!

But a little closer look might show that every guy in the room was sneaky smart and damn competent and brutally handsome! They hated to lose or fail to accomplish the mission and seldom did. They were the laziest guys on the planet until challenged and then they would do anything to win. They would fly with wing tips overlapped at night through the worst weather with only a little red light to hold on to, knowing that their Flight Lead would get them on the ground safely. They would fight in the air knowing the greatest risk and fear was that another fighter would arrive at the same six o'clock at the same time they did. They would fly in harm's way and act nonchalant as if to challenge the grim reaper.

When we went to another base we were the best Squadron on the base as soon as we landed. Often we were not welcomed back. When we went into a Bar we owned the Bar (even if it was a No Name Bar). We wore our commander's name tag … all of us. We were lucky to have the

Best of the Best in the military. We knew it and so did others. We found jobs, lost jobs, got married, got divorced, moved, went broke, got rich, broke something, and the only thing you could really count on was if you really needed help, a fellow Pilot would have your back.

I miss the call-signs, nicknames, and the stories behind them. I miss the getting lit up in a bar full of my buddies and watching the incredible, unbelievable things that were happening. I miss the Kangaroo Courts and the victim's poor aim when trying to hit a Judge. I miss the Roach eating contests and the ALMAR Fart Offs. I miss the Mess Nights where an Aviator would cut the candles in a candelabra in half with his dull sword and where Generals introductions were routinely screwed up. I miss the Crew Chiefs saluting as you taxied out the flight-line. I miss the lighting of the Afterburners, if you had them, especially at night. I miss the going straight up and straight down. I miss the cross countries. I miss the dice games at the bar for drinks. I miss listening to bullshit stories while drinking and laughing till my eyes watered.

I miss three-man lifts. I miss the dreadful Choir. I miss Yuma nacho-eating contests along with hotly fought Buffarillo contests. I miss naps in the Squadron with a room full of pilots working up new tricks to torment the sleeper. I miss flying upside down in the Grand Canyon and hearing about flying so low boats were blown over. I miss coming into the break Hot and looking over and seeing three wingmen tucked in tight ready to make the troops on the ground proud. I miss belches that could be heard in neighboring states. I miss putting on ad hoc Air Shows that might be over someone's home or farm in faraway towns.

Finally I miss hearing DEAD BUG being called out at the bar and seeing and hearing a room of men hit the deck with drinks spilling and chairs being knocked over as they rolled in the beer and kicked their legs in the air, followed closely by a Not Politically Correct Tap Dancing and Singing spectacle that couldn't help but make you grin and order another round!

I am a lucky guy and have lived a great life! One thing I know is that I was part of a special, really talented bunch of guys doing something dangerous and doing it better than most. Flying the most beautiful, ugly, noisy, solid aircraft ever built. Supported by ground troops committed to making sure we came home again! Being prepared to fly and fight and die for America. Having a clear mission. Having fun.

We box out the bad memories from various operations most of the time but never the hallowed memories of our fallen comrades. We are often amazed at how good war stories never let the truth interfere and they get better with age. We are lucky bastards to be able to walk into a Squadron or a Bar and have men we respect and love shout out our names, our call-signs, and know that this is truly where we belong. We are Fighter Pilots. We are Few and we are Proud.

I am Privileged and Proud to call you Brothers.

Push It Up! & Check SIX!

Clyde Romero

In Victory you deserve Champagne

In Defeat You Need It!

***

In 2006 I returned to Okinawa (and Kadena) as a civilian to take a job as a contract instructor pilot in the F-15C Mission Training Center (flight simulator). I was returning to do what I truly love to do … teach young Eagle drivers to be the best fighter pilots in the world.

In December of that same year, I received a call from my sister Joy, in California. Dad was dying. My father, the man who had taught me so much, including the love of flight, was quickly approaching the end of his life and was about to enter a hospice. I flew back the next day from Japan and made it to California in time. I was able to spend several days with Dad in the hospice and he passed away peacefully.

A few years prior, when author Steve Davies completed his book *F-15C Eagle Units in Combat*, he graciously sent me a copy for my contributions. After reading the book from front to back, I mailed it to my father with the inscription on the inside cover: "Dad, thank you for teaching me how to fly." I couldn't think of any better way to say "thank you" to him.

We often take our parents for granted until it's too late, but I was fortunate to have had a chance to express my appreciation to both my parents. Mom would follow our father in 2014. Our parents were proud of all three of their children and our accomplishments. In the end I understood the best way we can show our appreciation to our parents (other than just telling them) is to live noble lives as human beings and just do the best we can.

My own experience as a parent to Sakura and Lucas taught me that.

***

I have my own mantra of what it feels like to be a fighter pilot, but somebody else wrote it. When we moved to the Middlefield house during my 7th grade, my Nona (grandmother) bought a portable color TV for my brother Mark and me to watch in our large shared bedroom. I can remember many nights (mostly on weekends or during the summer) staying up to watch the Johnny Carson Show, but normally falling asleep somewhere before the end.

These were the days before "cable," and the three major networks usually signed off sometime shortly after midnight or 1am. I would always, for some reason, wake up just as the sign-off piece would start up.

Most stations played the "Star-Spangled Banner," or something like that, but the NBC affiliate for the Stockton area played something very special that I would never forget …

… it would start with a stirring symphonic orchestra, as a beautiful F-104 Starfighter would blast off into the blue sky and start an aerobatic show, to the narrated words of pilot/poet John Gillespie Magee, Jr.

John Gillespie Magee, Jr. was an Anglo-American pilot for the Royal Canadian Air Force in World War II. He would die tragically in a mid-air collision over England in 1941, but the legacy of the uplifting drama of his life and the life of every pilot would live on in his epic poem, *High Flight*:

> Oh! I have slipped the surly bonds of Earth
> And danced the skies on laughter-silvered wings;
> Sunward I've climbed, and joined the tumbling mirth
> of sun-split clouds,—and done a hundred things
> You have not dreamed of—wheeled and soared and swung
> High in the sunlit silence. Hovering there,
> I've chased the shouting wind along, and flung
> My eager craft through footless halls of air …
> Up, up the long, delirious, burning blue
> I've topped the wind-swept heights with easy grace

Where never lark nor even eagle flew ...
And, while with silent lifting mind I've trod
The high un-trespassed sanctity of space,
Put out my hand, and touched the face of God.

***

Douglas "Disco" Dildy was one of the three combat aviation authors to whose works I contributed my DESERT STORM experience. Disco had contacted me a couple of years after I had completed this manuscript, as it sat idle on my computer at home. I had made a firm commitment not to contribute again to another author who wanted to tell "my story," but with Disco it was a bit different

First, he was a former Eagle Driver, so I knew he had the knowledge and background to make sure the account was accurate, realistic, and not a "Hollywood" version. Second, and probably more important to me, he was working with a co-author, Tom Cooper, who reportedly had connections to former IrAF pilots who could provide their side of the story and what they were actually trying to accomplish on January 19, 1991. That's what I REALLY wanted to know. I have not included all of those specifics in this book, but I can encapsulate here the important things I learned. After the slew of Night One and Day One aerial victories by my squadron and other Coalition fighters over the IrAFs initial defense, the IrAF basically stood down for 24+ hours. Losing some frontline fighters and experienced fighter pilots so quickly, without much in return, may have given IrAF pause for thought. So, the IrAF command's intent, at first opportunity, was to plan a coordinated, multi-axis, well-timed tactic using decoys and deception to lure USAF F-15 CAPs into a trap. The overall objective was to "bag" an Eagle and demonstrate that the mighty, undefeated F-15C could be taken down and that IrAF pilots could compete with the Best.

When I learned of this, it all fell into place. The tactic that appeared to me as a decoy was actually intended to be that. It just didn't work. And the fact that we saw so much activity that day, and that Rico Rodriguez and Mole Underhill engaged and shot down their MiG-29s almost simultaneous with those for myself and Cherry Pitts, just further confirmed the IrAF's intent.

As I finished up my contributions to Disco's book, I asked him a favor. Was there any way for him to find out what happened to the Foxbat pilots that Cherry and I had shot down. My assumption had always been that Cherry's observation of his pilot ejecting possibly meant he had survived, and the extreme explosion of my Foxbat most likely meant that my pilot had not. But I wanted to know for sure ... if possible.

Disco said he would do his best to dig out that information with Tom Cooper's assistance, but could not guarantee much. It seems that large numbers of the IrAF pilots had left Iraq out of fear of Saddam's retribution, and later to avoid the sectarian violence that has ravaged the country since then, and that many were in hiding or did not want to be contacted.

The months passed and I had pretty much given up on ever knowing when I received this email from Disco …

> Kluso—The book manuscript is at the editor now. I did have to "pull it" (for edits) to insert some new information.
>
> One of the most important was that we have learned the names of the two Iraqi AF Foxbat pilots that you and your wingman (Cherry) fought and their fates (at least during ODS).
>
> … These were not recce [Reconnaissance] pilots (as I may have told you was reported [and I didn't believe it]), but were the cream of their AF and their squadron.
>
> They fully intended to trap you guys.
>
> The guy flying the Foxbat you shot down was Captain Sa'ad Nehme. Nehme was the flight lead, from 97 Squadron.
>
> He did eject and survived the engagement, … although he was seriously injured.
>
> The guy flying "Cherry's Foxbat" was Lieutenant Hussein Abdul Sattar. He too ejected but was not so fortunate (reason unknown).
>
> Captain Sa'ad Nehme
>
> Lieutenant Hussein Abdul Sattar

So now you know the rest of the story.

Before that mission, and before each combat mission, I would chant "Nam Myoho Renge Kyo" three times while sitting in my jet. I did it at that time as much for "good luck" as anything else—fighter pilots are *very* superstitious people. Captain Nehme should not have survived the explosion of my missile, but somehow he ejected before or as the missile arrived, and did survive.

From my 20 years of Buddhist practice I now understand that my simple *Daimoku* ("Nam Myoho Renge Kyo"), said over 25 years before, was setting in motion a great battle. This battle was fought to change my own Karma and to confront the puzzle of life events, leading me to begin my Buddhist practice and experience my own human revolution. In the process I sought to change a heart (my heart) … and change the world.

It's still a work in progress. I also chant daily during my silent prayers for my surviving Foxbat pilot (Capt Nehme) and now for his wingman who perished (Lt Abdul Sattar).